Realist Evaluation

Realist Evaluation: Principles and Practice offers a comprehensive exploration of contemporary realist evaluation, showcasing how skilled practitioners navigate diverse fieldwork contexts.

Authored by experts spanning academia and evaluation backgrounds across five continents in fields including climate change, criminology, health, and international development, the book provides a rich tapestry of perspectives. Covering participatory approaches, digital and visual data collection, interpreter-mediated interviews, and innovative methods like refuse data analysis, the authors delve into contemporary social research methodologies while addressing issues such as power, insider/outsider research, the nature of evidence, critical and scientific realism philosophies of science, and confirmation bias in qualitative research. Practical advice is provided in areas such as developing a topic guide, combining a realist review with an evaluation, and managing large, multi-site cross-national projects. This collection underscores the creative nature of the realist imagination, highlighting ongoing innovations by scholars and evaluators.

With contributions from an outstanding group of internationally renowned experts in realist evaluation including Nick Tilley, a key figure in the development of realist evaluation alongside Ray Pawson, this is the ideal text for students, researchers and professionals including policy makers, professional evaluators, and those at organisations such as thinktanks and NGOs, who require an accessible guide on how to use realist evaluation methods.

Ana Manzano is an Associate Professor in Public Policy at University of Leeds, UK.

Emma Williams was an Associate Professor in the Realist Research, Evaluation and Learning Initiative at Charles Darwin University, Australia until mid-2024 and now is an independent research and evaluation consultant.

"Many years ago, Charles Wright Mills implored us to remember that doing social research was not a matter of blindly following set designs and routinised procedures. It requires a generous application of the sociological imagination. In Manzano and Williams's collection we discover the same creative motif. In example after example, we gain insight on the resourcefulness of the realist imagination."

Ray Pawson

Realist Evaluation

Principles and Practice

**Edited by Ana Manzano
and Emma Williams**

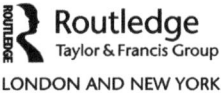

Routledge
Taylor & Francis Group

LONDON AND NEW YORK

Designed cover image: Andriy Onufriyenko/Getty Images

First published 2025
by Routledge
4 Park Square, Milton Park, Abingdon, Oxon OX14 4RN

and by Routledge
605 Third Avenue, New York, NY 10158

Routledge is an imprint of the Taylor & Francis Group, an informa business

British Library Cataloguing-in-Publication Data
A catalogue record for this book is available from the British Library

ISBN: 978-1-032-59978-6 (hbk)
ISBN: 978-1-032-59977-9 (pbk)
ISBN: 978-1-003-45707-7 (ebk)

DOI: 10.4324/9781003457077

Typeset in Optima
by KnowledgeWorks Global Ltd.

Contents

Figures and Tables

Figures

Tables

Contributors

Dr. Ibukun O. Abejirinde (MD, MSc, PhD) is an applied health researcher whose research programme focuses on understanding and enabling the role of digital technologies to strengthen health systems and advance health equity within Canada and globally. A medical doctor by training, she applies a trans-disciplinary approach that is anchored in community/patient partnerships and lies at the nexus of systems thinking, theory-driven inquiry and implementation science, to answer questions on 'what works, for whom, in which contexts, how and why?'. Dr. Abejirinde is a scientist at the Institute for Better Health, Trillium Health Partners, where she works collaboratively to help advance its Learning Health System Action Framework. She is also an Assistant Professor at the Dalla Lana School of Public Health, University of Toronto, and an Adjunct Scientist at Women's College Hospital Research Institute.

Dr. Troy Allard is an Associate Professor in the School of Criminology and Criminal Justice at Griffith University and a member of the Griffith Criminology Institute. He has expertise in youth justice and focuses on serious and persistent offending and 'what works' to reduce this offending. He is co-lead of the Queensland Cross-sector Research Collaboration (QCRC), an ongoing partnership between Griffith University and Queensland Government that promotes ongoing use and oversight of the 1983, 1984 and 1990 linked longitudinal birth cohorts. He has considerable experience evaluating innovative programmes and using complex administrative data to promote effective and efficient policies and practices. Dr Allard's research outputs include one edited book and over 70 peer-reviewed articles, book chapters and reports for funding bodies. These outputs inform decision-making processes and are used by those developing, justifying or evaluating interventions and programmes.

Dr. Tracey Carr, an early career researcher at the University of Saskatchewan, College of Medicine, Department of Community Health and Epidemiology, uses realism in her health services implementation research programme. She has worked with Dr. Gary Groot from the beginning of his academic career in 2016, first as a post-doctoral fellow and subsequently as Dr. Groot's research associate. Prior to working with Dr. Groot, she completed a post-doctoral fellowship in Sociology at the University of Saskatchewan where she received training in realist synthesis.

Tom Cornu (MD, MPH) is a public health researcher at the Institute of Tropical Medicine, Antwerp (Belgium) and the University of Antwerp, Belgium. His research interests include individual, community and health system resilience and the interlinkage between nature and health, in which research, realist evaluation and synthesis are the overarching approaches.

Sara Dada is a global health researcher and advocate, focusing on maternal health and community engagement. Since completing her MSc in One Health at the Royal Veterinary College and London School of Hygiene and Tropical Medicine as a Fulbright Scholar, Sara has conducted and led research projects focusing on communications and community engagement to empower communities and build capacity in Sierra Leone, Kenya, India, Tanzania, and Zambia. Sara has supported organisations such as the World Health Organization, Women in Global Health, and GOAL Global on research and advocacy projects relating to communications, community engagement, and participation. She has published peer-reviewed articles on subjects ranging from maternal and child health to vaccine hesitancy to community engagement and has been invited to present her innovative research on community engagement and realist methods in global health at numerous conferences, panels, and webinars.

Prof. Sonia Dalkin is a Professor of Applied Health and Social Care Research in the Faculty of Health & Life Sciences at Northumbria University in the UK. Sonia has expertise in complex intervention evaluation and realist approaches, providing training in realist evaluation and synthesis throughout the UK and internationally. In 2018, she co-authored *Doing Realist Research* and launched the Northern Realist Research Team Hub (NoRTH). NoRTH comprises an experienced team of researchers based at Northumbria University with established regional, national and international links, who have expertise in and are regularly using and developing realist approaches to research. Her most recent research aims to address the requirements outlined by the Medical Research Council Framework for the development and evaluation of complex interventions. This methodological development research aims to formulate Realist Economic Evaluation Methods (REEM) and associated guidance, to better understand and evaluate the costs and consequences of complex interventions.

Dr. Brynne Gilmore is an Assistant Professor of Health Systems at University College Dublin's School of Nursing, Midwifery and Health Systems. She is an applied health researcher who uses a theory-driven evaluation methodology, realist evaluation, to understand and improve health systems, specifically at the community level in low- and middle-income countries. Most of her previous work involves research partnerships with NGOs in

Africa using operations research and implementation science to support strengthening community-based health interventions. Within this, Dr. Gilmore explores the use and development of realist evaluation and synthesis methodology for health systems research in various contexts. She has research experience in Uganda, Tanzania, Kenya, Sierra Leone, Lebanon, Turkey and Ireland.

Dr. Gary Groot is a Professor at the University of Saskatchewan, College of Medicine with a joint appointment to the Departments of Community Health and Epidemiology and Surgery. While the Department of Surgery is his clinic home, CH&E is his research home where he weaves health equity, implementation science, patient-oriented/community research and realist philosophy throughout his health services programme of research. Dr. Groot uses a realist philosophical approach in most of his numerous research projects as he finds that it is more intuitive and leads to more impactful results. He teaches a realist graduate course on realist research at the University of Saskatchewan and has trained many graduate and post-doctoral fellows in the realist approach.

Dr. Catherine Hastings' interdisciplinary research concentrates on explaining issues of social justice and inequality alongside developing and evaluating policy and programme responses for social change. Catherine's current study, the Legal Needs Project funded by a Macquarie University Research Fellowship, investigates how, why and in what context types of legal needs develop for marginalised and disadvantaged populations in Australia. The philosophy of critical realism informs her research. Her methodological research aims to extend how social science research and complexity-informed evaluation methodologies may operationalise critical realism to deliver more transformative findings. Dr, Hastings received the Vice-Chancellor's Award for Academic Excellence for her PhD (Sociology) on the causal mechanisms of family homelessness in Australia. In addition to her academic work, she undertakes applied social research and evaluation for government and not-for-profit organisations.

Dr. Pragati B. Hebbar (MDS, PhD) is a dentist by education and currently a public health researcher and the Assistant Director of Research at the Institute of Public Health, Bengaluru (India). She carried out research and policy engagement on issues of tobacco control, road safety and non-communicable diseases. She contributes to teaching in courses and work-shops such as the online implementation research course and realist evaluation workshop series. Currently, she is leading a REALISE Lab (Realist Evaluation Advancement Lab for Implementation Strategy Explanations) supported by the DBT/Wellcome Trust India Alliance Intermediate fellowship.

Dr. Jo Howe is a Chartered Psychologist working as an academic healthcare post-doctoral researcher in the United Kingdom. She has a decade's worth of direct experience in realist evaluation and realist synthesis, gained from different areas of healthcare. She has collaborated on national and international projects with colleagues across the healthcare landscape including stroke, serious mental illness and parenting. Additionally, she owns The Realist Hub, which provides free online-training seminars for those interested in learning more about realist methods. Dr. Howe also offers realist training, 1:1 mentoring for students and research groups as well as formal collaboration via The Realist Hub.

Dr. Sebastian Lemire, Ph.D., is an evaluation expert with decades of experience designing and managing evaluations of education and workforce development programmes. He has extensive experience with a broad range of evaluation approaches, quasi- and non-experimental designs, qualitative and quantitative data collection and analysis methods, as well as systematic evidence reviews. Dr. Lemire is an award-winning author of over 40 peer-reviewed articles and book chapters on a broad range of methodological topics, including alternative approaches for impact evaluation, theory-based evaluation and evaluation capacity building. He currently serves on the editorial advisory boards of *Evaluation* and the *American Journal of Evaluation*. He is a current board member of the American Evaluation Association and a former board member of the European Evaluation Society and the Danish Evaluation Society.

Prof. Maura MacPhee is a Professor Emerita in Nursing from the University of British Columbia-Vancouver. She is a health services researcher with a special interest in realist methods. Prior to entering the world of academia, she was a paediatric nurse specialist at Denver Children's Hospital and a professional practice director at Boston Children's Hospital. Over the past two decades, she has been studying quality practice environments in different healthcare sectors with a focus on nursing. Her areas of expertise are leadership/healthcare administration and workload management. She has had international research/teaching affiliations with colleagues in Hong Kong, Taiwan and Brazil. She is currently engaged in realist syntheses and evaluations with research teams in the UK and Canada.

Prof. Ian Maidment is a Professor in Clinical Pharmacy and joined Aston University (United Kingdom) in February 2012. Prior to this, he worked in NHS Dementia/Mental Health services for 18 years, eight years at a senior level. He has also worked within community pharmacy, the acute sector and led R&D in an NHS trust. He has led three research projects, funded by NIHR/UKRI, using a realist approach: MEMORABLE (medication management in older people on complex regimens living in the community), PERISCOPE (role of community pharmacy in COVID vaccination) and MEDIATE (medication optimisation with people living with severe mental illness). He is currently leading a NIHR study using a realist approach; RESOLVE is focused on the non-pharmacological management of antipsychotic induced weight gain in people living with severe mental illness.

He has also provided methodological advice in diverse areas including osteoporosis treatment and disclosure of sexual violence and abuse.

Dr. Ana Manzano is an Associate Professor in Public Policy at the University of Leeds (UK), specialising in theory-driven and realist evaluation methodologies. She has significantly contributed to enhancing realist evaluation practices by writing extensively on data collection techniques, including realist qualitative interviews and focus groups; and contributed to the RAMESES II reporting and quality standards as a co-investigator. She has worked on large realist evaluation studies in Africa, Asia, and Europe, bringing a global perspective to her knowledge. Additionally, she serves as an associate editor for the journal *Evaluation & Program Planning*.

Prof. Bruno Marchal (MD, MPH, PhD) is Professor and head of the Complexity and Health Unit, Department of Public Health, Institute of Tropical Medicine, Antwerp (Belgium). He is a health systems research expert and an internationally recognised expert in realist evaluation.

Charles Michaelis is the Director at Strategy Development Solutions, and has thirty years of experience in assisting government and the public sector to evaluate policies and programmes relating to climate change. He has worked on energy efficiency policies in developing and developed countries and has also worked on renewables and demand side response. He has conducted more than 100 evaluations of industry, buildings, lighting and appliances policies, and was involved in the Compass evaluation, a portfolio-level evaluation of the UK's International Climate Finance (ICF) programmes.

Dr. Ferdinand Mukumbang is an Assistant Professor at the Department of Global Health, University of Washington, specialising in health policy and systems research with a specific focus on implementation sciences. Dr. Mukumbang is also interested in the development and implementation of strategies to decolonise global health, his work in this area relating to addressing issues of health inequities in global health. Regarding methodological advancements in implementation sciences, he is particularly interested in the development and adoption of realist-informed research methods – critical realist theorising, realist evaluation and realist synthesis and reviews – for evidence-based theorising in health care and global health to unpack implementation outcomes. He has published several methodological papers in this regard.

Dr. Steffen Bohni Nielsen, PhD, is Director General at the National Research Centre, Denmark. Formerly, he was partner at PricewaterhouseCoopers, Denmark. He has also held executive positions in national and local government and in an international management consulting firm. He is a member of the Danish Research and Innovation Council and serves on several boards. He serves on the editorial advisory board of the *American*

Journal of Evaluation. He is the author of several peer-reviewed articles and books on diverse topics such as public management and leadership, results-based management, artificial intelligence, Big Data, evaluation capacity building, theory-informed evaluation and realist evaluation.

Dr. Susan Rayment-McHugh is a Senior Lecturer in Criminology and Justice at the University of the Sunshine Coast (Australia) and Co-Leader of the Sexual Violence Research and Prevention Unit. Her research advances understanding, prevention, and responses to sexual violence and abuse, including place-based and contextual approaches to prevention, and the assessment and treatment of youth with harmful sexual behaviour and adults who have sexually offended. This applied research agenda builds on nearly 30 years' of experience as a clinical forensic practitioner. Susan is a member of the University's Indigenous and Transcultural Research Centre and an Associate Editor for the *Journal of Sexual Aggression*.

Dr. Sam Redgate is a Lecturer in Public Health at the Faculty of Health & Life Sciences at Northumbria University in the United Kingdom. With a research background rooted in prior UK Local Authority public health and social care commissioning. Dr. Redgate leverages applied practical knowledge to shape her approach to service design, implementation, delivery, and evaluation research. Dr. Redgate uses realist approaches to enhance the explanatory potential of her research, and practical application of the findings. She has substantial experience applying realist approaches across a variety of research disciplines, including public health, social care and education. Dr. Redgate is part of the Northern Realist Research Team Hub (NoRTH).

Dr. Prashanth N. Srinivas (MD, MPH, PhD) is a medical doctor and public health researcher working on health policy and systems research. His primary interest is in social determinants of health, primarily among Adivasi (indigenous) populations in southern India, where he has set up a long-term learning site for research and action on indigenous health. He is currently the Director of the Institute of Public Health Bengaluru (India) and teaches at various Indian and international institutions.

Prof. Nick Tilley has taught or conducted research at Coventry University, Nottingham Trent University, The University of Minnesota, Griffith University, the Home Office, and most recently University College London. He is an elected Fellow of the Academy of the Social Sciences (FAcSS) and has been awarded an OBE for services to policing and crime reduction. The Tilley Award for police problem-solving is named in his honour. He is an honorary professor at UCL, an emeritus professor at Nottingham Trent University, and a visiting professor at Huddersfield University. He is the author or editor of 15 books and more than 200 chapters and journal articles, mostly to do with evaluation methodology, policing, and crime prevention.

Dr. Nadege Sandrine Uwamahoro coordinates maternity waiting home realist research for the Mozambique-Canada Maternal Health Project. She is a public health researcher specialising in health systems strengthening and health behaviour change interventions in low and middle-income countries. Most of her research and practice has aimed to advance equitable access to quality and person-centred healthcare services for marginalised populations, including young people living with HIV, refugees, and pregnant women in rural, hard-to-reach settings. A proponent of participatory and theory-driven research and evaluation approaches, Dr. Uwamahoro's mission is to create new forms of exchange between research and practice to promote accessible, respectful, and person-centred care in health systems across southern Africa and beyond. She has research experience in Denmark, Malawi, Mozambique, and the United Kingdom.

Dr. Sara Van Belle (MA, PhD) is a senior researcher at the Department of Public Health, Institute of Tropical Medicine, Antwerp and currently holds a senior research fellowship of the Flemish Science Fund. She is a political scientist with a large research portfolio in policy analysis, governance and accountability, and an internationally renowned realist evaluation expert.

Emma Williams has had a long career in evaluation, research and programme development in Canada and Australia, moving between academia, public service and private practice. She is a Credentialed Evaluator with experience in realist, observational and participatory evaluations on topics such as throughcare, family violence, service access, employment, environmental issues, and international development. She has also conducted innovative research in areas such as urban planning and language acquisition, and has a special interest in ethics and child empowerment. Until mid-2024 she was a member of the RREALI (Realist Research, Evaluation and Learning Initiative) team at Charles Darwin University, and now is an independent research and evaluation consultant.

Dr. Geoff Wong is an Associate Professor in Primary Care at the Nuffield Department of Primary Care, University of Oxford, United Kingdom (UK). He has been conducting realist syntheses and realist evaluations in the health sector (and more recently in social care and education) for almost two decades. He led the development of the quality and reporting standards and training materials for realist syntheses and then realist evaluations in the RAMESES I and II projects respectively. He also regularly provides training on realist syntheses and realist evaluations, to MSc and DPhil (PhD) students and colleagues on projects he is collaborating with. Clinically, he still works as a General Practitioner (Family Physician) in the UK's National Health Service.

Acknowledgements

Initially, we approached the daunting task of editing a book with caution, fully aware of its complexities. However, we did not anticipate how deeply enjoyable the process would turn out to be.

Since embarking on the journey of conceptualising this book a few years ago, our team of editors, publishers, and contributors has navigated through numerous significant life events. These include the arrivals of new babies, encounters with loss, experiences with crime, divorce, battles with chronic illnesses, extensive international travels, and various other personal challenges, undoubtedly many of which have remained unspoken. For these reasons, we extend our deepest appreciation to the chapter contributors for their remarkable effectiveness, and promptness in their communications, and to our publisher, Eleanor, for her enthusiasm and trust in our vision for this book.

Ana would like to express her gratitude to the female theory-driven evaluators who continue to serve as her role models since she started delving into the world of evaluation twenty years ago: Carol Weiss, Patricia Rogers, Nicoletta Stame and Gill Westhorp. She also extends her thanks to her colleagues at the School of Sociology & Social Policy for cheering her up along the way and for their invaluable advice on all aspects related to writing a book and beyond (Roxana Barbulescu, Ipek Demir, Ieva Eskytė, Joanne Greenhalgh, Ruth Holliday, Kahryn Hughes, Maria Rovisco, Karen Throsby and Katy Wright).

To Ray Pawson for encompassing the definition of mentoring. Always being there to discuss ideas, answer questions, review first drafts, and for sharing his wisdom generously. Special thanks to Emma for the early morning laughs during all those online meetings in my pyjamas, for her insightful guidance, and for facilitating the most efficient and enjoyable co-editing process imaginable.

To her children Sam and Olivia for keeping her simultaneously sane and insane during the writing and editing process.

Emma would like to express her gratitude to Ray Pawson for giving a bureaucrat (as she then was) a vision years ago of a very different way of thinking about programmes, to Nick Tilley for helping her understand how realist ideas could be applied, and to Gill Westhorp for years of rigour and collegiality and setting the bar high, and from whom I have learned so much, even – or especially – when we disagreed.

To the evaluators who, each in their own way, eased the isolation of a person working thousands of kilometres from colleagues: Kim Grey with her dispassionate kindness, John Stoney with his warmth and insight, Liz Meggetto with her sass and technical know-how, Cara Donohue with her gentle probes to go deeper, and Kerryn O'Rourke, who supported self-belief.

And above all thanks to Adam, whose support has been steadfast every day for 26 years, and to Ana, whose patience, humour, and unfailing spirit made this experience one of far more sunlight than shade.

This book is the product of an online connection forged between Emma (Australia) and Ana (United Kingdom) during the COVID-19 pandemic, illustrating the enduring connectivity and enthusiasm within the international realist community of researchers. It serves as a platform for discussing struggles, innovations, and the exchange of invaluable tips and tricks of the trade. We hope this book helps realist researchers in their own fieldwork adventures.

Introduction

The context of realist data collection

Ana Manzano and Emma Williams

The central topic of **Realist Evaluation: Principles and Practice** is how realist practitioners respond to the infinite contexts of fieldwork. The book examines how realist evaluators are constructing and testing causation claims in a variety of fieldwork macro-meso-micro contexts, using diverse data collection approaches and instruments. Although there are areas where all contributors agree, it is not a book about consensus and we, as editors, have not aimed for representativeness; disparate views and practices are valued. Scholars and practitioners in the field continue to grapple – often productively – with the absence of specific guidance for stages of realist work such as data collection and analysis. The authors in this book, as they reflect on their fieldwork experiences, engage with contemporary discussions in social research methodologies, including participatory approaches, digital data collection, interviewing through interpreters and confirmation bias in qualitative research.

To borrow a joke by Prof. Frans Leeuw heard at a European Evaluation Society Conference a few years back, Manzano and Williams are old enough to remember when 'realist evaluation' was referred to as 'realistic evaluation', a terminological metamorphosis we witnessed in amusement. *Realistic Evaluation* is the title of the book published in 1997 by British social scientists Prof. Ray Pawson and Prof. Nick Tilley. They openly played about with the words 'realistic' and 'real' because they were seeking to understand how programmes work in specific contexts and settings, focusing on the 'real world' complexity of social interventions. The approach is intended to be pragmatic (realistic) because it informs policy and practice by producing knowledge that is practically applicable to improving social programmes and their implementation. Realist evaluations differ from other types of theory-driven evaluation approaches because of their explicit focus on identifying causal processes by examining how programme outcomes are caused by underlying mechanisms within specific contexts. This philosophy penetrates formal and/or informal data collection tools to help substantiate causal claims. That is, realist evaluators and researchers design fieldwork activities to theorise, test those theories, refine and test again in an iterative process for the purpose of cumulative enquiry.

DOI: 10.4324/9781003457077-1

This book focuses on principle-aligned realist fieldwork practices, drawing from the foundational work of Pawson and Tilley (1997), since bolstered with the publication of reporting and quality standards for realist evaluation and synthesis (Wong et al., 2014, 2016), often referred to as 'the RAMESES standards'. There are different flavours of realism, and Pawson and Tilley's version is 'scientific realism' or more often 'Pawson and Tilley style realism'. One could argue that a 'Ramesesian realism' has now surfaced, not solely due to its published guidelines but also owing to the continuous discussions and resources generated by the realist community, which significantly influence practice and theory.

Prior to the publication of the RAMESES standards, having witnessed debates about the necessity and form of realist guidance, Manzano and Williams recall intense discussions regarding the level of prescriptiveness desired. While some realists vehemently opposed standards, others argued for guidance with a sufficient level of generality that could adapt to diverse contexts. The compromise eventually materialised in the form of the RAMESES guidance documents, embodying a balance between useful structure and adaptability to known and unknown heterogeneous fieldwork contexts. Almost a decade later, the success of the RAMESES standards is undeniable: they have become widely adopted and have significantly propelled the application of realist theory and methodology. However, as the RAMESES authors foresaw, research contexts evolve over time, and the application and methodology evolve in tandem.

This lack of strict procedures captures the essence of the realist interconnected iterative fieldwork/analysis process; it unfolds as a dynamic journey. Flexibility and adaptability are paramount, as is the need for creativity and imagination. The only road to mastering realist fieldwork entails doing it. It is in real-world scenarios that researchers can meaningfully apply theoretical concepts, experiment with techniques and confront challenges first-hand. Dealing with multiple authentic (sometimes annoying) complex situations enables deeper understandings of complex concepts such as context, mechanisms, outcomes, and Context-Mechanism-Outcome configurations, which display the relationship between them. The real world of fieldwork is rarely straightforward, often presenting known and unknown contextual specificities, changing circumstances and unexpected obstacles that foster learning. We have attempted to replicate some semblance of that reality for readers by showcasing real-life examples within the contributors' chapters in this book. Some of the contributors are novices, others highly experienced. They are based in five continents, and they work in disparate fields, including climate change, mental health, criminology and international development, but every chapter aims to pass on the knowledge obtained through fieldwork experiences.

In this introduction to contributors' stories, our aim is threefold. Firstly, we provide a succinct overview of how realist evaluation has carved out a significant niche within the broader landscape of programme evaluation methodologies. Secondly, we examine the intricate relationship between context and method, focusing on how they intertwine and influence one another in multifaceted ways. Thirdly, we address fundamental terminology prevalent in realist evaluation studies and used in this book. By clarifying these concepts, we aim to prevent repetition in our chapters and facilitate comprehension for novice readers, ensuring a solid foundation of essential knowledge for all readers.

The history of realist evaluation in the programme evaluation landscape

In the early 1990s, theory-driven evaluation became popular in the evaluation community (Chen, 1990). This approach understands that in any social programme there is a 'programme theory' (i.e., a hypothesis) based on assumptions, conceptualisations and expectations about how the programme designers expect the intervention to work; by making these assumptions explicit, a better understanding of programme implementation complexities is achieved. Pawson and Tilley explicitly saw realist evaluation as belonging to this evaluation approach by following sociologist Robert K. Merton's call to middle-range theorisation. Pawson's and Tilley's (1994) writings about realist evaluation had started at the beginning of the 1990s in criminal justice evaluation with an article in the British Journal of Criminology called '*What works in evaluation research?*', where they identified the 'pressing need' to incorporate the scientific realist strategy into evaluation. In this paper, they also introduced their trademark 'Context-Mechanism-Outcome' configurations (abbreviated as 'CMO configurations' or 'CMOCs') as practical patterns to support hypothesis testing and refining in evaluation studies. Realist evaluation examines programme complexity by assuming that every single programme feature noted in implementation guidelines contains a set of hypotheses ('theories') about how that feature will contribute to programme outcomes and trying to understand why this operates differently across time, spaces, participant characteristics such as professional background, socio-economic status, personality, etc.

Realist evaluation has achieved mainstream recognition primarily in Europe thanks to Pawson's and Tilley's work. They concentrated on methods – thus extending the basic idea of realist generative causation into ideas on research relationships, data collection (e.g., the 'teacher-learner cycle' and 'realist theory-driven interviews') and retrospective review (realist synthesis). As this book demonstrates, when those methods are applied in sites across different continents, they continue to evolve, although retaining realist principles. In the United States, where realist evaluation is a little less popular, Henry et al. (1998) and Mark et al. (1998) shared the same philosophical roots but focused more on users/implementation/values with their main contributions being about evaluation being a process of 'sensemaking' and 'social betterment'. Following the publication of *Realistic Evaluation*, several books sought to apply realist approaches to specific areas of social enquiry. These include evidence-based policy (Pawson, 2006b), qualitative research (Maxwell, 2012; Emmel, 2013), quantitative research (Byrne, 2002) and broad data collection debates (Emmel et al., 2018). Evidence of adoption is reinforced by publications in specific fields, including the Edwards et al. (2014) edited collection in business studies, and too many reports and journal papers to note here. At the time of writing, there are six published reviews of realist evaluations (Marchal et al., 2012; Ridde et al,, 2012; Salter & Kothari, 2014; Lacouture, et al., 2015; Lemire et al., 2020; Nielsen et al., 2022) demonstrating the academic reach of this evaluation approach.

Where theory meets practice: Context and method in realist evaluation

In the real world of fieldwork, theory meets practice in many heterogeneous and convoluted ways because context and method are connected in many interrelated ways (Miller, 1997). Data collection techniques and choices matter; interviews cannot do what observations or focus groups can. However, while decisions about what techniques to use are important, the messiness of real-world fieldwork means those decisions are only half of the story embedded in the dialectical processes within which research is organised and researchers get the job done. New questions will come to mind, topic guides will be completely reworked, etc. Prescriptive methods suggest solutions and structured frameworks based on predefined criteria and/or models, assuming these will encourage clarity and efficiency when researchers make fieldwork choices. The trouble is that they are based on assumptions about the uniformity and feasible categorisation of research circumstances. Realists in both theory and practice acknowledge the key importance of contextual circumstances in fieldwork: micro, meso and macro contexts. An ever-present micro context is human volition, expressed through individual preferences, emotions, common sense, intuition, creativity, etc. during fieldwork interactions. Meso contexts such as organisations, language and culture are the subject of multiple chapters in the book. Realists also recognise that temporal contexts may render static prescriptive models obsolete; some recent macro level context developments such as the COVID-19 pandemic and Artificial Intelligence (AI) demonstrate how long-established models may quite suddenly need to be rethought. For example, at the time of writing, the transformative potential of AI technologies in research includes data collection through focus groups with AI-based focus groups using virtual personas generated by sophisticated language models. These virtual personas can act as participants or even as moderators. Could they ever be programmed to think as realists? (Williams, 2021) In summary, to rephrase one of our favourite realist mantras: *What worked for this British junior researcher with this participant in this fieldwork scenario on a sunny Sunday before the COVID-19 pandemic, may not only not work but prove inadequate or even counterproductive for this senior Bangladeshi researcher managing a large team of researchers doing focus groups through interpreters on a wet Wednesday post COVID-19 pandemic.*

Recognising the complexities involved in fieldwork decision-making processes while embracing flexibility and creativity are essential steps toward navigating the intricacies of realist fieldwork encounters, as with any others. This is why this book does not aim to provide satnav/GPS-style directive instructions for navigating the complexities inherent in infinite real-world research settings. As realists we understand that there is no tool or rule adequate to deal with the myriad of specific contexts in which evaluation and research are conducted, and to satisfy the breadth of expertise in our readers, ranging from novice researchers embarking on their first fieldwork adventure to professors of evaluation. Instead, chapters provide vivid descriptions of context-specific complexities and explain how different practitioners adjusted to them, while making sure their practices remained true to realist ontology and epistemologies. The book does not provide rules but does provide useful principles and models to apply in practice.

Introducing the book chapters

The contributors are experienced researchers who, rather than relying on recipes or handbook advice, reflect on their experiences, their assumptions and concerns within each of their projects. While addressing practical methodological issues, they also highlight problems, contradictions and suggest solutions that worked for them in their nuanced social contexts. This is all done within the realist framework, which involves collecting and interpreting data iteratively with a focus on causality and theory-testing. This holds consistent across research topics (e.g., crime, environment, health), settings (e.g., geographical areas), target populations, specific data collection methods, previous research experience, the audience to which research is reported and so on.

Allard, Rayment-McHugh and Tilley's Chapter One examines the nature and role of evidence, drawing parallels with the types of evidence used in courts and the use of scientific or physical evidence. They examine the idea of 'science' and the realist framework, along with the need to focus on the mechanisms that are hypothesised to be related to specific outcomes. Finally, using crime-related evaluation examples, they consider alternative sources of data to test hypotheses and their pitfalls – recorded crime data, victimisation surveys, observational data and interviews – before highlighting the potential benefits of using unobtrusive measures such as refuse data.

In Chapter Two, **Manzano** proposes a realist perspective on respondent and researcher bias. The chapter provides a brief history of bias, highlighting that 'bias' is a term rooted in the positivist research paradigm. Confirmation and social desirability biases in qualitative data collection are examined by critically engaging with the scientific literature dedicated to understanding why participants may withhold or distort information when interacting with researchers. Subsequently, the issue is explored of researchers' beliefs affecting data collection and interpretation. Finally, Manzano suggests some guiding principles for dealing with confirmation and social desirability bias in theory-driven realist interviews and focus groups.

Chapter Three presents **Nielsen and Lemire's** comprehensive review of realist evaluation analytical strategies. Realist evaluations are characterised by iterative processes wherein analysis and data collection are interwoven. Accordingly, realist evaluators must pay particular attention to the analytical strategies applied throughout the realist inquiry process. Informed by a comprehensive review of published realist evaluations, this chapter examines the analytical strategies and techniques applied by realist evaluators. The article concludes with a discussion on how to advance analytical rigour in future realist evaluations.

Chapter Four by **Wong et al.** examines the practicalities of combining realist reviews with realist evaluation, an increasingly common practice, offering benefits such as using primary data from realist evaluation to address gaps in the programme theory developed in the review. However, this approach tends to increase project cost, duration and complexity. When undertaking a combined project, practical considerations arise, including staffing, sequencing, data collection and analysis.

Michaelis in Chapter Five explores how quality was conceptualised and managed in a large cross-country realist evaluation, using as a case study three large realist portfolio evaluations of the UK's international climate finance. The portfolio evaluations each involved a combination of primary and secondary research. The chapter describes lessons relating to team composition, roles and training, research tools including interview guides and coding frameworks, capacity building, quality assurance processes and maintaining a large team's focus on the realist approach.

Howe's Chapter Six is the first in a series of chapters focusing on realist interviewing. She provides a practical guide for the realist novice who may be embarking upon realist interviews for the first time. The chapter highlights the importance of study design and discusses considerations necessary to gain ethical approval so that researchers have the flexibility they need to collect data whilst staying true to the iterative and evolving nature of realist research. Real-world examples of interview questions are outlined; explanations offered as to how realist interviews can be directed, and questions articulated when conducting research with vulnerable participants and professionals.

Van Belle et al.'s Chapter Seven focuses on realist interviewing as a methodological instrument and its potential to engage with 'context', and to manage the inevitable power dynamics between researcher and participant. The authors present the experiences of researchers with realist interviewing in the context of global health research. They then compare realist interviews with dialogic approaches informed by other paradigms and currently used in global health, such as interpretative interviewing, narrative inquiry and participatory action research.

Gilmore and Sandrine's Chapter Eight focuses on the practical and theoretical challenges of collecting realist data in unfamiliar settings and explores effective mitigation strategies, specifically highlighting the role of stakeholder engagement. It draws on the authors' first-hand experiences conducting global health-oriented realist evaluations across four African countries (Kenya, Mozambique, Tanzania and Uganda) as foreign researchers. Particularly, the chapter addresses challenges often encountered by researchers with an outsider perspective within global health and cross-cultural research.

Particularly in the years since COVID-19, interviewing using online video platforms such as Zoom, Teams or Skype has become common. In Chapter Nine, **Williams** outlines factors that should be considered when determining whether and how to conduct online audio-visual interviews in realist research and evaluations. The cognitive demands of realist interviews and differences between realist interviews and other types of interviews are discussed, and also how and why video realist interviews may differ from face-to-face realist interviews, particularly in some linguistic and cultural contexts. Challenges and opportunities of online interviewing to realist investigators are noted, and recommendations are provided.

In Chapter Ten, **Groot and Carr** present a brief history of patient-oriented research (POR) in Canada, while outlining key contexts and mechanisms from Zibrowski et al.'s programme theory to explain empowered patient-centred research (Zibrowski et al., 2021). They describe how they engaged with patient partners in two realist evaluations in which the patient partners had markedly different backgrounds. They reflect on areas where interactions aligned with Zibrowski et al.'s programme theory and areas where they identified potential refinements to the theory. They conclude with an emphasis on trust as the fundamental mechanism in POR realist research, and note that there are multiple dimensions of trust that are relevant to POR.

Redgate and Dalkin's Chapter Eleven outlines how the use of topic guides can assist researchers to enact realist principles within the field when collecting qualitative data. It focuses on ensuring the topic guide is theory-driven and adheres to generative causation. A comparison of realist vs. non-realist topic guides is provided together with the implications these differences imply. The underpinning epistemological considerations of the realist topic guide are made explicit, aided by a visual conceptualisation of the key considerations, reflecting on how they influence approaches to question and topic guide development.

In Chapter Twelve, **Hastings** offers a critical realist-informed perspective on the design of interviews in applied social science research including realist evaluation. The chapter starts by discussing the similarities and differences between scientific and critical realisms. It provides practical guidance on developing the kinds of interview questions that will generate the rich ontological 'deep' data that, with appropriate retroductive theoretical analysis, will enable answers to realist-inspired research and evaluation questions. It also provides ingredients and a method for developing an appropriate interview approach to meet the specific needs of a project within the principles of critical realism.

Finally, in Chapter Thirteen, **Mukumbang and Dada** introduce a realist photovoice technique as a potential innovative method in the toolbox of realist researchers. They explore its potential contribution to enhancing programme theory co-elicitation between the researchers and stakeholders while addressing power inequities in researcher-participant engagements. Using images as metaphors and allowing study participants to guide the conversations provides a unique strength to realist photovoice techniques for eliciting, testing and confirming programme theories.

Realist evaluation jargon oversimplified

As it is often the case with edited books, readers may pick up the book to read a particular chapter and miss important definitions and debates in other chapters. To fill gaps in knowledge, a brief realist glossary is provided in Table 0.1. We understand that the readership of this book may vary, from those new to fieldwork and realism to experienced realist evaluators keen on understanding the evolving conditions and expectations of fieldwork and exploring innovative options. Acknowledging the abundance of jargon in evaluation science, we offer below operational definitions of key concepts mentioned across this book's chapters. These definitions are no-doubt contested so we drew from a blend of reputable authorities and personal preferences, recognising the ongoing debates within the field. The reader should remember that there is more than one type of realist evaluation and more than one construct of key concepts in realist evaluation such as 'mechanism' (Westhorp, 2018).

Table 0.1 Definitions for key terms used throughout the book

Concept	Definition
CMO/CMOC	CMO configuration (sometimes written as CMOC) stands for Context-Mechanism-Outcome configuration. It is the basic causal explanatory framework for realist evaluation and realist reviews. Stated as a sentence, it means 'In this context, this mechanism generates this outcome.' It is a tool to help remember what needs explaining: all outcomes are a result of interactions between contexts and mechanisms. Other variations are used, such as ICMAO (Intervention-Context-Mechanism-Actor-Outcome) (Greenhalgh et al., 2017a).
Contexts	Context describes those features of the situations into which programmes/interventions are introduced that affect the operation of programme mechanisms. The settings into which programmes are introduced do not, in and of themselves, constitute context in the realist sense. However, things about the way those settings operate can (Greenhalgh et al., 2017g).

(Continued)

Table 0.1 (Continued)

Concept	Definition
Critical realism	Critical realism is a philosophy of science that suggests that the world is an open system with a constellation of structures, mechanisms, and other entities responsible for the observable patterns of events (Mukumbang et al., 2023, p. 513). Scientific realism and critical realism are the two prominent forms of realism. Pawson and Tilley (1997) situate realist evaluation in scientific realism although Mukumbang et al. (2023) illustrated that both scientific realism and critical realism make contributions to realist evaluation. The difficulty here lies in the presence of two distinct 'critical realisms': the one proposed by Bhaskar (2008) versus Campbell (1988) who focuses more on methodological approaches.
Formal or substantive theory	The theories that operate in different domains or disciplines. Examples might include incentives theory in economics, attachment theory in human development or constructivist learning theory in education (Greenhalgh et al., 2017d).
Mechanisms	Programme mechanisms describe how it is that programmes and interventions contribute to outcomes (Greenhalgh et al., 2017e).
Middle-range theory	These are theories that involve 'abstraction, of course, but they are close enough to observed data to be incorporated in propositions that permit empirical testing' (Merton, 1967).
Outcomes	'Realist evaluation uses the term 'outcome' to include short, medium and long term changes, intended and unintended, resulting from an intervention. The only difference between the terms 'impact' (as defined above) and 'outcome' (as used in realist evaluation) is that 'impact' implies changes 'for people and their lives'; whereas 'outcome' includes change for people and their lives but can also include other kinds of changes (for organisations, workers, governments and so on)' (Westhorp, 2014, p. 3).
Programme theory	It is the description, in words or diagrams, of what is supposed to be done in a policy or programme (theory of action) and how and why that is expected to work (theory of change) (Greenhalgh et al., 2017e).
RAMESES	Abbreviation for the Realist And Meta-narrative Evidence Synthesis: Evolving Standards studies (RAMESES I and II) which provide standards for conducting and reporting realist synthesis, research and evaluation.
Realism	Realism sits somewhere between constructivism and positivism, closer to post-positivism in ontology; closer to some forms of constructivism in epistemology. What distinguishes realism is its particular understanding of how causation works. The basic idea is that things that we experience or can observe are caused by 'deeper', usually non-observable processes (mechanisms) (Greenhalgh et al., 2017c).
Realist evaluation	Realist evaluation is, as the name implies, a form of evaluation, conducted on realist principles. Data is collected mainly but not exclusively from primary sources. This can include field research, interviews, focus groups and documentary analysis (Greenhalgh et al., 2017a).

(Continued)

Table 0.1 (Continued)

Concept	Definition
Realist research	Realist research is a collective name for research that is underpinned by the principles of realist philosophy. (Greenhalgh et al., 2017d). It may be conducted as part of a realist evaluation or conducted as a stand-alone realist primary or secondary research project.
Realist interview	Realist interviews are theory-driven interviews, meaning that theory should be used explicitly and systematically throughout the interview process. Realist interviews are semi-structured and qualitative in nature: participant views are explored through conversations (Greenhalgh et al., 2017b).
Realist synthesis/ realist review	Realist synthesis – also known as realist review – is a form of literature review. Realist review can use published peer-reviewed articles, evaluation reports, other grey literature, existing data sets (for example census information) and in some cases, interviews and other primary data collection to supplement the literature (Greenhalgh et al., 2017a).
Scientific realism	Scientific realism posits that our scientific theories are true or false based on the best scientific knowledge. We should consider our scientific theories true–the entities they postulate as real, not merely as 'useful' (Chernoff, 2007). Theoretical explanations in scientific realism go beyond the observable world captured through anthropocentric approaches and other observational measurements to accommodate knowledge about the unobservable (Mukumbang et al., 2023). It is one of the underlying philosophical bases of realist evaluation.
Teacher-learner cycle	'A distinctive process in realist interviews used to develop programme theory, that usually involves teaching participants the particular programme theory under test for them to teach the interviewer back by refine it, consolidate it or discard it' (Greenhalgh et al., 2017b).
Theory-driven evaluation	'Any evaluation strategy or approach that explicitly integrates and uses stakeholder, social science, some combination of, or other types of theories in conceptualizing, designing, conducting, interpreting, and applying an evaluation' (Coryn et al., 2011, p. 201). Other terms used for this: theory-based evaluation.
Theory of Change	'A theory of change explains how the activities undertaken by an intervention (such as a project, program or policy) contribute to a chain of results that lead to the intended or observed impacts' (Better Evaluation, 2024). Other terms related to this: results chain, logic model, programme theory, outcome mapping, impact pathway and investment logic.

1 Testing realist hypotheses

The value of diverse evidence, including unobtrusive measures

Troy Allard, Susan Rayment-McHugh, and Nick Tilley

Introduction

In this chapter, we consider the nature and role of evidence, arguing that there is a clear need for hypotheses to be tested using more than one type of data (triangulation), with specific data sources and indicators selected based on the highly specific type/s of information needed to answer realist hypotheses. First, we consider the nature and role of evidence, drawing parallels with the types of evidence used in courts and the use of scientific or physical evidence. Second, we examine the idea of 'science' and the realist framework, along with the need to focus on the mechanisms that are hypothesised to be related to specific outcomes. Third, using crime-related evaluation examples, we consider alternative sources of data to test hypotheses and their pitfalls – recorded crime data, victimisation surveys, observational data and interviews – before highlighting the potential benefits of using unobtrusive measures. Finally, we introduce refuse (rubbish) data as an unobtrusive measure that can add to our understanding about the impacts of programmes/interventions, using a project evaluating the impact of police patrols as an example. We briefly outline the programme and the realist context–mechanism–outcomes (CMOs) that were developed, explaining how refuse data was used with other data to address the hypotheses. We conclude by noting that while there are limitations with using physical evidence such as refuse data, it is an important additional data source that can help confirm, refute or refine realist hypotheses.

The nature and role of evidence

Science deals in evidence relating to regularities and their causes. Courts of law deal in evidence relating to specific events. However, the logic of evidence use is similar. The comparison is instructive. Courts test the theory that X committed a crime against Y. In adversarial systems the prosecution seeks to corroborate the hypothesis that X did it and presents evidence accordingly. The defence seeks to cast doubt on or, at best, falsify the theory, and presents evidence accordingly. In practice, both the prosecution and the defence will

DOI: 10.4324/9781003457077-2

also deploy a range of rhetorical skills to prop up their arguments. Judges and juries are then asked to come to a verdict. The system is far from perfect. Conclusive 'proof' is rarely, if ever, possible. Hence the reference to proof 'beyond reasonable doubt'. Moreover, there is strong pressure to come to a verdict in the practical business of meting out justice. The fallibility of verdicts reached is brought out in successful appeals.

Forensic scientists deal in physical evidence, for example, fingerprints, DNA profiles, toolmarks, soil, insects and shoe prints. They are opportunistic in the evidence they collect and analyse – anything that speaks to the case. The evidence can be used 'inceptively' to inform the investigation by building a picture of the course of events surrounding the crime; for example, who was where, when were they there, whether they had fired a gun and from what direction, whether a bullet came from a given gun and so on. Forensic evidence can also be used evidentially by the prosecution or defence to support a hypothesis that A did it or to cast doubt on that hypothesis.

Forensic evidence is rarely sufficient on its own to establish guilt (provide evidence for the hypothesis that X did it) beyond reasonable doubt. It is normally part of a package. However, forensic evidence can sometimes be sufficient to falsify the hypothesis beyond reasonable doubt[1]. Statistics cited by the Innocence Project suggest that 570 people convicted in the United States were exonerated because of DNA evidence, between 1989 and 2022 (University of California, 2023).

Andrew Malkinson provides a recent example from the United Kingdom. Malkinson was convicted for rape in 2004 and given a 17-year prison sentence, presumably because the case as presented at the time was taken by the jury to be proven beyond reasonable doubt. Malkinson protested his innocence at the time and continued to do so. In 2007, a DNA profile, neither matching Malkinson's nor that of the victim's then boyfriend, was found on the victim's vest. The location on the vest accorded with the victim's account of what happened during the incident. It was not until 2023 that the case was referred to the court of appeal and Malkinson's conviction was overturned. The DNA profile provided crucial evidence falsifying the original hypothesis that Malkinson did it.

The evidence used in criminal investigations and trials is fallible. Evidence from forensic science is widely taken to be especially strong. Those presenting it are treated as experts, giving their opinions dispassionately. This is not to say that their conclusions are incontestable and unchallenged. Interpretations can be and are questioned. However, the unspoken underbelly of theory underpinning the 'facts' presented is seldom articulated or subject to critical scrutiny. For instance, the supposed uniqueness of fingermarks, shoeprints, toolmarks and the science behind DNA profiling and the operation of the DNA database are taken as read. Forensic scientists, lawyers and investigators are, of course, mindful of the potential for challenges from probing interrogation from counsel in court, and (ideally) try to make sure that what they say is well founded and that uncertainties are acknowledged.

Science and the realist framework

Science is about patterns (regularities) and changes in regularities. What mechanisms produce regularities and changes in regularities? Some science focuses on identifying[2] regularities, some on explaining them, some on changes in regularities and some on variations in regularities. In social science, regularities may relate to behaviours (for example, crime patterns) or states of affairs (say morbidity or mortality rates). The empirical scientist has to adduce evidence that speaks to all this: regularities (and their changes), states of affairs (and their changes) and tests of theories that aim to explain the regularity and any changes in it. Sometimes a new regularity is identified as a consequence of a theory. The theory predicts the regularity (or a regular change in a known regularity) and this new regularity (or regular change in it) can be novel, interesting and useful. Applied science looks for interventions that will reliably produce changed states of affairs that accord with intentions.

Realist evaluation research tests theories that a given intervention activates one or more mechanisms that produce a predicted regular pattern of changes in regularity, and the contextual requirements for the intervention to activate the mechanism/s. The more precise and idiosyncratic the prediction the better, because precision and idiosyncrasy reduce the scope for (although never eliminate) alternative explanations. In Popperian terms, precise predictions facilitate falsification by enabling lots of potential ways of being wrong (see Popper 1959, 1972). Courts test very specific hypotheses: a particular person committed the crime.

It is often the case that alternative explanations are proposed and then crucial experiments (or crucial data) are sought to provide evidence to arbitrate between them. This can be the case in courts and criminal investigations, where a fixed number of suspects are in the frame but crucial evidence is sought to arbitrate between them. We should add that Popper's comments on fallibility should be remembered. Science and scientists can and do get things wrong. They have their own cognitive biases. Proofs are never possible. In the world of science, it is a critical and sceptical community of fellow scientists who provide checks (Collins, 1985; Merton, 1973; Popper, 1959; Tilley, 2009). In courts contending counsel, judges and juries fallibly do the same.

A key source of fallibility in all empirical science relates to evidence. We have hinted already at the theoretical embeddedness of data in reference to fingerprints and DNA. Popper famously put it in the Logic of Scientific Discovery (LSD) when he stated that,

> The empirical basis of objective science has nothing 'absolute' about it. Science does not rest on a solid bedrock. The bold structure of its theories rises, as it were, above a swamp. It is like a building erected on piles. The piles are driven down from above into the swamp, but not down to any natural or 'given' base; and if we stop driving the piles

deeper, it is not because we have reached firm ground. We simply stop when we are satisfied that the piles are firm enough to carry the structure, at least for the time being.

(Popper, 1959, p. 111)

In LSD, Popper was writing mainly about the physical sciences. In the social sciences, there is a rich history of critiques of assumptions that data of one sort or another unequivocally speak to facts plain and simple, that can be used to prove, corroborate, confirm or falsify a theory.

Alternative sources of 'evidence' and pitfalls

Recorded data

Durkheim's (1897/1951) use of cause of death records to test his theory of suicide has been subjected to repeated scrutiny (Atkinson, 1968; Taylor, 1982; Douglas, 2015). The statistics are socially constructed. Decisions have to be made about probable cause of death (suicide, homicide, natural causes, accident), or there is an open verdict. The decisions involve judgements where the evidence is often equivocal. The category chosen arbitrates between alternative possible theories that are consonant with the available evidence, and the choice may reflect folk theories or be swayed by the consequences of selecting one category or another.

Recorded crime data are notorious for the biases created by reporting and recording decisions and opportunities (Maguire, 2007; Tilley & Tseloni, 2016). Not all crime is reported and of that reported not all is recorded. Reporting and recording crimes require decisions and opportunities. Crimes may not be recorded because they are not noticed, they are not known to be crimes, they are thought too trivial, the police are thought unlikely to do anything about them, they are embarrassing, there are fears of recriminations from perpetrators, the effort to report is too great and so on. Reported crimes may not be recorded because there is no realistic chance of detection, the person reporting the crime is not believed, levels of recorded crime are a performance indicator, filling out the paperwork is too time-consuming and so on. Moreover, when an incident is recorded the category used can be moot, and the victim's belief that they have suffered one type of crime may not accord with that of an attending police officer.

Increases in recorded crime may be a sign of police success. If police become more trusted by victims that they will be taken seriously and action will follow, those victims are more likely to report incidents. More recorded crime may also be a sign of failure, where police preventive efforts have been inadequate. Increases in crime may have nothing to do with police action, where new crime opportunities emerge, for example, from the Internet. On top of that, definitions of crimes change over time and vary by place. These biases vary by place and time making comparisons tricky.

Victimisation surveys

Victimisation surveys are used to try to avoid biases in recorded crime data, but they have their own problems. Respondent recall, especially within the time period about which they are asked, is fallible. Sample sizes are never large enough to capture relatively rare crimes. Where individuals are questioned, some key categories of crime targets, such as businesses, voluntary and public sector organisations, are typically omitted although there are sometimes specialist surveys targeting these. Crimes without individual victims, such as much corporate and environmental crime, are omitted. Non-response undermines the strength of inferences that can be drawn from findings (and response rates have been falling, see Office for National Statistics [ONS], 2023). Repeat incidents against the same victims involve tricky counting decisions, especially when very high numbers are reported by some respondents. Crime surveys are also very expensive and are no panacea.

Observational data

Observational data, including the direct observation of behaviour in context, can also provide important insight into regularities, enabling testing of realist hypotheses. Observations can be undertaken in a wide range of settings and across time. This method has been employed across multiple disciplines, including education, health, psychology, criminology and anthropology (McCall, 1984; Walshe et al., 2012). It may be particularly useful with children, whenever communication challenges may limit engagement with other research methods, and in relation to complex issues that are difficult to report or describe, or where implicit bias or social desirability may impact responses (McCall, 1984; Walshe et al., 2012).

Direct observation may be undertaken in natural or contrived settings (using confederates), and through either structured or unstructured approaches (Bryman, 2012). This type of data may be more reliable than interview or survey data, given behaviour is observed 'in situ', and it does not rely on participant recall, perceptions or interpretation (Bryman, 2012). However, this may depend on the extent to which the observations are unobtrusive (unnoticed by those being observed), and thus whether observed behaviour may be reactive (or not) to the observer (McCall, 1984). Observational research can be difficult to implement, often requiring researchers to spend time in the field. Data may be impacted by sampling decisions, observer fatigue or by gaps in attention, or the extent to which an observational schedule is adhered to (Bryman, 2012).

Interviews

Data elicited in interviews are likewise fallible. They involve the respondent constructing the wants and intentions of the interviewer, choices over interviewees, decisions about what to disclose, presentation of self in interviews, perceptions of the interviewer, decisions about whether or not to participate, decisions about whether or not to tell the truth. Interview data are clearly socially constructed. Interviews do not display plain facts. They involve artful behaviours by interviewer and interviewee alike. Although there is a rich literature on interviewing and interview strategies to try to ensure that respondents are able to speak accurately to the researcher's interests, including contributions by realists, there is no way of escaping the infusion of the social in interviews. And those taking part in interview encounters may follow an agenda at variance with that of the interviewer. The famous story of extended and extensive research with 'Agnes' illustrates how artful responses even during successive, prolonged interviews can lead the interviewer to erroneous conclusions about the respondent's life and identity. In the case of Agnes, information collected during interviews was influenced by the interviewer's expectations and assumptions, as well as the respondent's desire to present themselves in a certain light; and this had to do with her biography, biology, behaviour and social and sexual identity (Garfinkel, 1967, p. 116–15 and p. 285–288).

The need for and use of unobtrusive measures

In courts and in criminal investigations, efforts to dissemble the interviewer are normal, which counsel attempt to penetrate in cross-examination. Where possible, physical evidence is sought to corroborate or cast doubt on what is said. This is where forensic scientists come in. They look for evidence to arbitrate between competing accounts of what happened and who did it in criminal cases. The forensic evidence itself is, of course, fallible. Take the residue left on the shooter's hand after the discharge of a firearm, which could be used to suggest who fired the shot in a crime where this is contested. French and Morgan (2015) report a neat experiment where they use standard measures of gunshot residue on the hands of the original shooter and on those who shook hands with them ('secondary transfer') and then on those who shook hands with that person ('tertiary transfer'). They also looked at the transmission of gunshot residue to those in the vicinity. They report findings that transmission did, indeed, occur in all cases. This does not mean that gunshot residue is of no evidential value, but it is fallible – not a clincher!

'Unobtrusive measures' comprise data sources sometimes used in the social sciences either instead of or in addition to data collected from relevant interview and questionnaire respondents. The classic pitch for their use is Webb et al.'s *Unobtrusive Measures*, originally published in 1966 (republished as a Sage Classic in 2000). Webb et al. include in unobtrusive measures all that do not involve interviews or surveys, so archival evidence such as that provided in records is included. Here we are concerned with what they refer to as 'physical traces' and their 'erosion and accretion'. For social science, Webb et al. comment that 'physical evidence is probably the social scientist's least-used source of data, yet because of its ubiquity, it holds flexible and broad-gauged potential' (Webb et al., 1966, p. 35).

Webb et al. acknowledge the weaknesses in physical evidence for social science. It can be ephemeral. It certainly does not speak for itself. Its production is not under the control of the investigator aiming to test their hypotheses. There may be none that is of any use. It is socially created and may be artfully manipulated in ways that (deliberately or otherwise) mislead the observer. It may result in misleading conclusions when the material available for examination, collection or observation is atypical. Physical evidence has, thus, to be used critically. Moreover, it can rarely be depended on, on its own. Triangulation with other data, with different weaknesses, is normally advisable, as is the case too in forensic examinations designed to inform and test hypotheses in criminal cases.

What physical evidence cannot tell us directly is about underlying causal mechanisms, but we should not worry about this. Such mechanisms are ultimately unobservable. We may talk to people to elicit theories that speak to mechanisms. We may also try to test conjectures about mechanisms through artful interviews (Pawson, 1996; Pawson & Tilley, 1997). But we are not directly observing them.

In relation to regularities and changes in regularities, which are concerns of social scientists, physical evidence can be an important source. Moreover, in applied research physical evidence can contribute to tests of hypotheses: if this mechanism is activated in this context along the lines we conjecture, what observable physical patterns would we expect or what changes in those patterns would we expect? Where there are competing hypotheses, what different physical patterns would we expect that could (at least provisionally) arbitrate between them?

Webb et al. (2000) provide a host of examples, including:

- Rate of removal/replacement of tiles surrounding different museum exhibits as an indicator of their relative popularity.
- Wear on library books as an indicator of their popularity (or of chapters/pages most looked at).
- Weighing food trucks going into and out of hospitals (or hospital wards) to indicate the level of consumption of food.
- Changing alcohol consumption patterns by the discarded bottles and cans that are collected.
- Sexual preoccupation variations by place and gender from graffiti found in public toilets.
- Activity levels of children by wear on shoes.
- Noseprints on glass display cabinets to gauge their relative popularity.

Physical evidence has been used to test a classic hypothesis in applied criminology: broken windows (Kelling & Coles 1996; Wilson & Kelling 1982). Let's spell the general theory out.

Failure to remove physical signs of criminal and other antisocial behaviour creates an environment that permits further criminal and antisocial behaviour.

The addition of further physical signs that elicit no corrective response increases the permissiveness of that behaviour. Those who are rewarded in some way by criminal and antisocial behaviour (for example, seeing their graffiti on display or avoiding the costs of disposing of waste products lawfully) persist in it. Others, who would normally behave lawfully, no longer perceive the benefit of doing so. Because their previous lawful behaviour makes no noticeable difference to the environment, they are likewise drawn into criminal or antisocial behaviour: criminal and antisocial behaviour is normalised. Behaving antisocially and criminally is a rational choice where rewards exceed costs for antisocial behaviour and where costs exceed benefits for prosocial behaviour. A spiral of decline follows from persistent failures in any area to correct signs of disorder.

An experiment was conducted in New York City as a partial test of the theory (Sloan-Howitt & Kelling, 1990). Subway cars (underground carriages) were festooned with graffiti. The graffiti were not routinely removed. Few were caught creating them. Graffiti artists could see their work on display. They were able to show it off to others. Creating graffiti was low risk and produced high rewards. They comprised a visible achievement. Drawing graffiti was normalised for those with an interest in producing it. Graffiti proliferated. The theory was tested through a subway car cleaning regime.

The results of the New York City experiment corroborated the theory. Gradually, graffiti ceased to reappear as more and more of the subway cars were brought into the cleaning regime and fewer and fewer carried visible graffiti. However, the results didn't *prove* the theory. But then nothing could do so. Readers will be able to think of lots of other potential (realist) hypotheses that could explain the pattern observed. Moreover, any of them may be correct. The point is that in the experiment the outcome pattern was as predicted from the application of a theory relating to underlying mechanisms. It behoves others to show empirically that an alternative theory is better! Had the outcome not been as expected, it would be equally possible to make ad hoc adjustments to the theory to accommodate the aberrant results, but that would be to weaken the theory by making it unfalsifiable. Of course, the ad hoc adjustments might also be warranted but these would need to be tested through further empirical research. In general, the more precise the theoretical prediction, the less scope there is for alternative theories, although their possibility is never eliminated.

Webb et al. (1996) comment:

> It is not often that an investigation tests a theory so precise in its predictions that the appearance or absence of a single trace is a critical test of a theory. Most of the time physical evidence is more appropriate for indexing the extent to which the activity has taken place…The more visible weaknesses of physical evidence should preclude its use no more than should the less visible, but equally real, weaknesses of other methods…

(p. 51–52)

Of course, forensic physical trace evidence is often used to help test rather specific hypotheses. At least it can provide quite compelling evidence to falsify a range of alternative hypotheses. In criminal investigations, physical evidence is rarely sufficient to make a case, but it can sometimes (fallibly!) falsify hypotheses or eliminate potential suspects.

Webb et al.(1966) use the term 'outcroppings' to refer to a range of implications that a theory might have. Although not using the term, Farrell (2013) refers to a number of conditions that a satisfactory theory for the global drop in crime must satisfy – outcroppings that must be satisfied empirically, if the theory is to be plausible. He adjudicates between competing hypotheses to explain the crime drop by examining whether or not these necessary outcroppings are satisfied by the theory (Farrell, 2013; Farrel et al., 2015). A weakness of the test of broken windows using the New York experiment is that there are no further outcroppings that would help test the theory. Moreover, for realists in particular, whose theories will specify mechanisms relating to the reasoning and resources at the disposal of those whose actions are at issue, further tests would be needed to try to elicit more direct evidence on this. The need for multiple sources of evidence that test hypotheses in diverse but independent ways is endorsed by Webb et al. (1966) who refer to triangulation as a method of gaining a fix on a phenomenon of interest from different vantage points.

Selecting indicators to test realist hypotheses: the impact of police patrols on youth sexual violence and abuse

We now turn our focus to a project that we undertook and highlighted the need for multiple indicators and the value of unobtrusive physical evidence – in the form of refuse data. Between 2013 and 2018, we contributed to a community prevention initiative, which aimed to reduce the prevalence of youth sexual violence and abuse (YSVA) issues that had been identified in two communities (Smallbone et al., 2013; Tilley et al., 2014). While the larger project included distinct activities and interventions that targeted specific aspects of the problem in specific domains (youth networks, home, school, public spaces, service system), here we focus on our realist evaluation of the targeted police patrols that were implemented in public spaces.

Prior research indicated that the abuse was largely occurring when young people were socialising late at night, in local parks and other public spaces, without adult supervision (Smallbone et al., 2013). These locations were poorly lit, with thick vegetation that restricted visibility or access to passing traffic and limited natural and formal surveillance. Desensitisation to violence and concerns for personal safety were further barriers to community guardianship, while peer subcultural social norms supported under-age and abusive sexual behaviour. In addition to sexual violence, young people also engaged in fights and substance misuse in these locations (Rayment-McHugh et al., 2021).

One intervention involved using targeted police patrols in selected parks and public spaces identified as 'hot spots' for abuse, to increase guardianship in at-risk locations (Allard et al., 2019). Locations and timing of these police patrols were informed by prior observational research that had identified specific parks and times as being most problematic for concerning youth behaviour, including YSVA (Smallbone et al., 2013). The patrols were planned in consultation with the local police service, to reflect operational demands and capacity (Allard et al., 2019). At each selected location, patrols were undertaken for 15 minutes, at randomised times during 'hot times' for concerning behaviour, because evidence indicated that this length of time maximised diffusion of benefits (Koper, 2006; Sherman et al., 2014). Police were asked to walk through each site to enhance visibility and to initiate conversations with young people and other community members present in these locations.

Developing realist hypotheses

To assess if the intervention was working, for whom, and how, we developed a series of CMO configurations for the police patrols. As displayed in Table 1.1, we viewed the context as being potentially different based on the gender of the young person, so explored CMO configurations separately for girls and boys. We hypothesised that the police patrols could produce change through a range of mechanisms, including if young people perceived the patrol outcomes as being potentially damaging to their reputations, avoided going to locations they perceived as 'risky', were uncertain about the risk of getting caught or overestimated the risk, or if they viewed the patrols as a provocation and became defiant. Depending on which mechanism/s were activated, alternative outcomes included young people reducing problem behaviours in the specific location/s that were patrolled, changing behaviours in the patrolled locations and similar settings (diffusion of benefits), going to less risky locations that were not patrolled to engage in problem behaviours (displacement), increasing their pro-social use of the area, or increasing unwanted and problem behaviours.

Identifying and selecting data sources

We considered a range of data sources and indicators, in light of the strengths and limitations of each. For illustrative purposes, we focus here on the CMOs relating to all likely offenders in Table 1.1 and why we selected these data sources and indicators to assess outcomes. As the police patrols were time-limited, only ever operating a very small proportion of each 24-hour day in practice, randomisation through the 15-minute patrols occurring 'anywhere, anytime' was hypothesised to result in uncertainty about the level of risk (general deterrence), thereby reducing the problem behaviours at times when the patrols were not 'active'.

Table 1.1 Context-Mechanism-Outcome configurations for police patrols

Context	Mechanisms	Outcome	Data
Girls valuing community/ family reputation (with stable families) Younger girls, inexperienced in offending/YSVA	Fear of loss of reputation (especially if told parents will be informed of antisocial behaviour)	Change behaviour in backtracks and/or go to other less risky location	Recorded data (patrol records) Recorded data (police crime records) Observational data Interviews
Girls indifferent to community/family reputation (living away from home or in unstable families) Older girls more embedded in offending/sexual behaviour	Risk avoidance	Go elsewhere for criminal/ antisocial behaviour	Recorded data (patrol records) Recorded data (police crime records) Observational data Interviews
Boys valuing community/ family reputation (with stable families) Younger boys, inexperienced in offending/YSVA	Fear of loss of reputation (especially if told parents will be informed of antisocial behaviour)	Change behaviour in backtracks and/or go to other less tempting location	Recorded data (patrol records) Recorded data (police crime records) Observational data Interviews
Boys indifferent to community/family reputation (living away from home or in unstable families) Older boys more embedded in offending/YSVA	Risk avoidance	Go elsewhere for criminal/ antisocial behaviour	Recorded data (patrol records) Recorded data (police crime records) Observational data Interviews
All likely offenders	Uncertainty over whether high or low risk at any given point (given random times and places of patrols)	Lower levels of crime and antisocial behaviour at all times in backtracks	Recorded data (police crime records) Observational data Interviews Unobtrusive measures (refuse)
All likely offenders	Overestimation of risk (residual deterrence)	Reduced crime and incivility after and during patrols at backtracks	Recorded data (police crime records) Observational data Interviews Unobtrusive measures (refuse)
Non-youth/non-offenders	Greater sense of security, with fewer signs of incivility	Higher rates of non-offender backtrack use	Observational data Unobtrusive measures (refuse)
Highly criminally involved angry and resentful boys and girls with no reputation to lose	Defiance/ provocation	Aggressive response to patrols	Interviews

To test these CMOs, we included four main data sources that might contribute to our assessments and a range of indicators. The main types of behaviours we were trying to reduce related to youth sexual violence and abuse, a (relatively) rare, sensitive and difficult to measure type of behaviour that often goes unreported or undetected because it occurs in private or unsupervised areas.

We used **recorded crime data**, which included reported sexual and violent offences that occurred in the public parks and spaces throughout the community. As anticipated, such behaviours in these public parks and spaces appeared to be rarely reported, particularly for this subcultural group, and reporting patterns may change over time. These factors cast some doubt as to our ability to use recorded crime data as a valid and reliable measure of youth sexual violence and abuse behaviours and to assess if these change over time. Officially recorded crime data therefore provides part of the picture – but it provides a narrow, limited and often distorted picture.

Observational data were used to assess whether young people were congregating in the parks and public spaces, and indicators about the types of behaviours observed at certain times/days were recorded, including the number of young people drinking alcohol, using drugs, and engaging in sexual activity. These observations were conducted randomly at different times/days, but limitations in the design (funding and safety requiring two researchers present) meant that observations were difficult to undertake, subsequently limiting the number of randomised observation points and its usefulness as a data source to assess change over time. It was also problematic that those observed were aware of the observation, which could have impacted the recorded behaviour.

Interviews with individuals who use the public spaces and parks were proposed as a data source that could help us assess the extent that individual youth and adults had changed their usage of the areas and their reasons for doing so (estimation of risk, greater security), as well as their perceptions about whether there had been changes in youth sexual violence and abuse in the area over time. Unfortunately, due to ethical issues, we were not able to access this community sample, which meant that we could gain little insight into how the mechanisms were working in the various contexts to produce outcomes. Interviews with professionals involved in some way in patrol implementation provided important insight into the patrol experience and perceptions (albeit biased) of patrol success. However, this could not directly test explanations for any changes in youth behaviour associated with these patrols.

We were, however, provided an opportunity to use an innovative data source to help us assess outcomes.

We used **refuse data** to help us assess if there had been changes in behaviours that could potentially be related to youth sexual violence and abuse. We formed a partnership with the local Council which collected refuse on a regular basis when public spaces and parks were mowed, ensuring that environments were neat and tidy, rather than conducive to antisocial behaviour. Council staff recorded refuse volume and the types and number of collected items that were indicative of alcohol consumption (e.g., bottles), drug us-age (bong parts, scissors), and sexual behaviour (condoms, lubrication). This information was typically collected every two or four weeks, and we could examine it longitudinally to assess if changes had occurred over time.

While the refuse data have been examined in depth elsewhere (see Allard et al., 2019), it is important to highlight that, like all data, the contexts where it is collected and how it is collected are critical. Refuse data is seasonal and impacted by events, with increases in antisocial refuse during the peak of the dry season and while students are on summer holidays in Australia (25th June to 10th July in this case). Refuse data may also be impacted as predicted by 'broken windows' theory – with untidy and uncared-for environ-ments conducive to and producing antisocial behaviour. As an unobtrusive measure, it is a valuable source of additional information that can help assess-ments of behaviours occurring in public spaces and parks.

While telling us nothing about the underlying causal mechanisms, the re-fuse data was a valuable source of additional information that could be used with recorded crime and observational data to help assess outcomes. The refuse data revealed patterns indicative of changed behaviour within these parks and public spaces. More 'alcohol' type refuse indicated increases in alcohol consumption, for example. More 'sexual behaviour' type refuse in-dicated a potential increase in the engagement in sexual behaviour in these public spaces. However, this data could not measure who engaged in alco-hol use or sexual behaviour in the park (e.g., youth or adult), or whether the sexual behaviour was consensual or not.

Because of the nature of the project and its focus on relatively serious, rare, underreported types of behaviours, no one source of data could adequately confirm or not our initial hypotheses. Despite limitations, however, the physical evidence that we collected using refuse data could be used with other types of available data to test whether the patrols produced intended outcomes. Indeed, the refuse data revealed behavioural patterns that were not evident in the of-ficial crime data, likely due to underreporting. In turn, interview data provided limited insights into patrol outcomes, given practitioners potentially biased per-ceptions of the initiative, yet provided important learnings about implementa-tion considerations and challenges. It is thus apparent from our work on this project that while refuse data can be used to assess outcomes, it needs to be supplemented with additional data sources, such as interviews and observa-tions, to understand the context and mechanisms responsible for producing outcomes. In short, some data are better suited to achieving particular purposes and researchers should bear this in mind when selecting appropriate sources.

Conclusion

In this chapter, we have argued that there is a need for researchers to use multiple sources of data to test their hypotheses and to be aware of the rela-tive strengths and limitations of each source. We reflected on a recent project where multiple sources were used to try and understand the impacts of police patrols on youth sexual violence and abuse – which includes behaviours that are difficult to assess. Data sources that were examined, along with their relative strengths and weaknesses, included officially recorded crime, observational, interview and refuse data. The strengths and weaknesses of each data source were examined, including our ability to collect the different types of data given the nature of the project. Refuse data provided indicators of several types of behaviours (alcohol usage, drug usage, sexual behaviour), and as such could be used to establish if these broad categories of behaviours occurred or changed in the locations over time. As it is unobtrusive and unaffected by researchers, it is an ideal outcome measure to complement other more direct measures, and ideally could be used with interview data that is particularly useful for teasing out and gaining in-depth understandings about contexts and underlying mechanisms.

Notes

1 Fingerprint evidence has a much longer history than DNA. It was first used to exonerate someone suspected of hospital theft in Japan in the 1870s, by Henry Faulds, a medical doctor who helped pioneer the use of fingerprints in criminal justice settings (Faulds, 1880).
2 Forensic scientists often identify patterns and regularities in evidence, such as recurring patterns in fingerprints, ballistics or DNA profiles to relate evidence to suspects or crime scenes.

2 A realist understanding of bias in qualitative data collection

Ana Manzano

Introduction

'Bias' is a term rooted in the positivist research paradigm, often erroneously attributed to data collected within the philosophical frameworks of constructivism and realism. This chapter aims to distance the realist position from some others by undertaking a critical examination of the term 'bias', and specifically of confirmation and social desirability bias in qualitative data. These biases often blame respondents and researchers for the lack of quality of their studies, suggesting that their data sources (respondents) may have not told them the 'truth'. This exercise is a necessary undertaking, as unfounded accusations of 'bias' can cast a lingering suspicion on any study, its data and/or the research teams, irrespective of the paradigm. This is also important because in the fierce battle of methodological hierarchy, 'bias' is often utilised also by qualitative researchers 'to establish a firmer footing on this hierarchy' (Galdas, 2017, p. 2). However, this can actually further weaken the standing of qualitative research when an ill-fitted bias judgement is misapplied to qualitative data.

There are many specific biases that are often attributed to qualitative data collection. These are broadly caused by the fact that the data collectors (researchers) and the data sources (participants) are human beings, and the data collection instruments (e.g., interviews, focus groups, ethnography) are based on human interaction. Consequently, because the researcher also serves as the research instrument that collects the data, those scientific observations are subject to the contamination of human volition. Generally, 'researcher-related bias' includes confirmation/myside and observer bias; 'participant-related bias' includes social desirability, recall bias and so on (See Table 2.1). Some qualitative researchers themselves propose many strategies and methodological checklists to fight 'against bias and enhance the reliability of findings' (Mays & Pope, 1995). Most of these strategies, however, apply quantitative understandings of bias, which do not account for the contextual quality considerations of different qualitative methodologies. As Williams et al. (2020, p. 10) noted: 'In this sense, it is akin to taking the entire field of "quantitative" study designs and applying a single method or tool for their quality appraisal.

DOI: 10.4324/9781003457077-3

Table 2.1 Common biases in researchers and research participants

Concept	Definition
Confirmation bias	'A subject's largely automatic and unconscious tendency to (i) seek support for her pre-existing, favored or not favored beliefs and (ii) ignore or distort information compromising them' (Peters, 2022, p. 1354).
Confounding bias	'Confounding is often referred to as a "mixing of effects" wherein the effects of the exposure under study on a given outcome are mixed in with the effects of an additional factor (or set of factors) resulting in a distortion of the true relationship' (Skelly et al., 2012, p. 9).
Differential courtesy bias	'The situation that would arise if clients found it harder to express negative views for certain types of questions than for others' (León et al., 2007, p. 26).
Information bias	'Information bias is any systematic difference from the truth that arises in the collection, recall, recording and handling of information in a study, including how missing data is dealt with. Major types of information bias are misclassification bias, observer bias, recall bias and reporting bias' (Bankhead et al., 2019, n. p).
Myside bias	'Mercier & Sperber (2017) and others prefer the term "myside bias" to "confirmation bias" because people don't have a general tendency to confirm any hypothesis that comes to their mind but only ones that are on "their side" of a debate' (Peters, 2022, p. 1351).
Observer/ interviewer bias	'The means by which interviewers can introduce error into a questionnaire include administering the interview or helping the respondents in different ways (even with gestures), putting emphases in different questions, and so on. A particular situation is when the measure of an exposure influences its value (for example, blood pressure) (apprehension bias)' (Delgado-Rodriguez & Llorca, 2004, p. 639).
Response bias	'A systematic difference between the answers provided by the survey respondents and their actual experiences'. 'Response bias is one of a group of biases collectively known as ascertainment bias and sometimes referred to as detection bias. Ascertainment bias is the systematic distortion of the assessment of outcome measures by researchers or study participants. This group of biases is a particular problem in clinical trials when the researchers or participants are aware of the treatment allocation' (Sedgwick, 2014, p. 1–2).
Selection bias	'Selection bias is induced by preferential selection of units for data analysis, usually governed by unknown factors including treatment, outcome, and their consequences, and represents a major obstacle to valid causal and statistical inferences' (Bareinboim et al., 2022, p. 2410).
Social desirability bias	'Social desirability bias refers to the tendency to present oneself and one's social context in a way that is perceived to be socially acceptable, but not wholly reflective of one's reality' (Bergen & Lebonté, 2020, p. 783).
Positivity bias	'Positivity bias may denote three phenomena: a tendency for people to report positive views of reality, a tendency to hold positive expectations, views, and memories, and a tendency to favor positive information in reasoning' (Hoorens, 2014, p. 4938).

In the case of qualitative research, checklists, therefore, offer only a blunt and arguably ineffective tool and potentially promote an incomplete understanding of good "quality" in qualitative research'.

This chapter starts by providing a brief history of bias and its conflated definitions as error and/or deviation from the 'truth'. These are connected to the rapid rise of the randomised controlled trial (RCT) as the gold standard research method in the 20th century. Then, confirmation and social desirability bias in qualitative data collection are examined by critically engaging with the science that agonises over participants not telling researchers the truth. Following from this, a realist understanding of bias is suggested by considering it an inherent and uncontrollable feature of research processes related to context. The realist position assumes that respondent's replies are always built on their assumptions about the assumptions built into the question. Respondents are smart rather than lazy or dishonest. Researchers are not that bad either. To illustrate this, the chapter follows on with a section on the problem of researchers' beliefs affecting data collection and interpretation and how this is reflected in the process of adjudication between rival theories. Finally, I discuss the implications of this paradigm positioning for theory-driven realist interviews and focus groups and I suggest some guiding principles to address the challenge of obtaining scientific data through people in individual and group interviews.

An abbreviated history of bias: Error or deviation from the truth?

Although the etymology of the word 'bias' is unknown, it seems to originate from the French word 'biais' meaning 'a slant, a slope, an oblique'. In the old game of bowls, this term referred to balls crafted with added weight on one side, prompting them to curve obliquely. From there, the figurative use of this word extended socially as 'a one-sided tendency of the mind', and 'undue propensity or prejudice' (Online Etymology Dictionary, 2023). In contemporary scientific contexts, 'bias' operates mostly as an uncontested term, despite different meanings and manifestations across disciplines (Vineis, 2002). While the term is widely accepted, the coexistence of meanings across specific fields arises due to differing theoretical and methodological frameworks, or objectives within each discipline. Unsurprisingly, bias definitions have changed over time, and nowadays, the word 'bias' has evolved to encompass two different but interrelated meanings: error and/or 'deviation' from the truth. This is a significant distinction as errors in scientific practices can be random or systematic (e.g., inaccuracies in measurement and analysis), but the connotation that those errors lead to a predictable deviation from a 'true' value, transcends its traditional connotation. Bias now incorporates the broader concept of 'deviation from truth', which may arise from unintentional cognitive biases such as inherent subjectivities and contextual cultural influences in researchers and participants. This expanded understanding firstly, redefines bias as a type of error that could stem from scientists' prejudices;

secondly, it reinforces a conceptualisation of scientific error drawn from the positivist research paradigm (Galdas, 2017), which searches for universal truths with their associated quantitative data collection practices.

Within this context, the use of the term 'bias' in science became more prominent in the 1950s as the RCT was deemed the 'gold standard' of study designs, precisely because of the supposed power that randomisation has to avoid measurement errors (bias) and offer us 'true' values. Interestingly, the concept of unconscious biases is based on the rational choice economics theory of cognitive human behaviour popularised in the 1950s, as systematic patterns of thinking are thought to deviate from a standard of rationality by taking shortcuts that can produce misjudgements (Buetow, 2019). Following the logic of rational choice theory, bias occurs because deviations from strict rationality occur. The implication here is that with proper instruction in the rules of reasoning, fallacious arguments can be avoided, and we get closer to the 'truth'. For instance, scientists only attending to information that supports their hypotheses (confirmation/myside bias) is considered an irrational deviation from the normative and rational behaviour that all scientists must follow (attending to all information whether this is supportive of their beliefs or not). Rational choice theory, despite its undeniable influence, is a neo-classical economic model with many flaws and criticisms (Tversky & Kahneman, 1988); at its simplest, it is an idealisation of actual behaviour, assuming that 'humans fit (and ought to fit)' a human rational-agent model where decisions are always well informed, in conformity with expected utility theory (Battersby, 2016). Unsurprisingly, humans are not well described by these rational-agent models since human reality and their social systems are more complex than the models suggest. In realist terms, the weakest link of rational choice theory is the insistence on the irrelevance of context.

The perception of which scientific errors are deemed most dangerous, as well as the recommended vigilance and countermeasures, vary in accordance with distinct historical contexts (Daston, 2005). For instance, during the early 17th century, discussing scientists' errors became commonplace. This period is often referred to as the time of a 'modern revival of academic scepticism' as newly invented research instruments such as the telescope and microscope challenged many explanatory systems and empirical claims, which were suddenly downgraded from eternal truths to embarrassing errors due to scientists' conjectures and beliefs (Daston, 2005). A few centuries later, the first taxonomies of scientific 'bias' (Murphy, 1976) were developed in the 1970s and biases started to multiply. Murphy had warned that biases could arise at each stage of scientific research and that a 'vicious circle of bias' can occur, defining it as a process and not just isolated errors. In 1978, in a symposium dedicated to case-control studies in epidemiology, Ibrahim and Spitzer (1979) proposed for the first time in the history of epidemiology the classification of biases into three broad categories: selection bias, information bias and confounding bias.

A year later, Murphy's predictions were proved right when Sackett (1979) proposed 35 types of bias for trials and 56 potential biases for case-control and cohort studies. As authors differed in their understanding of the function of randomisation, equally, the function and meaning of the concept of bias were also distinct. Some discussed statistical bias in connection with the notion of systematic error (as opposed to random error), while others referred to the psychological and subjective notion of bias, related to a sense of 'prejudice' (Brault, 2021). The latter was somehow unconscious, while systematic error was mostly due to professional incompetence, with researchers being regularly warned about the dangers of their 'unconscious' cognitive biases that could invalidate their studies (Brault, 2021).

The notion of 'bias' transitioned from laboratories to clinics and then into other fields, fieldwork and paradigms. The biases most often associated with qualitative data collection are social desirability (Bergen & Labonté, 2020), courtesy and confirmation bias; these biases have also been cited as limitations of theory-driven interviews (Gilmore, 2019; Vogel & Punton, 2017) recommended for use in the context of realist evaluation investigations (Manzano, 2016; Pawson, 1996), often referred to as realist interviews. While confirmation bias is a concern related to the researcher's approach and data interpretation (tendency to seek out and interpret information that confirms one's pre-existing beliefs), social desirability bias refers to the responses provided by participants during data collection. The next section examines the latter, that is the problem of people not telling researchers the 'truth' and the most common interventions to minimise these participant tendencies.

The problem of people not telling researchers the 'truth'

There is a colossal scientific literature dedicated to the study of why research participants do not tell the truth or the entire truth to researchers. An illustration of how scholars shame their participants is Winfred et al.'s (2021) paper 'The Lazy or Dishonest Respondent', published in the Annual Review of Organizational Psychology and Organizational Behavior. This example represents a thriving stop 'respondents' deceptions' science, which commonly distinguishes between those who deceive consciously versus unconsciously, and it examines, experiments on and suggests strategies to stop or reduce their deceptions.

Although bias studies overwhelmingly come from positivist academia, the worry of being deceived transfers to every paradigm. Constructivists and realist researchers also express preoccupation about their research participants either lying to them or suspecting that their answers are not being as truthful as they wished. The blame for this unwanted participant behaviour seems to be often attributed to various contextual factors, such as: the topics discussed (e.g., people are more likely to be untruthful when asked about certain things such as sensitive topics); the instruments used (e.g., some questions are more susceptible than others to trigger evasive or deceptive answers); the data collectors (e.g. people are more likely to lie in interviews than in surveys (Leon et al., 2021); the research participants (e.g. personality traits); the research setting (e.g., cross-cultural research (Johnson & Van de Vijver, 2003) the number of participants present (e.g., people are more likely to be dishonest in focus groups than in individual interviews) and so on. Typical strategies suggested to reduce this measurement problem attributed to the social desirability tendencies are summarised below. These seem to be mainly attempting to control the natural contexts in which research occurs:

a **'Eliminate the interviewee'** through survey self-administration. The assumption here is that if the 'noise' created by the presence of a human being (an interviewer) is eliminated, and people answer the questions as they read them out themselves in a paper or online, they will be more honest (Kreuter et al., 2008). The context in here to control is the human being per se.

b **'Question wording'.** If questions are redacted and presented to interview participants in a 'neutral way' (assuming that such a thing is possible), these are less likely to generate an evasive or untruthful answer. However, context strikes again as Leon et al. noted: 'questions may have different degrees of sensitivity in different countries and cultures, across social groups within the same country, and over time' (2021, p. 1025).

c **'Tell them to be honest'.** The assumption of this type of strategy is that if messages are given to participants to remind them to be honest in their answers, the truthful quality of their answers improves (Vésteinsdóttir et al., 2019). The issue here is that even if people would do as they are told (although, as we know, they often don't), respondents are well-known for not paying much attention to the instructions given in self-administered surveys, often skimming or skipping them.

d **'We will not tell anyone who you are'.** These types of interventions are used to encourage honesty by giving participants confidentiality assurances and by demonstrating that researchers have no way to know who they are. These range from simple confidentiality reminders to more sophisticated techniques used in surveys such as 'item count technique, or the list experiment', which protects the anonymity of participants by giving respondents a list of items and asking them how many, not which ones, they support (Glynn, 2013). Another one is the 'randomised response technique' (Warner, 1965), in which respondents employ a randomising method to add probabilistic misclassification to their responses and thus conceal their true answers from the interviewers (Kuha & Jackson, 2014).

e **'Measure how much they lie'.** Numerous scales have been developed to assess participants lying tendencies (also referred to as social desirability scales), accepting that since we cannot stop participants' dishonesty, at least we can try to guess the level of veracity in their answers. These scales try to assess the likelihood of people misrepresenting their reality (Loving & Agnew, 2001, p. 552). This concept seems paradoxical, as the misrepresentation itself becomes a part of their reality.

A further strategy that we will discuss later in the chapter is to contrast the information obtained from participants with other sources. However, before we delve into that strategy, it becomes imperative to address the elephant in the room – the inherent inaccuracy in all responses and the inability of many questions and answers to capture the complexity of human behaviour. Consider the classic example of inquiring about the weekly alcohol consumption of individuals. There are, of course, the well-known issues of people not remembering how much they consume, and the tendency to report less consumption to please the interviewer. But there is also the conceptual issue of assuming behavioural standardisation as such queries often presume a regular pattern of consumption that does not reflect the diversity of human drinking behaviour, and the variety of weekly social activities that human encounter. The only truly accurate response to inquiries about alcohol consumption comes from individuals who abstain from alcohol altogether, if they have done so. For the rest, potential inaccuracies are not only related to their bad memory and the stigma associated with excessive drinking but also with the varying dynamics and not-standardised patterns of consumption.

In summary, while there is a symbiotic relationship between the quality of queries and the reliability of responses, the pursuit of accurate data is a treacherous journey. As we will see in the next section, if some people are not truthful to researchers, these data cannot be dismissed as a methodological error. This phenomenon, instead, reveals useful information about the social reality of the participant, and of interactions between participants and researchers within the multiple uncontrollable research contexts.

Realism, bias and the truth

Implied in all the social desirability bias literature is that participants' behaviours can be socially desirable, socially undesirable or somehow neutral. This, in essence, suggests that human behaviours can be devoid of social influence, which is, of course, impossible. There is also another possibility, that is to consider that human beings are often not honest to themselves and/ or to each other and this is why we cannot be certain if our participants have told us 'the truth', their truth, half the truth or blatantly lied. It could also be that we may have misinterpreted their words or that we have asked them an impossible question. This is why our researchers' observations (interviews, surveys) are always selective (Popper (1963/1989). As Pawson (2024) remind us: 'Data derived from sensory observation or balanced observation ends with a proliferation of information rather than narrowing on the truth. The data used to proclaim bias and selectivity are themselves partial and selective. There is nothing as vacuous as data' (p. 123).

Realists understand that there is a reality that exists independently of our interpretations but that our apprehension of reality is always partial. Scientific theories are attempts to capture truths, but they are not the reality. They are incomplete, and subject to revision. Because while the reality is the state of things, truth is the correspondence of our beliefs, statements, interpretations of the reality to that actual state of things. Therefore, for realists, discussing bias is more than solely examining the feasibility of overcoming the limitations of human perception, including the psychological biases of researchers or participants. Rather, 'bias' has ended up as a general category that encompasses an 'iceberg' of a mass of factors (Mainland, 1958) that could mask alternative explanations of causation. The problem that realists have with bias is related to definitions of bias that situate the melting of the iceberg of biases as an effective pursuit of the holy grail of the scientific truth. Although bias is of interest of realist researchers because it may interfere with causal inference, realists understand that research errors could be considered socially constructed. As Pawson (2024) explains realists do not try to control all those contextual factors that may engender bias, instead understanding that 'No investigation is inviolable. We cannot be certain because errors can be made, further alternative explanations may be left unexplored and fresh, unanswered questions will have been created. The whole process is thus managed by external scrutiny, by peer review, by trial and error and by attempted replication. And then, before the dust has settled, there is a subsequent testing of rival explanations as proposed by independent teams' (p. 131).

Consequently, when we embark on our fieldwork activities, it is important to remember that realism is a philosophy of science that rejects 'the idea that objectivity depends on the production of hard data that is "factual", "given" and "beyond dispute"' (Pawson, 2024, p. 151). Although errors in research studies must of course be avoided as much as possible, realist researchers understand that bias as an uncontrollable context is an inherent aspect of social research and therefore, not an 'error of research'. For realists all data is data. That means lack of data is data, and negative data is data; contaminated data is data. Bias is therefore understood as inherent to all research processes, and efforts to try to control the uncontrollable are better dedicated to understanding why bias occurs and learning from this. For example, if research participants' honesty is doubted when asked about sensitive topics, positivists believe that they can control this fieldwork contextual feature with a combination of the techniques identified in the previous section such as careful phrasing, anonymity promises, etc. Realists instead, recognise the influence of social structures (context) in which research takes place and theorise about how these contextual features shape participants' responses during fieldwork. That is, these responses are indeed valid data. The level of 'honesty' in the answer does not discard their validity as human beings do not 'talk truth'. They talk and they sometimes get closer with their words to what they mean than others. This data is valid because realist researchers could, for example, theorise that the societal stigma associated with those sensitive topics (e.g., sexual behaviour, addictions) is a mechanism likely to operate in the fieldwork encounters. Consequently, they do not take interview data as face value, but contrast it with data from other nuggets of evidence such as secondary sources, mixed methods, follow-up interviews, etc. In this process, they learn more about how stigma operates in social encounters.

Context is inextricably enmeshed with the mechanisms through which things work. This means that context should not be understood as descriptive but as analytical (Boudon, 2014; Greenhalgh & Manzano, 2021). Like context, bias is not something detrimental per se but instead should be considered a source of insights in the pursuit of causal inferences. Bias is not just a nuisance; bias is also a constant and valuable source of information to analyse. This reconsideration does not imply a rejection of the need to be rigorous and accurate, but claims a different pathway to rigour.

Having established a realist perspective on bias, and how this is related to objectivity and truth-seeking behaviours, we move on to the issue of how researchers' individual contextual reasoning (supporting or contradicting favoured beliefs) affects generation and evaluation of scientific evidence.

The potential for researcher bias to affect qualitative data collection and interpretation

As theory-driven evaluation began gaining traction in the latter half of the 20th century, Carol Weiss (1997) noted some of the challenges associated with this evaluation approach, including the difficulty in identifying or constructing programme theories due to their unclear nature, confusion about their components and the existence of multiple possible theories to choose from and focus on. Furthermore, since realist evaluators search for nuggets of evidence (Pawson, 2006a) to support/refine/discard their tentative programme theories, the possibility of them striking gold with the evidence that confirm their programme theories seems possible. These issues are related to researchers' potential myside bias, which is the tendency to evaluate evidence consistent with their prior beliefs more positively than belief-inconsistent evidence (Drummond & Fischhoff, 2019, p. 478).

Researchers exercise judgments when determining research questions, selecting observations (data collection methods), interpreting data, etc. Rarely working in isolation, they tend to work in teams. Negotiations, consensus-building, practical considerations, research governance regulations, funding structures and feasibility play significant roles in many research decisions. For example, in commissioned evaluations, the evaluation client or commissioners often have considerable influence over which data to collect, how to make evaluation decisions and formulating recommendations. In summary, it is not only the micro-context of researchers' values, judgements and expertise (human reasoning) that shapes research processes, but also the meso-level contexts such as research governance and macro-level contexts like the broader research community and trends in which research processes occur. All these impact which observations we conduct, how and in what circumstances.

In theory-driven evaluations such as realist evaluation, we may pursue multiple stakeholder programme theories, which highlight the importance of which stakeholders are involved, how, why and for how long because this determines whose theory is developed, tested, discarded and refined. Hansen and Vedung (2010) noted in their review of theory-based evaluations that, in general, heterogeneous stakeholder programme theories are not kept apart; they are often merged by the evaluator into one unitary programme theory 'behind which all stakeholders may rally' (p. 297). This means that what is constructed is one unitary intervention theory of the evaluator, informed by relevant theory and negotiated with and agreed upon by the stakeholders. For example, when stakeholders of different types are gathered together for theory-building workshops, ideas of what the programme is meant to achieve are often radically different–the funder may have different ideas about programmes theories of action and theories of change from the agency delivering the programmes versus the staff–especially those who may work at some distance from head office and have been running the programme for years.

While the assumption behind this unitary fused theory of evaluator expertise with the stakeholders' first-hand knowledge is that it generates a more robust evaluation by integrating theoretical constructs with real-world experiences, this approach can sometimes lead to the evaluator's perspective carrying more weight, potentially overshadowing the heterogeneous input from various stakeholders (Manzano, 2024). In addition, this fused approach may not always be suitable for all evaluations, particularly in the case of large programmes or contested policy areas (e.g., drug legalisation, sex work). These situations often involve diverse perspectives and competing interests, which may be better served by maintaining separate stakeholder programme theories to capture the range of viewpoints and nuances involved. I would defer to Pawson's (2024, p. 140) 'Episode 23: Theory adjudication in social science' for an expanded explanation on how conceptualisations and academic disputes about "objectivity" come into play when we accuse researchers of myside bias. 'Theory adjudication' (Pawson, 2013, 2024) is related to the challenges in achieving objectivity in research by emphasising the iterative process of evaluating competing theories for relevance, rigour and reliability. Even when a study confirms a theory, it may not hold universally. Theory adjudication does not lead to absolute truth but it refines theories closer to it.

In summary, there are many problems with the notion of scientific consensus as truth; we have seen 'scientific truths' of the past revealed as errors when data collection instruments improved. Dissensus and scepticism reflect more adequately the process of how science advances. The decisions about what evidence counts as valid and what theory counts as plausible can be more or less rigorous, relevant and reliable, while researchers balance a huge plurality of values, interests and evidence. As researchers, we must acknowledge and not fight that diversity, accept that it exists and lean into it, always transparently. It will be the job of the rest of the academic community to challenge, ask difficult questions, judge and improve those, a process referred to as 'organised scepticism' (Merton,1942/1973). In the final section of this chapter, I discuss the implications of this paradigm positioning for theory-driven realist interviews and focus groups, and suggest some guiding principles to deal with the challenge of people obtaining scientific data through people in individual and group interviews.

Dealing with researcher and respondent biases in realist interviews and focus groups

The theory-driven interview as proposed by Merton and Kendall in 1946, and the realist interview as theorised by Pawson (1996) and Manzano (2016), deviated from the conventional advice for qualitative interviewing repeated ad nauseam in handbooks of qualitative research. This is mainly because of the interview focus on developing, testing and/or refining programme theory; and Pawson's (1996) 'teacher-learner cycle', where participants and researchers have interchangeable roles while they teach each other and learn together about the programme evaluated and the theories being developed.

Scientific methods are cultural and social artefacts, and it is normal and healthy that resistance occurs to normative social behaviour in scientists' communities of practice. Unsurprisingly, concerns regarding confirmation bias in the teacher-learner cycle within the realist interview have predominantly been highlighted by researchers involved in international development evaluations. These apprehensions were initially brought to attention by Punton et al. (2016). Their evaluation team expressed reservations about conducting realist interviews as they were worried about testing theories without encountering confirmation bias. These reservations were based on their previous contextual knowledge of doing fieldwork in low- and middle-income countries: 'In some settings in Africa and Asia, it is considered rude or inappropriate to disagree with an 'expert'. Moreover, in an international development context where many governments are dependent on international funds for their programmes, respondents may be accustomed to giving encouraging responses to evaluators' (p. 6). These evaluators' concerns were reiterated by their evaluation Steering Committee as part of the review process for their study report. In 2017, Vogel and Punton reported three confirmation bias mitigation strategies when interviewing in government settings in low-and-middle-income countries:

1   In the sampling strategy, by interviewing a range of participants including stakeholders external to the project, and cross-checking claims made by civil servants with their managers and peers.
2   During the interview, by approaching the same topic from different angles and with various respondents and by asking for specific examples to corroborate claims.
3   In the analysis, by triangulating between diverse primary and secondary data sources.

In addition, Punton and Vogel (2020) noted that different respondents have varying levels of capacity and interest in scrutinising 'how and why' questions characteristic of realist interviews. Gilmore (2019) also noticed that some of her interview participants offered little engagement in identifying appropriate programme theories and attributed this to the influence of power imbalances within realist interviews. The well-documented challenges of using interpreters when interviewing in a different language and/or culture of the researcher added an extra layer of difficulty when discerning CMOC elements. Translators often struggle to convey the full nuance and context of participants' responses, leading to potential loss of meaning in the translation process that is key when refining theories constructed with CMO configurations. In addition, Gilmore and Punton and Vogel's teams (e.g. research assistants) were novices to realist evaluation and realist interviews.

In response to all these contextual worries, the following seven guiding principles are proposed, not to avoid bias, but instead to ensure that findings from realist interviews and focus groups reflect the complexities of collecting data about human experiences, opinions and perspectives in different research contexts.

1 **There is no way of escaping the infusion of 'the social' in interviews.** We must acknowledge the limitations of self-reporting and individual and group interview data. As Allard et al. explain in Chapter One of this book: 'Interviews do not display plain facts. They involve artful behaviours by interviewer and interviewee alike. Although there is a rich literature on interviewing and interview strategies to try to ensure that respondents are able to speak accurately to the researcher's interests, including contributions by realists, there is no way of escaping the infusion of the social in interviews.' Interviews are 'true' and relevant only as they are fragments of evidence that can contribute to our interpretations and explanations tested and refined within and between other evidence fragments. The researcher must find other methods of investigation to build up theories from relevance to rigour (Pawson, 2013). Therefore, since the realist interviews are not beyond dispute, they should not be considered hard data. Neither are surveys. They all together contribute to progressive, cumulative knowledge.

2 **Participants are smart rather than lazy, dishonest or easily disempowered.** Many interviewers working in other contexts than research studies (e.g., police, journalists, social workers, etc.) know from their experiences that for interview participants, it is sometimes smart to be dishonest. However, it is not our role as researchers to forensically examine the honesty within the interview data because we are not there to judge, help or prosecute our participants. If interview data is triangulated with sufficient additional data to reveal discrepancies, the nature of these discrepancies can provide useful realist information. Although power differentials exist in all research encounters, the forms of resistance that participants find against researchers' ideas cannot be dismissed either. As the reader may have noticed, there is something uncomfortable about those 20th-century writings on the problem of social desirability and confirmation bias described

in the first section of this chapter. The portrayal of participants as lacking agency and the critical judgement to challenge intelligent scientists is inappropriate; it also contradicts the practice of many interviewers who have seen their ideas challenged, refuted and improved by participants in their theory-driven conversations. (See Howe's chapter in this book). However, as realists, we know that all depends on the contexts. As fieldwork contexts are infinite, in some particular contexts, participants' answers may be less likely to present to researchers the knowledge needed for the teacher-learner cycle to operate as intended. However, the teacher-learner approach assumes that participants are knowledgeable and places explicit value on their individual reasoning (O'Rourke et al., 2022), and it is a valuable tool for minimising power imbalances instead of promoting them.

3   **Respondent biases are not unique to realist interviews.** As Becker (1967, p. 245) noticed 'there is no position from which sociological research can be done that is not biased one way or another … the question is not whether we should take sides, since we inevitably will, but whose side we are on'. Viewing confirmation bias as an inherent challenge within realist interviews serves to diminish its novelty as an interview methodology. The desire to present oneself favourably could be considered a mechanism influenced by contextual micro-meso-macro social structures. Researchers need to scratch beyond the surface and be prepared to delve into the deeper causal mechanisms that may shape what is considered socially desirable in specific contexts as this varies across topics, populations and time periods. Realism epistemology is more conducive to do so than others because it aims to understand how these contextual factors influence participants' responses.

4   **Reflexivity with an analytical purpose is useful.** Realism acknowledges that researchers bring their perspectives into the research process, but this is a methodological consideration rather than a challenge to the reality (and the truth). The programme theory of reflexivity as a bias reduction intervention claimed by constructivism is that if researchers acknowledge and make explicit (public disclosure) their biased tendencies, this magically minimises errors by acknowledging the existence of multiple co-constructed realities. However, for realists, reflexivity is necessary but not enough. Realists, instead, are interested in reflexivity with an analytical purpose, considering it a useful tool to understand how researchers' contexts interact with participants' contexts and how these interactions influence data collection, interpretation and causation claims. In summary, while constructivists use reflexivity to contextualise and interpret the data within a broader socio-cultural contextual framework, realists use that knowledge of the researcher/participant contextualised interactions to further understand the generative mechanisms that lead to causation in their topics under investigation.

5   **Normalise an interview environment where participants are teachers.** It is good that realist researchers have doubts about whether their participants

may have agreed with their theory too quickly, without engaging in deeper or more critical thinking. For this reason, it is useful to frame questions acknowledging that there are diverse viewpoints, encouraging participants to express their thoughts, even if they differ from the perceived norm. It is also important to be explicit from the start about using the teacher-learner cycle; and how this research environment is different from others that participants may or may have not encountered. As an example of this practice, this paragraph from topic guides used in the realist evaluation of the BCURE Programme (Vogel & Punton, 2018, p. 90): 'We'd like to talk to you about your perceptions of the XX programme. As you know, we're not just interested in what is happening, but also in your ideas about how and why things have changed, or not, over the past few years. We'd like to share our initial ideas with you during the interview and get your thoughts.' O'Rourke et al. (2022) explained how their interview introduction 'invited women to exercise agency' aiming to minimise cultural power imbalances in their realist evaluation of a doula programme in Australia and emphasising that there were no right or wrong answers to the realist interview questions. Gilmore (2019) also included in her interviews a short discussion asking the participants about their experience with the programme before moving on to more explicit conversations about theory-testing.

6 **Remember organised scepticism.** Realists build rigour with a strategy based on 'organised scepticism' (Merton, 1942/1973). They use diverse data sources to enhance the reliability of the research by cross-verifying information with other participants, with the same participant during the interview and with follow-up interviews and with other primary and secondary data collection methods. But this process does not end with the incorporation of multiple perspectives and triangulating nuggets of evidence. The wider scientific community as a collective is responsible for further testing, discarding and refining our research findings as these are always provisional.

7 **Focus groups are similar but different.** Although the six previous principles apply to interviews and focus groups, data collected in focus groups have specific contextual limitations (Manzano, 2023). To mention a few, discussions of sensitive or controversial topics may be compromised because participants may be hesitant to open up due to concerns about confidentiality and anonymity. Group settings often limit the depth of responses, leading to a more superficial understanding of participants' perspectives. Participants with physical and communication access needs may face challenges in participating in focus groups. Culturally responsive focus groups should consider language and cultural identities. In some cultures, alternative methods like sharing circles based on open-structured storytelling may be more appropriate, as focus groups may not align with cultural preferences. Individuals comfortable with public speaking are more likely to be recruited for focus groups, and discussions can be dominated by vocal individuals or group opinion leaders. Status differences among participants

and/or researchers and participants may influence the dynamics of the discussion. Although many textbooks talk about focus group facilitators 'controlling the group', realist evaluators aim for deliberation instead, assuming that when different people are in the same room, they will say different things and they will not necessarily agree. It is not consensus that is pursued but disputation, contradictions and disagreements (Manzano, 2022). Encouraging disputation and not consensus is more likely to provide evaluators with examples, exceptions and contradictions that will provide a rich sub-set of possible causal explanations to be tested.

Conclusion

This chapter has examined the contrasting perspectives of positivists, constructivists and realists regarding bias, while providing a historical overview of how fear of bias has become omnipresent in research practitioners across paradigms. Positivists advocate for stringent bias control aiming for objectivity and neutrality. In contrast, constructivists tend towards a more passive acceptance of bias, acknowledging their inevitable presence without actively intervening. However, the realist perspective offers a nuanced understanding of bias in qualitative data collection that considers bias as a source of valuable information. Realists recognise that biases are inherent in human perception and interpretation, and instead of seeking to eliminate them entirely, they navigate through complexity with an awareness of their influence as a part of striving for clarity and rigour in their data collection and analysis strategies.

3 Nothing as practical as an analytical strategy in realist evaluation

Findings and recommendations from a comprehensive review

Steffen Bohni Nielsen and Sebastian Lemire

Introduction

At the European Evaluation Society conference in 2002, Ray Pawson dubbed his keynote address 'Nothing as practical as a good theory' (2003). The phrase, originally coined by Kurt Lewin and since reiterated by Carol Weiss, was an argument for the centrality of theory in understanding whether and how programmes work (Weiss, 1995). Over the years, and parallel to a similar growth in theory-informed evaluation at large (Coryn et al., 2011), realist evaluation has gained momentum as an alternative to experimental designs – a counter to so-called 'black box evaluations' (Pawson & Tilley, 1997).

The main question driving realist evaluation is to uncover how programmes work, for whom and under what conditions through the elicitation of a programme theory (Pawson & Tilley, 1997). The realist evaluation approach is grounded in generative causation, whereby a sequence of unobserved entities – so-called mechanisms – are activated in specific contexts to generate one or more outcomes. Moreover, the approach recognises that an outcome is sometimes produced by a complex combination of causes – or causal packages – so a configurational approach to understanding and explaining how and why interventions work is imperative. Accordingly, realist causal analysis focuses on identifying 'the configuration that links the outcome to mechanism(s) triggered by the context, often combining quantitative and qualitative data' (Van Belle et al., 2016: n.p.).

In line with this thinking, realist evaluation structures the data collection and analysis around Context–Mechanism–Outcome (CMO) configurations. These CMOs are intended to capture the generative processes (mechanisms) that in a specific setting (context) contribute to one or more psychological, attitudinal and behavioural changes (outcomes) among intervention participants. As Pawson and Tilley (1997) explain, 'outcomes are explained by the action of particular mechanisms in particular contexts, and this explanatory structure is put in place over time by a combination of theory and experimental observation' (p.59).

Since Pawson and Tilley's publication of *Realistic Evaluation* in 1997, there has been an exponential growth of published realist evaluations, especially in

DOI: 10.4324/9781003457077-4

the area of public health and health (Lemire et al., 2020; Nielsen et al., 2022). The growing volume of publications has been followed by books (Emmel et al., 2018) and several conferences dedicated to the topic of realist evaluation. Speaking to the formalisation of realist evaluation, quality standards for realist evaluations have been published as part of the RAMESES Projects, covering both methodological quality and reporting standards for realist evaluations and realist syntheses (Wong et al., 2014; Greenhalgh et al., 2016; Wong et al., 2017).

Emerging from the growing literature on realist evaluation, several reviews of realist evaluations have over the years been published. Some reviews have focused on the application of realist evaluation in particular domains, such as the application in health systems research (Marchal et al., 2012) or knowledge transfer (Salter & Kothari, 2014). Other more methodology-oriented reviews have focused on the practical challenges of using realist evaluation (Ridde et al., 2012), data collection methods used in realist evaluation (Manzano, 2016; Renmans & Pleguezuelo, 2023), how mechanisms have been conceptualised and applied in realist evaluations (Lacouture et al., 2015; Lemire et al., 2020), underlying ontological and epistemological variations in the conceptualisation of context (Greenhalgh & Manzano, 2021; Nielsen et al., 2022), as well as variants of realist evaluations, such as realist trials (Nielsen et al., 2023).

The present review both builds on and reaches beyond previous reviews of realist evaluations by focusing specifically on the analytical strategies applied in realist evaluation. To our knowledge, as at the time of writing, there is no systematic examination of the analytical strategies used in realist evaluation. Based on a comprehensive review of published realist evaluations, we aim to open this analytical black box by identifying and illustrating the analytical strategies commonly used in realist evaluations and discussing how these are related to the research designs and data collection methods employed. Informed by the findings of our review, we discuss how to advance analytical rigour in future realist evaluations.

The chapter is structured in four parts. In the first part, we describe the iterative process of refining CMOs, as initially intended by Pawson and Tilley (1997). In the second part of the chapter, we describe the review methodology. In the third part, we present the findings from our review; focusing on how realist evaluators formulate initial CMOs; collect data on CMOs; and analyse, test and refine CMOs based on findings. In the fourth part, we conclude our chapter with a discussion on the need for further attention to analytical strategies and how these relate to data collection strategies in future realist evaluations.

The realist cycle – Iterative refinement of CMOs

Pawson and Tilley (1997) introduced realist evaluation as a logic of inquiry structured around iterative rounds of testing and refining CMOs, which typically involve multiple rounds of data collection and analysis.

In their review, Salter and Kothari (2014) found that realist evaluations typically consist of four phases: (1) formulation of the initial programme theory articulated as CMOs, (2) collection of data on the CMOs, (3) data analysis and testing of the CMOs and (4) formulation of a refined set of CMOs based on the findings. As Salter and Kothari (2014) note, this realist inquiry cycle is intended to be iterative, with each cycle further refining the CMOs. Table 3.1 provides an overview of the four phases and the main activities within each phase. In the third column, we have added common data collection methods and analytical techniques applied in each phase. In the fourth column, we also provide published practice examples that provide inspiration and guidance pertaining to each phase of the realist inquiry cycle.

In the remainder of this chapter, we will examine how realist evaluators conduct each of these four phases as described in published realist evaluations, awarding particular attention to phase three where analytical strategies come to the forefront. Before advancing our findings, we provide a brief description of the review methodology.

Table 3.1 The four phases of a realist evaluation

Phase	Activities	Data collection and analytical tools	Exemplars
1 Formulating initial programme theory and its CMOs	1 Formulation of initial programme theory 2 Development of potential CMOs 3 Generate testable hypotheses for CMOs	1 Research literature analysis 2 Document analysis 3 Stakeholder consultation 4 Programme theory construction	Vareilles et al. (2015) Westhorp (2013)
2 Data collection	1 Collect data appropriate to test hypotheses for CMOs	1 Research Design 2 Quantitative data collection methods 3 Qualitative data collection methods	Manzano (2016) (qual) Oroviogoicoechea and Watson (2009) (quant)
3 Data analysis and hypothesis testing	1 Data analysis centred on testing hypotheses	1 Statistical analytical techniques 2 Qualitative analytical techniques 3 Mixed-methods convergence	Von Thiele Schwarz et al. (2017) (quant) Martin and Tannenbaum (2017) (mixed)
4 Refining the CMOs	1 Assess on empirical findings and verification of hypotheses 2 Refine CMOs	1 Programme theory revision	Martin and Tannenbaum (2017) Vareilles et al. (2015)

Source: Adapted from Salter and Kothari (2014).

Review methodology

The present review of analytical strategies in realist evaluation emerges from a broader review of published realist evaluations (Lemire et al., 2020; Nielsen et al., 2022; Nielsen et al., 2023). A detailed description of the search strategy and terms, screening criteria, coding framework and procedures, among other aspects of the review methodology, is available in Lemire et al. (2020) and Nielsen et al. (2022).

The review was based on an electronic and manual search for realist evaluations published between 1997 and 2017 – the two decades after Pawson and Tilley's ground-breaking publication. The review identified 195 published studies with case examples of realist evaluations, of which 126 realist evaluations presented one or more CMOs. The focus of the present chapter is on the analytical strategies used for refining CMOs thus examining exclusively the 126 realist evaluations with one or more codable CMOs and the analytical strategies that could be discerned from these studies.

Table 3.2 provides an overview of the basic characteristics of the 126 cases with CMOs. As the table shows, realist evaluations are primarily from Europe (91 realist evaluations), of which most (69 realist evaluations) are from the United Kingdom alone. Realist evaluation appears to have gained traction within the (public) health sector, within which 94 (75%) of the realist evaluations are published.

The 126 case applications were coded according to a pre-specified coding framework structured around the characteristics of the realist evaluations (i.e., year, country, sector, study design, data collection methods [how data is collected; e.g., survey, interview], and data sources [from whom data is

Table 3.2 Characteristics of 126 realist evaluations (1997–2017)

	Count	*Percent*
Geography		
Europe	91	72.2
Australia	11	8.7
Africa	8	6.3
North America	7	5.6
Asia	6	4.8
South America	3	2.4
Sector		
Health (medicine/public health)	94	74.6
Social welfare	11	8.7
Other (public government, civic, tourism)	10	7.9
Education	5	4.0
Criminal justice	3	2.4
Environment	3	2.4
Employment	0	0.0
Total	126	100.0

Source: Adapted from Nielsen et al. (2022).

collected; e.g., programme staff, recipients or policy-makers], as well as types of mechanisms, context factors and outcomes presented in the CMOs). In addition, information on analytical strategies applied in the realist evaluations was extracted and coded for further analysis. We categorised the analytical strategies according to the label and description provided by the authors. Finally, we recorded whether CMOs were refined.

No review is without its limitations. One limitation of the present review is that it solely pertains to published realist evaluations that use explicit CMOs. These published applications represent a smaller subsample of all realist evaluations conducted during the time period. Some examples of realist evaluation without CMOs can be identified in the published literature (Pawson et al., 2011; Pawson et al., 2014). Second, the timeframe of the review (1997–2017) may have caused us to miss important publications that address some of the analytical gaps we identified, for example, Pattyn et al.'s incisive application of Qualitative Comparative Analysis (QCA) and process tracing in a realist evaluation study (2022).

As such, the published subsample of realist evaluations may differ in important ways from some currently published and non-published realist evaluations. For this reason, generalisation of findings beyond the boundaries of the sample should be approached with caution. Despite this limitation, the position we take is that the present review provides important and useful insights into how realist evaluations are designed and implemented.

Findings

This section presents the review findings structured in accordance with the four phases in the realist evaluation cycle of inquiry: (1) formulation of the initial CMOs (informed by a programme theory), (2) collection of data on the CMOs, (3) data analysis and CMOs testing and (4) refinement of CMOs based on the findings.

Phase 1: Formulation of initial CMO configurations

In our earlier review, we identified CMOs in two-thirds (65%) of the 195 published cases of realist studies (Nielsen et al., 2022). In these 126 cases, we identified 517 CMOs, averaging 4.1 CMOs per evaluation. Over three-quarters (77%) of the realist evaluations contained five or fewer CMOs. Another 18% contained between six and ten CMOs (Table 3.3). The number

Table 3.3 Number of CMOs in study distributed research design (*n* = 126)

	1–5 CMOs	6–10 CMOs	11–15 CMOs	16 or more CMOs
Experimental	11	3	0	
Non-experimental	84	20	2	4
Quasi-experimental	2			
Total (%)	97 (76.9)	23 (18.2)	2 (1.6)	4 (3.1)

Source: Adapted from Nielsen et al. (2022).

of CMOs varied noticeably across the realist evaluations, with as many as 23 CMOs identified in one evaluation. There is no clear variation across designs. Typically, the studies do not report on whether, how or why the number of CMOs initially developed and eventually tested differ.

As formulating the programme theory, and thereby uncovering CMOs, is pivotal in realist evaluation, we first describe how realist evaluators defined and operationalised each of the main concepts comprising their CMOs.

Mechanisms

In realism there are different constructs of mechanism (Westhorp, 2018). Pawson and Tilley (1997; 2008) proposed at least three different conceptualisations of mechanism: (1) as a programme component, (2) as participant reaction to programme component and (3) as an explanatory account (Lemire et al., 2020). Astbury and Leeuw (2010) furthermore describe mechanisms as underlying and hidden. In their review, Lemire and colleagues found that 46% of the studies did not include an explicit definition of mechanism (2020).

In our earlier review of realist evaluation, we examined the mechanisms included in 126 realist evaluations (Lemire et al., 2020). They contained a total of 904 mechanisms. (See Table 3.4). Most mechanisms were in the form of programme components (39%), participant psychological reactions (31%) or participant behavioural reactions (21%). Interestingly, the types of mechanisms examined in the evaluations – the actual CMOs around which the evaluation was structured – did not necessarily correspond with the definition of mechanisms offered by the author(s). That is, a realist evaluation defining mechanism as a programme component in the methods section might include a broader range of mechanisms in the subsequent CMO configurations, such as participant reactions to programme activities.

Table 3.4 Mechanisms in realist evaluations (*n* = 126)

Mechanism type	Frequency	Percent
Programme component	351	38.8
Participant psychological reaction	277	30.7
Participant behavioural reaction	185	20.5
Contextual conditions	78	8.6
Other	13	1.4
Total	904	100.0

Source: Database on published realist evaluations, 1997–2017.

Context

Nielsen et al. (2022) expanded on this analysis and examined how another key term, context, was conceptualised and operationalised by realist evaluators. The authors found that in 126 case applications with CMOs, 48%

contained an explicit definition of context. This finding aligned well with a contemporary review by Greenhalgh and Manzano (2021), which found that 45% of realist evaluations include explicit definitions.

Table 3.5 Contextual factors in realist evaluations
(*n* = 126)

Context type	Frequency	Percent
Individual	138	16.2
Interpersonal	53	6.2
Institutional	310	36.5
Infrastructure	124	14.6
Intervention features	180	21.2
Other	45	5.3
Total	850	100.0

Source: Adapted from Nielsen et al. (2022).

Table 3.5 shows at what level the actual context factors were operationalised. Nielsen and colleagues (2022) noted a broad dispersion at different levels, with institutional (37%) and intervention features (21%) representing the most common levels.

In both reviews of context and mechanism conceptualisations in realist evaluations, the authors noted that methodological challenges remain, insofar as analytically distinguishing programme components, mechanism and contexts from each other both conceptually and operationally seems difficult for realist evaluators (Lemire et al., 2020; Nielsen et al., 2022).

Outcomes

Obviously, the number and types of outcomes depend on the programme being evaluated. On average, the 126 realist evaluations included five outcomes. Bearing in mind that most realist evaluations are conducted in the health and social service domains (see Table 3.2), it is no wonder that most outcomes pertain to human behaviour, knowledge, mental and physical health (see Table 3.6). A notable share of outcomes relates to changes in

Table 3.6 Outcomes in realist evaluations (*n* = 126)

Type	Frequency	Percent
Outcome psychological change	105	15.4
Outcome knowledge/understanding	75	11.0
Outcome skill/behaviour change	180	26.4
Outcome health change	28	4.1
Outcome programme change	252	36.9
Outcome other	43	6.3
Total	683	100.0

Source: Database on published realist evaluation, 1997–2017.

programme (37%), which may be an immediate or intermediate step towards longer-term outcomes measured on programme participants, and/or the programme's target population.

Considered collectively, the findings for the first phase of the realist cycle suggest that many realist evaluations have not defined the key constructs comprising the analytical template – the CMOs – for realist evaluations in the published articles. The mechanisms and context factors included in realist evaluations do not always align with the definitions of the terms provided in the article.

In most cases, realist studies include ten or fewer CMOs.

Phase 2: Data collection

A central premise for realist evaluation is that the analysis of the programme theory should drive all phases of the inquiry. As realist evaluation is 'methods neutral' (Van Belle et al., 2016), one could expect variation in research design, methods for data collection and data analysis across realist evaluations. Additionally, multiple rounds of data collection would be expected as the programme theory is translated into CMOs and further tested and refined in an iterative fashion.

Variation in research design seemed somewhat limited across realist evaluations. Almost all the realist evaluations involved non-experimental designs (87%), with only a few using an experimental (11%) or quasi-experimental design (2%) (see Table 3.3). The prevalence of non-experimental designs is perhaps not too surprising given the initial introduction of realist evaluation as an alternative to experimental designs. Indeed, realist evaluation and experimental designs are considered incompatible in some realist evaluation circles (see Nielsen et al., 2023).

The data collection techniques in our sample primarily relied on qualitative data (49%) or mixed methods data (44%) (Table 3.7). As expected, given realist adherence to method pluralism, realist evaluations display a wide variety of data collection techniques and sources. However, interviews and surveys are common. Moreover, a sizeable proportion of all realist evaluations (37%) involved only one round of data collection, deviating from the

Table 3.7 Type of data collection methods in realist evaluation (*n* = 126)

	Frequency	*Percent*
Qualitative	62	49.2
Mixed methods	56	44.5
Quantitative	8	6.3
Total	126	100.0

Source: Database on published realist evaluation, 1997–2017.

intended iterative rounds of data collection initially intended to be included in the realist evaluation cycle to refine the programme theory (Table 3.9), a point we return to later in this chapter.

Phase 3: Analysis and testing of CMOs

Given the diversity in data collection methods, one could expect similar variation in data analytical techniques. Table 3.8 illustrates the analytical techniques mentioned by realist evaluators when analysing CMOs. Notably, 58 of 126 cases (46%) did *not* explicitly report the analytical techniques they applied. By far, the most commonly reported analytical technique is thematic analysis followed by framework analysis, both of which are qualitative coding and analysis techniques. It is notable that explicitly stated analytical techniques and the chosen research design do not always seem to align. For example, one would expect an experimental design (realist trial) to rely on quantitative analytical techniques. This may be due to emphasis in the published account where multiple lines of inquiry were included in the study and results using the experimental design are published elsewhere (Nielsen et al., 2023).

Table 3.8 Types of analytical techniques applied in realist evaluation cases (*n* = 126)

Analytical technique	Type of research design			
	Experimental	Non-experimental	Quasi-experimental	Total
Unspecified	4	54		58
Thematic Analysis	5	39	1	45
Framework Analysis	3	8		11
Qualitative Comparative Analysis		2		2
Structural Equation Modelling	2			2
Causal Loop Diagram		1		1
Cognitive Mapping, Constant Comparative Method		1		1
Concept Mapping and Framework Analysis		1		1
Delphi Technique		1		1
Explanatory Effects Matrix		1		1
Linked Coding Approach		1		1
Statistical Multivariate Analysis		1		1
Systematic Text Condensation/Statistical analysis			1	1
Total	**14**	**110**	**2**	**126**

Source: Database on published realist evaluation, 1997–2017.

In the following section, we will outline the analytical techniques applied. The section is structured based on the prevalence of the analytical strategy in the realist evaluations.

Thematic analysis

Thematic analysis is a qualitative analytical technique, which is used across a range of epistemologies and research questions. Thematic analysis can be used for identifying, analysing, organising, describing and reporting themes found within a body of text, such as existing literature, administrative texts and interview transcripts (Nowell et al., 2017). As thematic analysis does not rest on a specific methodological and procedural prescription as some other qualitative approaches do, it offers a more accessible form of analysis which is useful for in-depth description of a phenomenon. However, it may be more suitable for initial theory development rather than for testing and refining CMOs, as the latter process requires additional systematic techniques (e.g., the Linked Coding Approach), which are not inherently part of thematic analysis. This holds true for the Explanatory Effects Matrix as well. Both the Explanatory Effects Matrix and the Linked Coding Approach will be discussed later in this section.

Framework analysis

Closely related to thematic analysis, the overall purpose of Framework Analysis is to identify, describe and interpret key patterns within, and across, cases. As such Framework Analysis is an inherently comparative form of thematic analysis, which applies an organised structure of inductively and deductively derived themes (i.e., in a matrix or visual diagram) to conduct cross-sectional analysis (Goldsmith, 2021). The technique has the advantage of lending structure to thematic analysis. As is the case with thematic analysis and concept mapping, it is highly flexible and may be applied under many different circumstances, but lacks systematic steps and transparency needed for configurational causal analysis. As such, the technique seems most appropriate for formulating CMOs than to test concrete hypotheses.

Qualitative comparative analysis

Qualitative Comparative Analysis (QCA) is a case-based approach to causal analysis that uses Boolean algebra as a set of logical procedures in order to minimise the configuration of conditions (i.e., combinations of contexts conditions) that distinguish the cases with a specific outcome (Ragin, 2000). It uses minimisations of qualitative data into binary or interval (quantitative) data that are then computed to arrive at generalisations about the factors that generate a certain outcome. Renmans (2023) has developed and tested a specific version of QCA in realist evaluation. QCA uses a systematic set of steps and is supported by software. It is particularly useful for testing and refining

CMOs as it tests different configurations of conditions (contextual factors) that are tied to a particular outcome.

Structural equation modelling

Structural Equation Modelling (SEM) is a particular variant of Multivariate Analysis, which is widely used in the social sciences. It provides a flexible framework for developing and analysing complex relationships among multiple variables that allow researchers to test the validity of theory using empirical models (Beran & Violato, 2010). Its ability to test theoretical models makes it especially useful for theory-informed evaluations that apply quantitative data. It has also been applied in realist evaluations (Von Thiele Schwarz et al., 2017) and other types of theory-based evaluation (Lemire et al., 2023). As with statistical multivariate analysis in general, it is particularly useful for quantitatively testing CMOs and hypothesised causal processes.

Causal loop diagram

Rooted in systems thinking, causal loop diagrams are best described as a form of visualisation of complex relationships. In a recent review, Baugh Littlejohns et al. (2021) documents its applications using mixed methods. Examples in realist evaluation include Byng et al. (2005), who used causal loop diagrams to depict more complex interactions between individual CMOs. As a visualisation tool it can be applied when formulating, testing or refining CMOs. See Lemire et al. (2023) for examples of causal loop diagrams.

Cognitive mapping

Cognitive mapping is a qualitative and phenomenologically informed method of recording how different actors perceive reality. Parlour and McCormack (2012) used the techniques to collate data from converging lines of inquiry for the final analysis. The technique is essentially a visualisation of links between meaning units and does not offer a systematic procedure for analysing the proposed links. Therefore, the technique seems more appropriate to elicit CMOs through the collation of stakeholder perspectives.

Constant comparative method

In the Constant Comparative Method (CCM) every new data unit is compared with previous data to identify similarities and differences within the meaning unit. Saturation is achieved when further empirical data do not add further insights compared with previous data. CCM seems most appropriate for testing and refining CMOs as it pursues a within-case or across-case comparison of data for a proposed relation between meaning units such as CMO configurations (see Parlour & McCormack, 2012). According to Malterud (2012), the synthesis procedure in Systematic Text Condensation (discussed later in this section) is comparable to the Constant Comparative Method (Glaser & Strauss, 2017).

Concept mapping

Closely related to cognitive mapping, concept mapping is a visual strategy for displaying concepts, and relationships between concepts, that are typically linked by connecting lines (De Ries et al., 2022). Concept maps can be applied at each step of the research process and can be particularly useful as part of thematic analysis (Ward & Haigh, 2017). There are examples of using concept mapping in conjunction with quantitative data and analysis (Mehdipanah et al., 2013) and programme theories (Lemire et al., 2023). The technique can be used to formulate CMOs through the identification of potential contexts and mechanisms, but also to test CMOs.

Delphi survey

The Delphi Survey is a technique used to obtain a consensus of opinion from a panel of stakeholders (Fisher & Downes, 2008). Delphi Surveys use questionnaires in multiple rounds to identify and consolidate a consensus position. Researchers can report findings on a specific question (or set of questions) that are based on the knowledge and experience of experts in their field (such as propositions as about mechanisms and contexts). Participants are able to see the results of previous rounds – including their own responses. Marginal positions are asked to reflect on their assessment and reposition their own opinions accordingly (Barrett & Heale, 2020). As such the technique often drives towards a consensus. It has been applied in realist evaluation (Fisher & Downes, 2008) and theory-based evaluation more broadly (Lemire et al., 2023) and can be useful for both the initial development and testing of CMOs.

Explanatory effects matrix

Explanatory Effects Matrix is a technique developed by Miles and Huberman (1994) and aims to order the (causal) relations in a particular domain in the shape of a chart linking certain concepts (e.g., mechanisms, context factors) with outcomes. According to its creators, it is useful for initial exploration of causation in a particular domain. It has been applied in a realist evaluation by Kovacs and Corrie (2016). As it is recommended for exploration of causation, the technique seems most appropriate for formulating CMOs.

Linked coding approach

Linked Coding Approach (LCA) is a qualitative analytical technique developed specifically to analyse and test CMOs (Jackson & Kolla, 2012). Essentially, textual data are coded for individual meaning units (a discrete C, M or O identified in a prior step). In text sections dyads, triads or more complex strings may be coded. As such textual data can be analysed for implicit and explicit CMO connections as represented by different sources. The approach can be used for eliciting, testing and refining CMOs.

Statistical multivariate analysis

Multivariate Analysis is a frequently used inferential statistical technique used to analyse data with multiple variables simultaneously. Multivariate analysis aims to understand relationships between these variables and explore patterns, correlations and interactions among them. Multivariate analysis encompasses a wide range of discrete methods, including regression analysis, multivariate analysis of variance, discriminant analysis, principal component analysis and factor analysis (Hutcheson & Sofroniou, 1999). It has been used in realist evaluation to test causal pathways in programme theories (Oroviogoicoechea & Watson, 2009). The various techniques hold multiple options for quantitatively testing CMOs and hypothesised causal processes.

Systematic text condensation

Systematic Text Condensation (STC) is a qualitative analytical technique which is used to identify and elicit themes. STC consists of four steps: (1) reading through the material to identify preliminary themes; (2) identifying and developing meaning units; (3) systematically abstracting meaning units; and (4) reconceptualising data and develop concepts and descriptions (Malterud, 2012). In one of the cases reviewed, coding was guided by the previously developed programme theory, but unexpected findings were also coded. Further, the authors used ordinal logistic regressions for the quantitative analysis of outcome data (Pals et al., 2016). The technique is used to elicit meaning units (nodes) that are linked. Such links can create and test configuration. As such it seems most appropriate for formulating and testing CMOs.

Considered collectively, we were surprised that we did not find any published examples of some different analytical techniques that we considered particularly amenable to realist evaluation and generative causation. These include Process Tracing (Bennett et al., 2019), Outcome Pattern Matching (Trochim, 1989), Contribution Tracing (Befani & Stedman-Bryce, 2017) and Logic Analysis (Brousselle & Champagne, 2011). We shall consider these further in the discussion below.

Phase 4: Refinement of CMOs

There is only general procedural guidance on how refinement of CMOs should be carried out in realist evaluations (Wong et al., 2016). Of the 126 realist evaluations in our review, 64% included refined CMOs. Most of these were in narrative and or table format. Moreover, the refinements of CMOs were mostly carried out by the evaluator alone, sometimes in collaboration with staff or other stakeholders. (See Table 3.9).

Table 3.9 Refined CMO reported in study (*n* = 126)

Refined CMO reported:	
Yes	**No**
81	45
(64%)	(36%)

Refined CMO developed by:	
Evaluator	**Evaluator with staff/stakeholder**
62	19
(77%)	(23%)

Refined CMO reported as*:			
Narrative	Table	Diagram	Other
78	37	21	3
(96%)	(46%)	(26%)	(4%)

Source: Database on published realist evaluation, 1997–2017.

* Does not sum to 126 (100%) as multiple options possible

Summarising across the phases of the realist inquiry cycle, our review findings reveal that many realist evaluations have not defined the key constructs comprising the analytical template – the CMOs – for realist evaluations. In most cases, realist studies include ten or fewer CMOs. The methodological diversity hailed by realists is evident in the wide variety of data collection methods and to some extent the analytical techniques applied in realist evaluations. Analytical strategies and the techniques applied are central to empirically substantiating theories and claims about the existence of CMOs. Ultimately the analytical strategy is central to providing a plausible explanatory account of why a programme works.

Discussion and recommendations for practice

In this chapter, we argue that an analytical strategy that includes the application of concrete analytical techniques is an indispensable tool for substantiating programme theories. This is the case for realist evaluations and for theory-based evaluation more broadly. Towards advancing analytical strategies in evaluation, evaluators should apply rigor in thinking. This implies knowing a broad range of methodological tools for evaluation design, data collection, analysis and inferring judgement, as well as making an explicit and reasoned application of analytical strategies to fit the specific purposes of the evaluation.

Some analytical techniques may be more fit-for-purpose at different stages of the realist endeavour. Based on our presentation of the techniques and concrete application in realist evaluation cases, we have summarised what we consider the most appropriate fit for the different analytical techniques

Table 3.10 Appropriateness of analytical techniques for developing/testing/refining CMO configurations

Analytical technique	Step of CMO configuration development			
	Formulating CMOs	Testing CMOs	Refining CMOs	Type of data
Cognitive Mapping	●	●		Qualitative
Concept Mapping	●			Qualitative
Constant Comparative Method		●	●	Qualitative
Delphi Technique	●		●	Qualitative
Explanatory Effects Matrix	●			Qualitative
Framework Analysis	●	●		Qualitative
Linked Coding Approach	●	●	●	Qualitative
Process Tracing		●		Qualitative
Systematic Text Condensation	●	●		Qualitative
Thematic Analysis	●			Qualitative
Statistical Multivariate Analysis		●		Quantitative
Structural Equation Modelling		●		Quantitative
Causal Loop Diagram	●	●	●	Mixed
Contribution Tracing		●		Mixed
Logic Analysis	●	●		Mixed
Outcome Pattern Matching		●		Mixed
Qualitative Comparative Analysis		●	●	Mixed

applied (and some promising but absent, in the sample we used for analysis). These are presented in Table 3.10. Following Salter and Kothari (2014), we have related them to the three stages wherein programme theory and CMOs are formulated, tested and refined. The table indicates that some techniques may be more appropriate for gleaning programme theories and establish (potential) CMOs, but less applicable for testing CMOs and providing a rigorous explanatory account that takes into account configurational causal analysis.

Other than applying analytical strategies for the right purposes, the data from our comprehensive review of published realist evaluation cases suggests that some lessons can be learned and principles for rigor in thinking in realist evaluation practice can be discerned. These principles should form a point of reference for the application of realist evaluation.

1 *Define key constructs – mechanisms, context and outcomes.* Too many realist evaluators report methodological challenges in distinguishing mechanisms, context and outcomes from another. Realist evaluators should consult established definitions and determine why and how said definition is most useful in their particular evaluation context. Clear and operable definitions promote transparency and provide a firm foundation for data collection and analysis.
2 *Ensure that sufficient CMOs are identified to test the programme theory.* Operatively, one may have too few or too many CMOs to create a convincing argument that a programme works in a specific way. The adequate

number of CMOs ultimately hinges on the complexity of the programme. Shaw and colleagues (2018) provide an insightful example of analysing CMOs moving from a macro to a micro level, skilfully showing how different mechanisms and contexts can be at play at different levels of the analysis and thereby some mechanisms at a higher level (i.e., policy level) may become context at a lower level (i.e., organisational level).

3 *Make explicit priorities for selected CMO configurations and hypotheses.* There is an unending range of possibilities as to what contexts may be imparted in CMO configurations, and one can speculate an infinite number of mechanisms. Often evaluators need to prioritise which ones are salient and should be the object of study. Tools and techniques to do so rigorously and explicitly are necessary (Lemire et al., 2012).

4 *Decide on an analytical strategy early on.* The ever-presence of theory implies that realist evaluators must be clear on what analytical techniques should be applied at different stages of the research so that they support a realist logic of analysis. These tools are essential in shaping fieldwork data collection, and formulating, testing and refining the CMOs. In recent publications, there are promising examples of applying conventional qualitative analytical techniques (Dalkin et al., 2021) and combining a realist logic of analysis with other techniques, such as QCA and process tracing (Pattyn et al., 2022).

5 *Converge and fit research design, data collection methods and analytical strategy.* The professed methodological plurality of realist evaluation means that many options exist. Design, data collection methods and instruments and analytical techniques should be logically and transparently aligned so they can support the theory testing and refining strategy. We recommend creating a protocol/methodology note early on, which details how and why each activity is conducted and how it is related to subsequent procedures of analysis and data collection that eventually leads to a refined programme theory. However, it is important for this protocol to remain flexible to accommodate fieldwork contingencies and the emergence of new theories.

6 *Triangulate sources and data collection methods.* Realist evaluators are focused on middle-range theories with context-dependent applicability. Realist evaluators should deftly collect data from multiple sources using multiple forms of data collection and analysis to strengthen the validity of their findings.

Returning to the initial clarion call of Ray Pawson, that there is nothing as practical as a good theory, we posit that there is nothing as practical as a good analytical strategy. Rigour in realist evaluation necessarily implies an explicit, reasoned application of an analytical strategy that purposefully deploys data collection methods and analytical techniques that enable the formulation, testing and refinement of said theory. Ultimately, this is the empirical testing ground of evaluation. As such there is nothing as practical as an analytical strategy.

Conclusion

In this chapter, we focused on the analytical strategies applied in published cases of realist evaluations. We found that (too) many realist evaluators struggled to define key constructs and specify the analytical strategy and techniques used to substantiate the programme theory and CMOs forwarded in their realist evaluation. We found that about nine of ten cases applied non-experimental research designs and used qualitative or mixed-methods. About six of ten applied one or more explicit analytical techniques. We then examined which analytical techniques were applied, and assessed whether the techniques we found were particularly appropriate at different stages of the realist evaluation cycle. Finally, we recommended a number of principles that we consider important towards advancing the practice of designing and conducting realist evaluations.

Acknowledgements

The authors would like to thank the editors of the book for useful and actionable feedback and Ingrid Bjerregaard Lauridsen for technical assistance with the data analysis.

4 Combining realist reviews with realist evaluations

Geoff Wong, Jo Howe, Maura MacPhee, and Ian Maidment

Introduction

In this chapter, we provide advice on combining realist reviews (also called realist syntheses) with realist evaluations. Below, we set out the main areas that require consideration, discuss each in turn and provide advice. We have drawn upon our experience of working on three UK-funded projects that deliberately sought to combine realist reviews with realist evaluations (Maidment et al., 2020; Maidment et al., 2022; Lindsay et al., 2023). We have also drawn upon our experience of working with doctoral students who conducted a realist review and a realist evaluation in their thesis. In addition, we have collaboratively reflected upon our combined decades of experience working on separate realist reviews or realist evaluation projects. We bring diverse clinical backgrounds: medicine (GW), nursing (MM), psychology (JH) and pharmacy (IM) in addition to methodological expertise. Our interdisciplinary approach adds further insights as we interpret the data. Whilst the projects we (and our students) have worked on are research projects that have been directed at addressing knowledge gaps in health, we have done our best to draw out methodological advice that we hope is more widely applicable.

At this point we want to point out that some of our advice is generic, in that it applies to research projects more widely, but some will be much more specific to situations when realist reviews and realist evaluations are combined. Where this is the case, we will make this clear. An important first bit of advice we would like to give right at the start is that many of you will have well-honed research skills. These skills may include how to: assemble an effective team, design research projects, write grant applications and manage projects well, including budget, personnel, stakeholder engagement and ethical considerations. Researchers will also likely have specific quantitative and qualitative methodological skills that may be invaluable to the project and possess the necessary expertise to effectively produce research outputs and disseminate them to a wide audience. In common with many realist projects, all of our combined realist review and realist evaluation projects have had patient and public involvement. The skills needed to make their contributions meaningful and respectful are not unique to realist projects. In summary,

DOI: 10.4324/9781003457077-5

when conducting a combined realist review and realist evaluation, never forget to draw on the skills you already have where they are relevant.

Developing a proposal for a combined realist review and realist evaluation

An initial question any researcher must ask themselves is: Why is there a need to combine a realist review with a realist evaluation in the first place? The most common reason for combining a realist review with a realist evaluation is because we know there are likely to be gaps in the literature that only primary data will be able to address. In other words, we have an indication in advance that what we will be able to find in the literature is unlikely to contain enough relevant secondary data for us to be able to sufficiently develop and refine our initial programme theory. Of course, this then begs the question as to how we know this is likely to be the case before we have even begun the review.

This is where two things can help. Firstly, for any research project (or DPhil/PhD) you are likely to have content experts as part of the team; as mentioned earlier we have found that having an inter-disciplinary team strengthens the content expertise. Amongst other knowledge that they bring will be an understanding of what type and how much research has been done in the field of interest. Draw on their knowledge to make your case. In addition, there is nothing to stop you from doing an initial exploratory search of the literature to confirm any suspicions that you and your project team colleagues may have. It makes sense to have a librarian or information specialist on your project team early on to help with the process of determining the existence of relevant secondary data. Whenever possible, if budget allows, a librarian can be a valuable team asset to do ongoing searches throughout the iterative process of document data collection for the review. Later, a librarian can also assist with searches for locating literature, particularly the non-academic grey literature, pertinent to substantive theories and comparative literature to include in reports and publications.

Our experience is that there are 'costs' to the project team and (if applicable) the funder when doing both a realist review and a realist evaluation. To illustrate, a realist review can be completed in 12 (at a stretch) to 18 months. But when both are undertaken, the time frame has ranged from 24 to 27 months in duration (or longer). For the sake of expediency, it is entirely possible to truncate processes within a realist review – for example, by having inclusion or exclusion criteria with a tighter focus, or by limiting the extent of the analysis. This is something we have done in a project on Recovery Colleges, where the focus was developing only an initial programme theory and the causal explanations were much more rudimentary, expressed only as 'If … then' statements vs. detailed constituent context-mechanism-outcome-configurations (CMOCs) (Birt et al., 2023). This allows a realist review to be conducted within a short period of time, but anyone doing this needs to be aware of the potential threats to the validity of their findings and highlight these in any publication or report.

When writing a grant application for a combined realist review and realist evaluation issues that arise can include the following. The grant can take longer to write as there is a need to justify to the funder why the combined approaches are needed, and to provide methodological details for the review and the evaluation. The project team is likely to need to be expanded to include members with expertise in both doing a realist review and realist evaluation. This may seem obvious, but it cannot and should not be assumed that picking up and undertaking a realist review or realist evaluation is easy – let alone when they are combined.

There will need to be coherence between both components – so that it is clear to the funder how one part links to the other. One very important consideration to bear in mind is that, with the exception of DPhil/PhD projects, each component may require different project team members throughout the time period. Added personnel and costs need to be considered for the review (e.g., information specialist) and for the evaluation (primary data collection through methods such as interviews and surveys). Mapping out who will be needed at different points along an extended time frame for the review and evaluation must be carefully considered with respect to optimising each team member's role (s) and the budget.

The implication here is that a strong justification is needed to convince funders that the extra expense is worth the knowledge gained. Because of these considerations, all the projects we have worked on which have combined a realist review with a realist evaluation have mainly used one-to-one interviews to collect the additional primary data needed. Most commonly these interviews are based on the principles of realist interviews (Wong et al., 2017). This does not mean that the realist evaluation component cannot use other data collection methods such as surveys, focus groups or focused observations. But we have found that the most efficient way of getting the in-depth data needed to understand 'why', 'for whom' and 'when' knowledge gaps in the programme theory tends to be interviews. The most important principles here when designing the data collection method(s) for the realist evaluation are to justify your choice of method(s) selected and consider the impact of your choices on the cost and duration of the project. This we would suggest is good practice in grant writing for any type of research project.

The project team's content and especially team members' methodological expertise is important, as it is one of the ways that funders work out that the team is likely to have the ability to successfully deliver a grant. As in any project, realist or not, it goes without saying that any team assembled needs to be able to work together, be reliable and actively contribute. When putting together a team, do make sure that anyone invited to a project will be someone all team members can work with and who will reliably contribute. Common pitfalls are adding in 'superstar' researchers who contribute little, 'impostors' (people who claim to be experts in a field, but this is not supported by their list of publications or projects they have worked on), and individuals who fail to respond to any drafts of the project proposal. The team also needs balance. For example, a research study on medication optimisation in primary care should contain primary care medical doctors, nurses and pharmacists without being too heavily weighted towards a single profession.

Another issue you need to address is coherence within any project proposal. Someone has to make sure that the realist review and realist evaluation make sense as a whole. We have seen multiple projects that use different analysis processes for the review and evaluation. For example, a project plans to use a realist logic of analysis for the review but a form of thematic analysis for the evaluation. Logically and coherently a realist logic of analysis should be used for both the realist review and realist evaluation. Another common issue is a lack of clarity as to how the outputs from the review link to the evaluation. The key here is to remember that both realist reviews and realist evaluations are theory-driven forms of research. Theory drives both sense-making of the data but also informs what data are needed. In a realist review and realist evaluation, the theory we want to develop is a programme theory about the intervention, programme or phenomenon of interest. This is what should link the realist review and realist evaluation – the output of the realist review is a better refined initial programme theory drawing on the secondary data from included documents (Rohrbasser et al., 2022; Jager, Papoutsi, et al., 2023a; Jager, Wong, et al., 2023b). This in turn is then further refined using the primary data collected from the realist evaluation. Box 4.1 summarises our advice for this section.

Box 4.1   Advice on developing a proposal for conducting a realist review and realist evaluation.

Ensure you have:

Provided a strong justification for why both approaches are needed to address your research question(s). This can be supported by drawing on the project team's content expertise and informal searches of the literature. We mean literature in the widest sense; the grey literature including service evaluations can be very valuable.

A project team that has the necessary content and proven methodological expertise that can work well together, with members that are reliable and actively contribute.

Explained how the realist review and the realist evaluation are linked. Usually, the link is that both contribute data for programme theory development and 'testing' (confirming, refuting, refining the programme theory).

The practicalities of running projects that combine a realist review and realist evaluation

Within this section, we provide some practical advice to researchers who have decided that there is a need to combine a realist review with a realist evaluation to answer their research question(s). Whilst each of the issues we discuss below is presented separately for the sake of clarity, in reality there are overlaps. In addition, we do not present them in any order of importance, but they should all be considered and addressed where needed.

Staffing

As in any project, the individual(s) conducting the research are a key consideration. An important decision that must be made early in the project – unless it is a PhD/DPhil project – is whether to have one or more people conducting the research. Is it better to have one person doing the realist review and another doing the realist evaluation? Unfortunately, there is no simple answer to this question as there are pros and cons to each approach. With a single person tasked to do both the review and evaluation, there are the following benefits. You only need to recruit one person and as staff costs usually make up the bulk of any realist project's budget, costs will be lower and hence a funder might view the project as more 'competitive'. With fewer people on the project, it can be easier to manage it (e.g. organising meetings or chances of personality clashes) and analysis issues (see below) are less likely to occur. When there are short timelines, integrating deliverables from two different members of staff can be challenging. A single person will be able to develop expertise on the topic in the realist review, which is likely to be essential for the evaluation.

There are, however, disadvantages in a single person. There is the potential challenge of overreliance on one individual for the duration of the project, such as if the person becomes unwell or decides to take up another job. Another consideration is how the researcher spends their time and the workload they have to deal with. In effect, the individual researcher has to split their time between the realist review and realist evaluation or try to do them both at the same time. (See Sequencing for additional discussion.) This runs the risk of both being done less well than intended because of the inability to fully immerse themselves in one or the other. Having the time to think and discuss emerging findings are valuable activities in realist reviews and realist evaluations. (See Analysis for more details.) One risk of having only a single researcher conducting both is that in order to meet the project's deadlines, no time is left for in-depth reflection, analysis and stakeholder discussions. We have also found that some researchers have personal preferences for what types of research they like to conduct. If a researcher has a preference for primary data collection (vs. conducting an evidence synthesis), then they may unintentionally neglect the realist review or half-heartedly conduct it. Should this occur, it will add to the challenges faced by the project lead – as it is yet another issue they will need to spot and rectify.

Having two or more individuals conducting the research can have benefits. An obvious one is in the potential resilience this brings as hopefully not all the researchers will decide to leave at the same time! Additionally, as already mentioned, having the time to think and discuss emerging findings are valuable activities in realist reviews and realist evaluations. So, for example, having two researchers will enable them to regularly share and discuss their emerging findings. When recruited or assigned their roles in the project, better matching could also be made between the type of research they prefer to do and the project's components. The benefits of having two or more researchers can also help the project progress more rapidly where tasks can be undertaken simultaneously – as long as the researchers are willing and able to be flexible in how they deploy their time. Examples of potential benefits of having two or more researchers, drawn from the projects we have worked on, include: writing protocols for publication; screening search results from a realist review; preparing ethical approval submissions; data analysis; and preparing project outputs. However, this is not always trouble-free and we discuss this issue in more detail in the Analysis section below.

We have configured the grading of the staff on the project in different ways and there does not seem to be a one-size-fits-all solution. One way has been to have a more experienced 'senior' researcher supported by a less experienced 'junior' one. As well as contributing to the conduct of the realist review and evaluation, we have also found that the more junior member of staff can support their senior colleague with the practical and other aspects. These include, but are not limited to, organising project team meetings, setting up interviews, reimbursing participants, producing newsletters and supporting other aspects of dissemination including conference presentations and proofreading documents. In other projects when the two researchers have similar research experience, the most important thing is that they can work together in a collaborative, supportive and flexible way. Effective collaboration seems to us to be far more important than the levels of experience they bring.

Having two or more researchers can also be very helpful with the ethical approvals process. When combining a realist review with a realist evaluation, ethical approval will be needed for the primary data collection. This can be an onerous and protracted process and sharing the load between the researchers can be helpful. In addition, with two or more researchers, one could be tasked with conducting the review whilst the other works on getting ethical approval. The latter task is something that we would recommend is started as soon as possible, so as to avoid any delays to the project.

Regardless of whether one, two or more researchers are working on the project, our experience is that a small but dedicated amount of funding set aside to provide administrative support can pay dividends. This is because an administrator can free up the researchers to focus on the research, as opposed to spending time on other tasks, such as organising meetings, reimbursements, booking rooms and so on.

One final issue that relates to staffing is about how well the whole project team functions as a team. This is a generic issue that applies to all research teams, but has greater importance when realist reviews and realist evaluations are combined. Those involved in the data collection and analysis need to be able to share, discuss and debate emerging findings. They also need to be able to argue for and make changes to the focus of the realist review or type of data collected in the evaluation where justified – for example, when there are emerging gaps in the programme theory that need to be filled. To do so requires a team culture that is respectful, listens, is reflective, humble and responsive. Far be it from us to tell people how to run their teams, but our experience is that time spent on developing, nurturing and sustaining such a culture is time well spent, as it not only supports analysis and other aspects of the team, but makes working on a project more enjoyable. Box 4.2 summarises our advice for this section.

Box 4.2   Advice on staffing.

Ensure you have:

Weighed up the pros and cons between employing one versus two or more people to undertake the combined realist review and realist evaluation.

Sufficient administrative support for the project (as this can free up researcher(s)' time).

Spend time building a project team that is respectful, listens, is reflective, humble and responsive.

Sequencing

There is a logical rationale to sequencing when a realist review and realist evaluation are combined – namely, realist review first followed by realist evaluation. The logic underlying this sequencing is that the available literature is first used to develop an understanding of the intervention, programme or phenomenon, captured in the form of a realist programme theory with its constituent CMOCs. Primary data are then used to test (confirm, refute or refine) the programme theory and CMOCs; as well as addressing any knowledge 'gaps' uncovered from the review. This sequencing builds on one of the central tenets of realist reviews and realist evaluations – namely that where possible we should be cumulating our understanding of the intervention, programme or phenomenon we are studying (Pawson, 2013). Doing the realist review first can also have additional benefits. For example, in one of the projects we have worked on, the realist review identified that much of the research in the field was very narrowly focussed on specific issues, favoured particular research methods and was mainly atheoretical. Knowing this helped us to understand not only where we needed to focus our primary data collection, but also informed where future research was needed and, importantly, what types of research methods were least likely to advance our knowledge. It is also important to remember that when there is an overlap between the review and evaluation, emerging findings from the primary data can also influence the focus of the realist review. From our experience, primary data collection starts at about 6 to 8 months into a 24-month+ project.

However, practicalities can get in the way of any intended sequencing. The first and foremost is the duration of the project. As already mentioned, it can be challenging to get funding for a project that is considered to be too 'expensive' and 'uncompetitive' because it costs too much and is too long. This means that it is often not possible to do sufficient justice to the realist review before embarking on the realist evaluation. In other words, the programme theory from the realist review may not be as well developed as you would like before having to embark on the primary data collection. We have found that a judgement needs to be made as to whether the developing programme theory is 'good enough' to inform what needs to happen in the realist evaluation. Our experience is that with a good analytical process (discussed below in more detail), it is often possible to identify quite early on in a project where there are clear knowledge gaps. This may be when the secondary data is simply missing or when additional data are needed on specific parts of the programme theory to provide causal explanations. An example of this is when the secondary data is atheoretical or mainly of a quantitative nature. The latter can create challenges because quantitative data tends to focus on outcomes. Quantitative data can be helpful to understand outcome patterns or what outcomes are important to the study intervention or programme. But qualitative data is often needed as well because it can provide more details on contextual factors and potential mechanisms.

One challenge that may come up is that as the project progresses, there may need to be a change in focus within both the realist review and/or evaluation. We have found this might arise because of (for example): feedback and advice from stakeholders, such as input from practitioners, service commissioners and patient and public involvement.

On this last point, in many of the projects we work on, we pay particular attention to our stakeholder voice with respect to our findings' implications for policy and practice. Our approach is to consider how issues, such as stigma from serious mental illness, will need to be addressed at a wider societal level and we also consider outputs from our work that will get impact sooner, such as more immediate and shorter-term guidance with recommendations that are more readily achievable. As we see these impact opportunities through our discussions with stakeholders, our team needs to be willing to make decisions, flexibly, on how we will continue with the project and primary data collection.

Mundane issues can have profound impacts on sequencing. For example, it may not be possible to recruit two researchers so that they can start at the same time. Staff may leave, become unwell and so on. These are more generic issues that affect all projects and not just realist ones. What this sometimes means is that the existing project team must be willing to do more to keep the project running. As we have emphasised in the Staffing section above, this is when we have found that having a cohesive team can help allay the stress and strain from staffing changes during the project. Box 4.3 summarises our advice for this section.

Box 4.3   Advice on sequencing.

Ensure you have:

Decided how you are going to sequence the realist review and realist evaluation, and paid specific attention to staffing requirements needed to support the sequencing.

Regular discussions within the project team to decide on the focus of the realist review and whether and when you have a 'good enough' understanding to inform primary data collection in the realist evaluation. Also consider if emerging findings from the primary data might indicate a change in the realist review is needed.

Flexibility. Your final sequence may not be your planned sequence. Be led by the data and consider your stakeholder feedback. Changes to staffing may also affect how you sequence the review and evaluation.

Data collection

The data needs to enable programme theory and CMOC development and then testing (refuting, confirming or refining). In a realist review, the secondary data come from documents so the key individual in this endeavour is a librarian or information specialist. It is beyond the scope of this chapter to cover their role in any detail and instead we direct those interested in learning more to the RAMESES project website (2024) (https://www.ramesesproject. org/media/RAMESES_II_Working_with_a_librarian.pdf) where relevant open access materials may be found. We always ensure that the contributions of the information specialist are fully recognised on any outputs.

With regard to primary data collection for the realist evaluation component, we have three bits of advice. Firstly, and obviously, the evaluation design should enable the gathering of data needed to develop and test the programme theory. Any research method could potentially contribute data that may be relevant for programme theory and CMOC development and testing. The key principle is to ensure that when any data collection method is used, it is conducted in a way that minimises any threats to the validity of the findings. This can be done by adhering as much as possible to what counts as high-quality practice in the method being used. To illustrate, in projects where we use realist interviews, we have employed what many would consider to be 'good' interview techniques (Maidment et al., 2020). These include settling in the interviewee, using appropriate body language, asking open questions and only probing with more specific questions when necessary.

Secondly, our experience is that interview data can be used to test CMOCs from the literature. The triangulation of data collected using different methods facilitate validation, for example, if the same CMOC is found in both the literature and interviews. Primary data can also lead to the development of new CMOCs not present in the literature, particularly if there is little existing secondary data on the subject. As an example of how primary data can inform the direction of the evaluation when secondary data are lacking, we draw on our REalist Synthesis and evaluation Of effective, community-based, non-pharmacologicaL weight management interVEntions for service users with psychosis who have experienced rapid weight gain from anti-psychotic medications (RESOLVE) (Maidment et al., 2022). One researcher conducted the review while another researcher carried out the interviews for the evaluation. The two researchers met weekly to exchange data findings. The review literature was primarily composed of randomised controlled trials (RCTs) of different weight management intervention programmes. These RCTs reported mixed results with respect to weight loss, clinical indicators and stakeholder survey findings, such as programme satisfaction and quality of life. The evaluation interviews added greater depth to the literature by exploring why some programmes had positive outcomes while others did not. Service users' reports of their biggest barriers to programme participation informed a return to the literature to locate more secondary data on potential strategies for overcoming the programme barriers identified by interviewees. The interviews, therefore, allowed us to confirm, refine and expand our initial review findings.

Finally, we have found that the types of interviews conducted in a realist evaluation to gather the necessary data can be cognitively taxing for researchers. The interviewer needs time to reflect on what has been said, thinking back to what is in the programme theory and adapting their questioning as needed. In addition, to enable diverse surfacing of interviewee ideas during the interview, the researcher may need to cede control of the interview guide and quickly adapt questions and prompts. These are skills that many good interviewers have, especially researchers with expertise in qualitative methods. However, given the possibility of the additional 'work' during interviews, we recommend limiting the number of interviews conducted in any one day. Another risk to multiple interviews in one day is the possibility of mixing up interviews. We have found that time must be factored in between interviews for writing out summary notes and reflections after each interview, to capture important elements. When interviews are spaced too closely together, researchers can get confused in their note-taking or lose valuable information. Box 4.4 summarises our advice for this section.

Box 4.4 Advice on data collection.

Ensure you have:

A project team with the right skill set. For example, a librarian or information specialist is an essential team member in a realist review.
Conducted any primary data collection using accepted quality standards for that data collection method.
A realistic timetable for data collection that does not overburden the researchers collecting the data. Allow time between episodes of primary data collection for note-taking and reflection.

Analysis

There is no one standardised method that researchers must use when analysing their data in a realist review or evaluation. Sensemaking of the data collected and developing CMOCs is a personal endeavour: different people have different ways of working and will approach this task in different ways. For example, some researchers on our team use Word documents, Excel spreadsheets and NVivo software to organise data from documents (review) and interviews (evaluation). What must be done is to develop a process and to apply this process in a consistent way across all the data. This is a process that should be gradually developed and applied with input from all the relevant members of the project team. One way we do check-ins with all our team members is for the researchers to regularly prepare (if needed with input from the wider project team) and present PowerPoint summaries of work to date. Simple visual slides can be an effective way of sharing progress on the review and evaluation.

The person(s) who are leading the project, that is, the project lead(s), should ensure that the analysis process is coherent, as should the researcher(s) doing the analyses and the realist methodologist(s). (It is essential that there should be at least one person with realist expertise on the project). This process of discussing and negotiating how the analysis is going is much easier when the project team functions well (See Staffing). Most importantly, whether there is only one researcher or many conducting the combined review and evaluation, all involved in conducting the analysis need to be satisfied with the process agreed upon at the beginning of the project or any later modifications that are needed. Mundane issues that need to be initially discussed, most of which are applicable to many research projects, include: who will do what; what software (if any) will be used to support analyses; how often will you meet; how will you code the data; how do you keep the codebook consistent and up to date; how will you share emerging findings; how will you write up your findings; and who will do these.

Regular team meetings between those involved in the analyses are important. As mentioned above, the 'core' analysis team (i.e., those most involved in the analysis) should meet up at least weekly using online meeting tools such as Microsoft Teams or Zoom. Virtual meetings are cost-effective ways of connecting team members from different geographic locations on busy schedules. In addition to weekly analysis meetings between researchers, we also recommend frequent, set meetings between the researchers and the project lead(s). Since the project lead is ultimately responsible for the successful delivery of the project, set meetings are necessary to ensure effective communications between key team members and the lead. We have also found that in addition to formal meetings with the lead, informal emails and/or phone conversations with the lead may be necessary if unexpected project issues arise. Otherwise, the following may happen: miscommunications and conflicts, rejection of hours of hard work, or sudden changes of direction or focus.

During our regular analysis meetings, we share CMOCs and emerging data, to ensure a 'fit' between the data and the Cs-Ms-Os we have developed. Because of multiple iterations, it is important to clearly label versions of CMOCs with accompanying data and data sources. Where a realist review has already produced well-developed and supported CMOCs, these often form the basis for the analysis of the data from the realist evaluation. For example, in one of our projects, we used the CMOCs from the realist review as a coding framework for primary data from the realist evaluation. The sharing of data at meetings enables different viewpoints to be brought to bear on the emerging findings. This can help to address the potential Achilles heels of any research approach where the interpretation of the data may be clouded by tunnel vision and confirmation bias. Where new data emerges that challenges our existing understanding, new CMOCs need to be developed and efforts made to recheck the secondary or primary data – to identify if anything has been missed or if new searches for secondary data or changes in primary data collection are needed. We have found that this sharing can help provide clarity to the researchers conducting the realist review and realist evaluation. For example, in our experience, team discussions have helped inform the need for new questions to ask in the realist evaluation, based on knowledge gaps in the realist review or through discussions with stakeholder groups. (See below.)

We have also found that these regular meetings are an opportunity to take stock on whether the project needs to be continued as is (for example, whether the sampling frame is still valid) and if the agreed data analysis plan and processes are working, or if changes need to be made. As an example, in one of our projects, when we were able to identify theoretical saturation with one of our participant samples, we agreed that we would devote the remaining time in the project to sample those participants with less representation. In one realist evaluation, where we were interested in integrated care needs for individuals with serious mental illness, we had sufficient interviews from mental health workers, but we lacked interviews with service providers who address the physical health needs of this population (Maidment et al., 2022). As a result, we changed our sampling frame. These regular meetings can also be a very helpful way for the project team members to support each other – for example, when challenges arise with opening sites, recruitment, analysis or team dynamics issues. At these regular meetings, ad hoc training and learning can also take place, for example to help a team member struggling to understand realist concepts, terminology or how to develop programme theory and CMOCs.

Related to the aforementioned Achilles heel is the benefit of involving stakeholders in the project. By stakeholders we mean anyone who is involved in or impacted by the intervention, programme or phenomenon under investigation. Within our projects, because they are situated in health, our stakeholders usually include some or all of the following: clinicians and/or practitioners; administrators; policy and decision makers; patients and family carers and the public. We cost and timetable in regular meetings with them, asking for feedback and advice on differing aspects of the project. At the start of the project their advice is used to identify aspects of a programme or intervention that we should consider within our review's initial programme theory. Later on, they assist by providing feedback and advice on emerging findings. For example, in our MEMORABLE study on medication management in older people, our initial CMOCs presented evidence of the burden associated with medication. After reviewing our literature findings, stakeholders with lived experience asked about training for family carers in key aspects of medication management to mitigate the burden (Lawson et al., 2021). Our secondary data found little research on this, providing avenues for further exploration in MEMORABLE, including a specific subset analysis and follow-on research. Nearer the end of the projects such as MEMORABLE, stakeholders play a key role in developing outputs, such as recommendations and reports, publications and documents aimed at policy and decision-makers or service users and the public. We have found that respectfully drawing on the input of stakeholders has helped us to identify areas that need further attention (as mentioned above) and has helped us to avoid groupthink with the project team. Box 4.5 summarises our advice for this section.

Box 4.5   Advice on analysis.

Ensure you have:

All discussed and agreed on, as early as possible, a data analysis plan and processes or any modifications needed later.

Regular meetings, pre-planned or ad hoc as needed, to share and discuss emerging data as well as take stock of how well the project is progressing and if changes are required. These meetings can also be used for other purposes, such as mutual support and ad hoc training.

Regular feedback and advice from a range of stakeholders – to inform and enrich the project.

Summary

Combining a realist review with a realist evaluation can be an efficient and effective way for developing a programme theory about an intervention, programme or phenomenon. However, this combination will make a project longer in duration, particularly as conducting a rigorous realist review and realist evaluation takes time. In addition, obtaining ethical approval may add to the duration. As such, combined projects will likely cost more, and require a broader set of skills compared to just doing one or the other. It is important to provide a strong and coherent justification for why the combination is needed. If it is needed, then there are practical considerations to bear in mind and address. Much of our advice applies to many other types of research and hence we urge you, where relevant, to draw on the existing skills you have for designing and managing projects.

In this chapter, we have covered the issues of staffing, sequencing, data collection and analysis. As in many research projects, we have found that having researchers with the right skill set is paramount. In terms of how many members of staff you need, there is no magic answer; the decision needs to be driven by weighing up the pros and cons we have highlighted in this chapter. Regardless of the number of staff there are, we have found that time and effort spent in developing a well-functioning team is invaluable. The researchers can then get on with the tasks of conducting the review and data collection and analysis in a thoughtful, supported and nimble way. Finally on the issue of sequencing, again there is no single best answer. Ideally, a realist review should precede the realist evaluation, but to minimise costs and ensure that findings are developed sooner, some overlap may be needed. Advanced planning of when this overlap should occur and attention to staffing levels can make the overlap less problematic – especially if there is only one researcher tasked with conducting either the review or the evaluation component of the research.

5 Managing abundance rigorously

Quality in realist evaluation with extensive qualitative data

Charles Michaelis

Introduction

Qualitative research comprises many different qualitative traditions based on different paradigms, with diverse philosophical assumptions. The area of 'qualitative data quality criteria' is controversial, with various positions and many classificatory suggestions available, which range from a total rejection of the notion of criteria, to those who propose similar criterion for quantitative and qualitative research. Consequently, although there are abundant quality criteria on when to use qualitative data and how to design, recruit, conduct and analyse interviews, there are no agreed standards for judging quality in qualitative research evaluations (Manzano, 2024). Rigour in a realist evaluation has been described as consisting of achieving immersion (i.e., spending enough time in the study to really understand what is going on), collecting data meticulously and analysing them systematically, thinking reflexively about findings, developing theory iteratively as emerging data are analysed, seeking disconfirming cases and alternative explanations and defending one's interpretations to researchers within and outside one's own team (Wong et al., 2012, p. 94). This chapter uses as a case study three large realist portfolio evaluations of the UK's international climate finance evaluation, which conceptualised quality in terms of obtaining relevant and rigorous evidence from each participant and using it to support the process of refining a theory of change. This required the process to be flexible and adaptive rather than consistent.

Background

The UK International Climate Finance and the Climate Change Compass evaluation consortium

International Climate Finance (ICF) is a United Kingdom (UK) government (HMG) commitment to support low - and middle- income countries to respond to the challenges and opportunities of climate change (HMG, 2018). It is part of the concerted global action to limit and manage the impact of climate change and, in particular, ensure that the global temperature rise will

DOI: 10.4324/9781003457077-6

stay well below 2C. It contributes to progress on the Sustainable Development Goals (SDGs) and delivers against the UK aid strategy.

The United Kingdom is firmly committed, alongside other high-income countries, to contribute to the mobilisation of US$100 billion of public and private climate finance a year, and ICF is a core component of the UK's contribution to this shared goal. ICF invested at least £5.8 billion between 2016 and 2021 in over 50 low- and middle- income countries and committed to doubling this investment for the 2021–2026 period (HMG, August 2023). ICF is managed jointly by the Foreign, Commonwealth and Development Office (FCDO), the Department for Energy Security and Net Zero (DESNZ), and the Department for Environment, Food and Rural Affairs (Defra). It works through diverse channels from private equity funds to small non-governmental organisation (NGO) grants to:

- change facts on the ground, delivering results that demonstrate that low-carbon, climate-resilient development is feasible and desirable.
- improve the international climate architecture and finance system to increase the scale, efficiency and value for money of climate spending.
- test out new approaches to delivering climate finance that have the potential to achieve bigger and better results in the future.

Since 2011, the UK ICF has had a global impact. Its programmes have:

- helped over 100 million people cope with the effects of climate change;
- provided nearly 70 million people with improved access to clean energy;
- reduced or avoided 86m tonnes of greenhouse gas emissions;
- avoided 413,000 hectares of deforestation; and
- leveraged nearly £7 billion of public and £6.9 billion of private finance for climate change (HMG, 2023).

HMG established the Climate Change Compass (Compass) consortium led by IMC Worldwide which supported the UK government departments responsible for ICF to improve generation, dissemination and uptake of results data, evidence and knowledge from across the ICF portfolio. The aims were to:

- help address a critical evidence gap on effective approaches to promote and support low carbon, climate resilient growth and development.
- support transparency, accountability and strengthened capacity for measurement-based performance management of international climate finance and results.
- encourage harmonisation and alignment of climate finance monitoring and evaluation activities, systems and agendas.
- facilitate, capture and synthesise lessons learned to inform future investments.

HMG decided to undertake three separate evaluations as opposed to one overarching evaluation to enable different programme strategies and approaches to be investigated. For each, evaluation programmes were grouped by similar intended outcomes. HMG chose to specify a realist approach to understand how and why different investments lead to different outcomes in different contexts and to provide insights to inform programme improvement and future policy decisions.

The strengths of the realist approach were seen to be:

- the approach delivers a deep and rich understanding of how contexts and mechanisms combine to cause different outcomes in different circumstances.
- realist theories of change are developed and tested at a middle level of abstraction and can then be applied across different programmes, in different locations and circumstances. This strong external validity was expected to enable lessons from the evaluation to be applied across the ICF and more widely.

Considering the intricacy of the large evaluation and the complexity of the subject matter, a mixed-methodological evaluation approach was adopted. This approach incorporated the use of both realist evaluation and process tracing (Beach, 2017, p. 17) in combination, enhancing the substantiation of our claims regarding causality and their correlation with outcomes. Process tracing has been used in other realist evaluations to guide the collection and assessment of data to test the contribution made by an intervention to outcomes (Bouyousfi & Sabar, 2022).

The case study: Three evaluation studies to assess International Climate Finance's integration, mobilisation of private finance and policy changes

Three evaluations were undertaken between 2017 and 2020; each evaluation addressed a key strategic issue for ICF (Table 5.1). The evaluations were all published in the form of a non-technical main report and a technical report (Foreign, Commonwealth & Development Office, 2023b).

Table 5.1 Total number of qualitative interviews across the three evaluation projects

	HMG	*Delivery partners*	*Beneficiaries and other stakeholders*	**Total**
Portfolio evaluation 1	24	-	-	**24**
Portfolio evaluation 2	11	67	65	**143**
Portfolio evaluation 3	15	33	63	**111**
Total	**50**	**100**	**128**	**278**

Portfolio evaluation 1 – Integration of ICF

The first evaluation, conducted between late 2017 and October 2018, addressed the question:

> In what circumstances and how has climate finance integration supported progress towards transformational change within the wider DFID[1] portfolio, and towards more effective delivery of climate change outcomes than would have been achieved without integration?

The evaluation drew on evidence from three sources:

- Analysis of data relating to DFID's 86 integrated ICF programmes since 2011.
- In-depth review of documents relating to 25 of the 86 programmes that had integrated ICF and nine programmes that did not, which enabled us to focus the primary research on the programmes most likely to be relevant for the evaluation.
- Interviews with 14 Senior Responsible Owners[2] and eight advisors.

Portfolio evaluation 2 – Mobilising private finance through demonstration effects

The second evaluation, conducted between late 2018 and December 2019 addressed the question:

> How and in what circumstances is ICF mobilising private finance into low carbon climate resilient markets through demonstration effects?

The evaluation identified 46 ICF-funded programmes that aimed to mobilise private finance through demonstration effects. 20 of these were selected for further investigation based on the availability of evidence, a balance between sectors, and geographical spread. This involved a more detailed document review along with interviews with 11 Senior Responsible Owners and 15 implementing partners. We also interviewed 14 members of the evaluation and/or syndication teams at eight Development Finance Institutions to explore their experience of demonstration effects and to understand whether they consider that their investments had a demonstration effect, and if so, for whom and how. We then revised the question theory based on these initial interviews and selected 10 of the 20 programmes to identify and explore wider demonstration effects through 103 interviews with programme partners, potential replicators and other investors.

Portfolio evaluation 3 – Support for policy change

The third evaluation, conducted between mid-2019 and June 2020 addressed the question:

> How, in what respects, and in what circumstances has the ICF supported change in global, national and sub-national policies relating to climate change?

We identified 27 programmes that a) had objectives to support policy change and b) were focussing on either forestry and land-use policy, or low-carbon development policy (including renewable energy policy). The first phase of the evaluation involved 27 interviews with HMG officials and other donors to identify the type of support for policy change that occurred, the claimed outcomes, and to start to test and refine our initial theories of how support works. At the end of this phase, the theories were revised, and five case studies were designed to test the revised theories. These case studies investigated three countries (Colombia, Indonesia and Uganda) and two international organisations (the Climate Investment Funds and the World Bank). 111 interviews were conducted with implementing partners, government officials and sector experts.

A strategy for delivering the portfolio of evaluations

The evaluations were conducted by Itad (2024), a specialist evaluation consultancy. The team for each evaluation included:

- A project director who was responsible for the overall quality of the work. Each evaluation had a different director.
- The team leader who was responsible for the management of the project and ensuring that the realist approach was implemented faithfully. The team leader role was performed by the same person for all three evaluations.
- An evaluation question lead who was responsible for day-to-day client relationships, data collection, analysis and who led the report writing.
- Up to six research analysts who were responsible for interviewing and analysis of their interviews.
- Subject matter specialists as required. For example, finance specialists were recruited for the second evaluation and a gender and inclusion specialist was recruited for the third.
- A realist methodologist was retained throughout the project. This person provided training to the team, assisted in the drafting of the Quality Assurance Framework (see below) and reviewed reports.

The team was mainly based in the United Kingdom with members in France, Australia and the United States. There were weekly team meetings online and monthly meetings in person attended by the UK-based staff.

HMG appointed a steering group as the key decision-making body for each evaluation, which included officials involved in the delivery of relevant ICF programmes and evaluation specialists from all three departments. Each evaluation had an HMG official who acted as project manager and who was the key point of contact between the steering group and the evaluation team. HMG retained two evaluators from their EQUALS (Foreign, Commonwealth & Development Office, 2023a) peer review panel to provide independent QA. They reviewed the overall QA Framework and the inception and final reports for each evaluation.

HMG requires evaluation providers to comply with their ethical guidance for research, evaluation and monitoring activities (Department for International Development, 2020). However, specific ethics approval was not required for the evaluation.

Evaluation quality framework and standards

A Quality Assurance (QA) Framework was developed to guide the three evaluations. This drew on and supplemented the RAMESES international realist standards (Wong et al., 2016) by explaining in detail how primary and secondary research would be undertaken and how data would be analysed. The Framework also set out how process tracing would be used and integrated with the realist approach.

The QA Framework was agreed with HMG and reviewed by their independent QA advisors. The Framework guided the development of the approach for each of the evaluations and helped to give wider stakeholders in HMG confidence in the robustness of the methods to be used.

Capacity building in the realist evaluation approach

The team leader, the question lead for the first evaluation, and the realist methodologist were the only members of the team with experience in realist evaluation prior to working on Compass. The rest of the team were introduced to realist methods in three ways:

- Everyone in the team was provided with a copy of Pawson and Tilley (1997) and they were paid for a day to read it.
- The realist methodologist conducted two training sessions lasting two days each prior to the first and second evaluations. The session for the second evaluation was attended by the client team.
- The evaluation teams discussed realist theory and how to put it into practice during the monthly meetings. This acted as a refresher and an opportunity to address issues that came up in the regular QA process.

The overall training approach involved in-depth sessions to provide an introduction to a subject followed by discussion during the regular team meetings to clarify issues and address any problems that arose. This worked well and helped to ensure that everyone in the team had the same understanding of what was needed from the project and how we were going to deliver it. The regular team meetings provided an opportunity for short training updates at relevant stages of the work. For example, we provided a reminder of realist interviewing principles when we were restarting data collection after a break.

We also had a training day with an expert in realist interviewing prior to starting data collection on the second evaluation. The learning and materials from this training were used to induct researchers who subsequently joined the team. The HMG staff who attended the training with the realist methodologist found it useful both in developing their knowledge of realist methods and in understanding how the project team were approaching the work. In addition, the team leader, question leads and research analysts were trained in technical aspects of the evaluations (such as finance) by the specialist members of the team. In general, training worked better in person than remotely, and it was harder to provide training to remote staff and to non-English speakers.

Developing theories of change for each evaluation project

Each evaluation project examined a portfolio of programmes each of which had their own theory of change. For example, for the first evaluation, the question explored 'how and in what circumstances climate finance had been integrated into development programmes and to what extent and why this had resulted in transformation within DFID'. Each of the programmes that we used for evidence had development objectives, for example, to assist with reconstruction from a natural disaster. The programmes had theories of change for how their objectives would be achieved.

In this example, we were interested in the integration of climate finance rather than whether the programme theory was correct. Therefore, during the inception stage, we developed what we called 'question theory' to distinguish it from the theory of change for individual programmes. In this example, this was a theory about how climate finance was integrated into development programmes and how that would result in transformation within DFID. This 'question theory' was then tested and refined through each evaluation.

The development of initial question theory involved:

1 Discussions with the steering group to elicit a rough initial theory and to identify which or which types of programmes were likely to provide us with relevant evidence.
2 A review of the literature relating to relevant programmes to extract their theories of change (all ICF programmes were required to have a theory of change, but these were not in realist form) and evidence relevant to those theories.

3 Identifying formal theory that was relevant to the question. For example, there is a significant body of work about policy change which was relevant to the third evaluation.
4 Drafting initial question theory in realist form, drawing on relevant programme and formal theory. This was then presented to the steering group for discussion.
5 The refined initial question theory formed the basis of the evaluation design.

ICF programmes report annually on progress and their results against a menu of 15 KPIs. These reports were used to select a sample of ICF programmes that were relevant to the question theory, and which had progressed to a stage where there was likely to be evidence to test the theory. Between 20 and 30 programmes were selected for each evaluation. For all three evaluations, we conducted interviews with programme managers and other key stakeholders to test the initial theory and to identify further documentary evidence. For the second and third evaluations, we refined the initial question theory at the end of the first phase and conducted a second phase of interviews with programme beneficiaries, partners and wider stakeholders.

The question theory was discussed at monthly team meetings. At those meetings, the team often identified emerging insights (such as the details of how specific mechanisms operated) or potential revisions (such as refinements to the contexts in which specific mechanisms operated) which were then tested in subsequent interviews. Additionally, we planned to use Slack, a messaging application for businesses, for internal team communications with a channel for each Context-Mechanism-Outcome configuration (CMOC) where team members could capture relevant thoughts and ideas. In practice, this was not used as members found team meetings a more accessible process for sharing their thinking.

Managing a large number of qualitative interviews

All the interviews for the first and second evaluations were conducted online and in English. The third evaluation included face-to-face interviews in Colombia, Indonesia and Uganda. The Colombian interviews we conducted in Spanish and the Indonesian interviews were conducted in Bahasa Indonesian. In recruiting research analysts, we relied on Itad's network and were looking for candidates with qualitative interviewing experience, skills at building rapport, interest in the subject of the evaluations and curiosity.

For the first evaluation, the interviews were conducted by the team leader and the question lead. Both were experienced realist interviewers and were deeply familiar with the project so there was no need for training. For the second evaluation, the interviews were conducted by the question lead (who had performed the same role on the first evaluation) and three research analysts. The research analysts were two freelance interviewers and one Itad staff member. All three had experience of qualitative interviewing but did not have experience of realist interviewing, so realist interview training was provided. For the third evaluation, we were able to retain the three research analysts from the second evaluation and recruited three more; a Spanish speaker to assist with the interviews in Colombia, a researcher based in Uganda to support the interviews there and a researcher based in the USA to conduct interviews in that time zone, who all received some training in realist interviewing.

A flexible approach to developing and using interview guides

The interview guides were initially developed by the question lead and refined by the team. For each evaluation:

1 We held a meeting of the project team to talk through the interview guide and ensure it addressed all aspects of the question theory that we wanted to cover.
2 Team members roleplayed the guides for each evaluation, taking it in turns to be interviewer and interviewee. This ensured that they were comfortable with the language in the guides and that the questions were clear and understandable.
3 When all the interviewers had conducted at least one interview and the team leader and question lead had listened to the recordings the team met to consider and agree improvements to the guides. This meeting also served to build consistency of approach across interviewers.

The interview guides were revised to reflect the revised question theory in phase 2 of the second and third evaluations. These included exploring outcome patterns in more detail and testing new hypotheses about mechanisms and the contexts in which they fired. Minor amendments were also made during data collection to explore insights that were identified by the team at monthly team meetings. These could include probing aspects of mechanisms or contexts to explore whether potential refinements to theory that had been mentioned by interviewees in the early stages of that phase of data collection were supported by others.

The teacher-learner approach used in realist interviews involves the interviewer sharing theory with the respondent and the two working together to refine it (Pawson, 1996). Before conducting the interviews, we had some concerns that interviewees from different cultural backgrounds may be unwilling to disagree with the theory described by the interviewer as it would be considered impolite or disrespectful to do so. However, in practice, we did not identify any reluctance on the part of interviewees to challenge or disagree with theory. Some members of the steering group were also concerned that the realist interviewing approach would 'lead' interviewees answers. (See Manzano's chapter in this book about researchers' preoccupations with confirmation bias in realist interviewing.) To address their concerns, we structured the questioning starting with an open question before sharing the question theory with the interviewee.

The questioning went along the following lines:

- Starting with an open question, for example, *'Please tell me how you made the decision to...'* and then probing around context.
- Confirming the theory articulated by the interviewee, for example, *'So you made the decision to ... in these circumstances...because...'*
- If participants had not provided their own theory, the interviewer asked for their response to the question theory being tested, for example, *'Based on what we have read/heard from other people it seems that people in these circumstances often made the decision like this...was it like that for you?'*

We experimented with different approaches for interview guides and found that the guides did not need to be highly scripted. For example:

- We found that interviewers were much more comfortable explaining theory using the phrases and specific examples used by interviewees rather than using the wording in the question theory. For example, in the second evaluation the question theory referred to private finance being mobilised. Some interviewees used the language of mobilisation, others talked about investment from the private sector and a third group talked about private finance being crowded in. Interviewers felt that using the same language helped to build rapport and avoided any risk that the interviewee would feel they were being corrected if the interviewer used different terms.
- Responses often did not follow the envisaged question order and it was better to allow the conversation to develop organically than to have a tightly structured order of questions.

This approach to questioning meant that the interviewers needed to be deeply familiar with the question theory and the interview guide as well as to have a capacity to think on their feet.

Participant recruitment and organising the interviews

For the first evaluation, respondents were introduced to the project team by members of the steering group. For the second and third evaluations, we were initially introduced to managers of the relevant ICF programmes. The programme managers introduced us to implementing partners.

There were three ways we identified respondents in the second wave of the second and third evaluations:

- Some respondents were introduced to us by programme partners.
- Where we could not obtain an introduction, we approached potential respondents directly. We found LinkedIn particularly effective as a route for connecting with potential respondents.

- On the second evaluation, some respondents who had invested in projects were able to introduce us to co-investors.

All the recruitment for the second and third evaluations was conducted by one member of the team. Her thorough understanding of the theories of change that we were investigating, and the methods being used enabled her to identify the right respondents. Her knowledge of the project helped her explain the project to potential respondents, effectively securing their participation.

The interviews in Colombia, Indonesia and Uganda were all conducted during a two-week mission to each country. This limited amount of time made it hard to travel to remote locations or to provide many options for timing to respondents. Some parts of Colombia could not be visited due to safety concerns. The research was conducted before the use of Zoom and Teams became widespread and some respondents did not have access to the technologies or were not permitted to use them by corporate IT policies. Where respondents could not use online technologies, interviews were conducted by telephone. A small number of UK interviews and all the case study interviews in Colombia, Indonesia and Uganda were conducted face-to-face. We found that it was easier to create rapport face-to-face and the interviews created richer data. Face-to-face interviews were seen as more burdensome than online/telephone by some respondents; even though they took the same amount of time, it was necessary to book a room and organise visitor passes.

Interview quality assurance framework: enhancing evidence through rigour

At the start of fieldwork each interviewer observed an interview conducted by the team leader or the question lead. After the interview the observer and the person who had conducted the interview discussed the interview, the reasons for particular areas of questioning and the key areas of learning from the interview.

Each interviewer then conducted an interview observed by the team leader or question lead. Following the interview, the team leader/question lead and interviewer discussed the interview and where the team leader/question lead was confident that the interviewer would conduct good quality interviews, they conducted further interviews unaccompanied.

At the start of each evaluation, the team leader listened to a sample of interviews and provided feedback drawn from those interviews to all interviewers. It was initially intended that the team leader would listen to all interviews. However, this proved to be too time-consuming and so instead we set up a process of peer review where each interviewer listened to a sample of other interviewers' work and provided feedback to them. Common areas of feedback were identifying opportunities where the interviewer could have probed further, spotting linkages to other interviews that the reviewer had conducted and sharing tips about good ways to introduce a topic or explain a concept.

This helped to ensure consistency and had the unanticipated benefit of sharing good practice and increasing knowledge across the interviewing team. The team leader and question lead continued to listen to a random sample of around 10% of interviews but did not provide feedback unless they identified serious issues. We had intended that interviewers would record their reflections after each interview with the intention that this would support the analysis process by ensuring that more recent interviews did not carry greater weight as they were fresher in the research team's minds. However, in practice, this did not occur due to work-related pressures.

All interviews were recorded with the permission of the respondent. They were then transcribed using automatic transcription software. The transcripts were of variable quality, and all required some work to ensure they were faithful to the interview itself.

Interviews with non-English-speaking respondents

Many of the people we identified for interviews in Colombia and Indonesia did not speak English. Others spoke enough English to conduct an interview, but we were not convinced that they understood the nuance in questions or were able to describe their actions and motivations in English as they would have been able to do in their native language.

That resulted in three choices:

1 Restrict the interviews to fluent English speakers.
2 Use interpreters for English-speaking interviewers.
3 Use bilingual interviewers.

We dismissed the first option as we would have been unable to interview some key respondents if we had limited ourselves to fluent English speakers. We worked with interpreters for interviews in Indonesia. We chose two individuals with a working knowledge of climate change issues who had a technical background. The interviewer trained them in realist methods and provided them with background to the subject of the interview and the reason the interviewee had been selected.

This approach worked to some extent; it helped to set the interviewee at ease and was effective in obtaining information about facts (what did you do, who was involved, what was the result, etc.?) but it was less good at exploring reasoning (why did you do it?) and context (why did you do it like this in these circumstances and like that in other circumstances?). This was because the interpreter was uncomfortable with asking what they saw as stupid questions or ones which the respondent would not be able to answer. The interpreters also tended to precis their translations so they often did not communicate the full richness of respondents' answers and there were often circumstances where an interviewee would speak for a minute or two and the translation was just one line. We had no evidence that the interpreters were being deliberately obstructive and believed that the problem was that we had taken them too far out of their comfort zones as technical interpreters. It is possible that this approach would have been more successful if the training had been conducted by someone more experienced in cross-cultural interviewing. Although the challenges with interpreters could have been addressed with more time, it was not feasible within the two weeks available for fieldwork.

Drawing on the experience in Indonesia, we tried a different approach for the interviews in Colombia. We were able to recruit a Spanish-speaking qualitative interviewer who was already known to the team leader and question lead. This individual already had some awareness of realist methods and we provided her with additional realist training and training in the subject of the interviews. The Spanish-speaking interviewer and the member of the team responsible for the Colombia case study conducted the interviews together. The case study author and the interviewer discussed the aims of the interview in advance and conducted a debrief afterwards. However, the interview was conducted completely in Spanish with no interpretation. The Spanish-speaking interviewer did the coding (see analysis section below) and translated coded nuggets into English. This approach seemed to provide a better interview experience for the respondent and much richer information was obtained. There were disadvantages in that it was more expensive to send two researchers from the United Kingdom to Colombia and it was impossible for others to review the interviews or the coding, limiting the effectiveness of QA.

Strategy for analysing large sets of realist qualitative data

Analysis for the first evaluation was conducted using MS Excel. Each CMO had a sheet in an Excel workbook and coded segments were collected there. With a sample of only 24 interviews, this was completely adequate. The second and third evaluations had much more data with well over 100 interviews each and we felt that Excel would not be sufficient for our needs. Following a review of analysis software for qualitative interviews we decided to use MaxQDA (2024). The coding framework was developed collaboratively by the whole research team. Initially, we coded segments by CMO and according to whether they were relevant to a context, mechanism or outcome. However, this proved challenging as segments often related to why a mechanism fired in a particular context (i.e., both C and M) or how a mechanism generated an outcome (i.e., both M and O). After much discussion and experimentation, we changed our approach to simply code segments as relevant to a particular CMO and left it to the synthesis stage to bring all the segments together and to revise the theory.

The research team did the analysis with each interviewer coding their own interviews. Concurrently with coding the interviewer corrected the transcript for the coded sections by listening to the recording, and, in the case of interviews in Spanish, translated the coded sections into English. In most cases, the interview was coded within a day or two of being completed, which ensured that the conversation was fresh in the interviewer's mind. The use of process tracing inculcated the good habit of asking whether we would be likely to see the same evidence if the theory was not true (referred to as 'uniqueness of evidence' in Beach, 2017, p. 10). We found this very useful in helping us to decide whether evidence really did support the theory of change or not.

The coding of a sample of interviews was reviewed by the team leader and the question lead at the same time as they listened to the interviews to assess their quality. Common issues that arose with coding included content that was relevant to the theory but which had not been coded, normally because the interviewer had missed it and, less often, speculation by the interviewee being coded as evidence. The emerging theory was discussed at the team's monthly meetings and for the second and third evaluations the coding framework was revised to reflect the emerging theory of change. This required segments that had already been coded to be re-coded to the new coding framework. Although this was time-consuming it enabled the team to keep track of how the theory was evolving. The research team worked together during day-long, in-person sessions to refine the theory of change, building on the discussions at team meetings. The refined theory along with the supporting evidence was reviewed by the question lead for quality and relevance.

What did we learn?

Flexibility and the value of an engaged client well-versed in the realist approach

It was important to have an engaged client who understood the realist approach and who was willing to get involved in the detail of data collection. There was no requirement for ethics approval which allowed us more flexibility than would otherwise have been the case. However, the client had to approve changes to the method in order to test emerging revisions to the theories of change – for example, by including a new group of interviewees or by adding questions to the interview guides.

The HMG project manager was closely involved in the evaluation and had a good understanding of realist methods. We were able to present ideas for changes to them and they were able to provide constructive suggestions and to secure approvals for changes.

The challenge of keeping the evaluation 'realist'

We all needed to work hard to keep the approach 'realist'. We found that it was easy to slip back into traditional approaches and thinking. We were able to keep the focus on the realist approach in a light-touch way by introducing reminders of the theory and practice during team meetings. We also had training sessions on specific subjects such as interviewing and analysis. Some of the training was provided by external trainers which helped to bring new ideas for how to implement a realist approach.

Everyone needs to know and own the theories of change

It was essential that every member of the team had a deep and thorough knowledge and understanding of all aspects of the theories of change. This influenced the quality of the work and the efficiency with which the Compass evaluations were delivered. For example:

- The person responsible for recruiting interviewees understood the aspects of the theory that their interviews would test and so she was well placed to check whether they were suitable respondents.
- Interviewers' deep knowledge of the theory enabled them to follow the respondents' thought processes and explore relevant aspects of theory as they arose in the interview. That helped the conversation to flow, put the respondent at ease and consequently secured richer, more relevant data.

It was most effective to involve the whole team at every stage of the work. Even if it was not an individual's particular responsibility it helped them to understand what was being done, for what purpose and how it impacted their work. Therefore, the whole team was involved in all the activities including theory development data collection design, interviewing and analysis. Because team members had an excellent understanding of the theories of change, they were able to contribute fully to discussions about potential revisions to the theories which enhanced the process of revising them and the quality of those revisions. Since the completion of the project, team members have said that this was valuable in supporting their personal development as evaluators, as it built an understanding of all aspects of a project and how each complemented others.

Delivering realist quality in interviews

The key aspects of delivering quality interviews were that the team had a shared understanding of quality in realist work and were motivated and empowered to deliver high-quality work. The investment in resources for quality such as the QA framework and the training helped to deliver the shared understanding that we needed. The regular feedback and meetings helped to ensure everyone on the team felt responsible for and committed to delivering quality as a team. This involved getting the right team with a shared understanding of realist quality and where everyone had responsibility for delivering quality, getting the interview guides and coding structures right and interviewing the right people in the right language.

Getting the right team with a shared understanding of quality

Working within the realist approach did not suit everyone. Some interviewers like more structure, others prefer traditional qualitative interviewing approaches. We had one or two interviewers on each evaluation who did not stay on the team for long. We tried to manage this in a sensitive and constructive way to avoid disrupting the team or damaging the confidence of the interviewers who were not suited to the work.

We found it was essential early in the evaluation to have a shared understanding of what good quality in realist evaluation looked like. For example, to ensure rigour, we only used evidence of interviewees' personal experience rather than where they speculated about the experience of others. We embedded this in the team through:

- The training where we reviewed documents together to agree on what would be acceptable as rigorous evidence and what would not.
- Designing and planning the interviews to ensure that we focused questioning on respondents' own experience.
- In reviewing interviews and coding we reminded interviewers of the importance of rigorous evidence.

The practice of asking whether we would be likely to see the same evidence if the theory was not true was valuable and could be adopted on realist projects more widely. We also worked to develop a shared understanding of the depth of insight that we were looking for. We took the advice of the realist methodology advisor to 'unleash our inner two-year-old' and keep asking 'why?' until we were satisfied that we had got to a full understanding of what lay behind particular decisions.

Because interviewers were reviewing each other's interviews there was constant sharing of approaches and ideas. That allowed us to quickly share and replicate good ideas and to address problems and challenges as soon as they arose. Frequent in-person meetings also helped to build that shared understanding of quality as we were able to spend time getting into the details together with the clarity of communication that is enhanced by being in the same room.

The team was small and focused and, as the evaluations progressed, everyone developed significant expertise and understanding of the subjects of the evaluations.

Each member of the team knew that the quality of the evidence and the way it was analysed was essential to the success of the project. Because we worked together in a collaborative spirit everyone felt able to suggest improvements to the methods, approaches and analysis. Competing theories, discussion and debate are at the heart of realist evaluation. We emphasised that no one person had a monopoly of knowledge and everyone had the right to question and challenge anyone else.

Getting the interview guides and coding framework right

The time put into developing the interview guides was essential to conducting a good interview. The role playing gave us confidence that the interview would flow as a conversation and that the interviewer was comfortable with the questions. The early quality assessment and review of the interview guides enabled us to fix any problems early on. We found that it was better to have a guide that provided a simple, flexible interview structure that the interviewer could keep in their mind rather than trying to anticipate every possible probe or line of questioning that could arise.

The coding framework was revised multiple times for each evaluation to ensure it reflected our thinking about the theories of change. This ensured that the theory was at the forefront of our minds throughout the work and simplified the synthesis as we had already given a good deal of thought to the revised theories of change before starting on the formal synthesis process. However, revising the coding framework was a resource intensive task requiring re-reading and re-coding evidence to which we had not initially anticipated allocating resources.

On the first evaluation we had not anticipated that it would be necessary to revise the coding framework and so approached the task with some reluctance. However, as the project progressed, we realised that revising the framework was an integral part of the work and planned for it as part of the analysis process. This meant that we did not invest too heavily in getting coding 'right' but instead made sure it was adequate and that we could remain as flexible as possible.

Conclusions

Delivering quality in this large realist evaluation is a complex process involving four key elements:

1 Everyone involved in the project, including the client, had a good understanding of realist methods and was committed to delivering the approach.
2 We recruited a team with the right skills and provided them with training in realist methods and the specific theories of change and technical aspects of each evaluation. The Quality Assurance Framework set out a structure to guide their work.
3 The interview guides and coding frameworks provided enough structure but were also flexible to allow changes to be accommodated as the theory evolved.
4 Frequent interaction within the team enabled refinement of the theory and the approach to be integrated into the work and ensured everyone on the team had a shared understanding of the theory and what realist quality looked like.

Notes

1 The UK's Department for International Development, now part of the Foreign, Commonwealth and Development Office (FCDO)
2 The government official responsible for the programme

6 Realist interviewing for novice realist evaluators

Jo Howe

Introduction

This chapter aims to provide guidance, reassurance and confidence for novice realist researchers. Drawing heavily on my own PhD journey, I have shared many challenges using examples from my thesis. Undertaking a realist evaluation can feel overwhelming, and methodological guidance for realist evaluations was limited when I started my PhD. Thankfully, more methodologically focussed academic papers, books, blogs and support networks exist now – including this book. I urge novice realist evaluators to seek out resources and also talk with peers to understand the decisions they are making.

The importance of study design should not be underestimated. I hope novice realist evaluators will appreciate that time designing the research, articulating realist research questions and deriving candidate programme theories will ensure appropriate data is collected during the evaluation. Ethical approval processes pose challenges to novice realist evaluators; therefore, I have outlined some necessary considerations during this stage to help retain flexibility during data collection and stay true to the iterative and evolving nature of realist research.

Data collection methods and tools are an important component of realist evaluations and also need careful consideration during the design stage. I have explained the reasoning behind the sources I included within my PhD and provided some advice to consider before embarking upon your first realist interview. Drawing upon methodological guidance from Manzano (2016), I have provided sample questions and guidance to elicit the theoretical stages of theory gleaning, refinement and consolidation.

Finally, data analysis can be daunting for novice evaluators. I offer some tips based on my own experiences which you can adapt and expand within your own research. I hope this chapter proves useful to those new to realist evaluations and realist interviewing.

Keep calm and carry on

Embarking upon a realist evaluation can be daunting, especially for novices. My research training and experience prior to my PhD was overwhelmingly positivist. I had completed a master's degree in brain imaging whilst

DOI: 10.4324/9781003457077-7

managing the delivery of a randomised controlled trial (RCT). However, these experiences drew me to implementation science, and during those first few months of the PhD, I stumbled across realism. Consequently, as a doctoral student, not only was I a nervous first-time realist interviewer undertaking my first qualitative project since my undergraduate days in the 1990s, but I was a first-time evaluator as well. I had a whole new language to learn; much of the terminology and philosophy I struggled with was not unique to realist research, but it is a huge undertaking for doctoral students to amass this amount of seemingly new and confusing material. I was worried I was 'getting it all wrong' and spent lots of time micro-analysing my interview technique. I wish I had known in those early interviews, that everything would be okay, I would settle into a groove, develop my own interview style and there would be far too much data to include within my PhD!

Getting comfortable with being uncomfortable

On reflection, I now appreciate that my psychological training had influenced many of my fears; something I also notice with others who have studied or trained in psychology. I was worried about asking leading questions, a notion contrary to psychology where we are taught not to do this. My fellow PhD colleagues from allied healthcare backgrounds did not have the same concerns as I did with asking realist questions. They told me that realist interviewing was not that different to taking a clinical history from patients. This was a lightbulb moment for me; the way I was approaching interviews was engrained in my psyche. The only way to move forward was to 'get comfortable with being uncomfortable', ask more direct questions and embrace the realist process. After all, the reason behind realist interviewing is to test, refine or refute programme theories (Pawson, 2006b; Wong et al., 2016); to do this effectively questions need to be more direct and targeted than those typically used in psychology.

Finding your support network

The best piece of advice I can offer novice realist evaluators is to prepare for the journey ahead. At the risk of sounding clichéd – if I can do this, so can you. Realist academics are often eager to engage in discussions about methods and share learning with newer researchers. Immerse yourself in the realist community; engage in realist conversations to cement knowledge and understanding of key concepts. At the time of writing this chapter, the realist community is active online on Twitter/X and via the RAMESES jiscmail; online methods focussed seminars are often advertised via these channels. When I first embarked upon scientific realism, I was so confused, the terminology had me tied up in knots. There are things people could have told me in 20 seconds that would have saved me months of confusion. For example, it took me about a year before I realised programme theories are akin to hypotheses in scientific research. When I learned that context, mechanism and outcome could change depending upon their analytical focus (such as when considering an implementation chain, the outcome of one Context-Mechanism-Outcome configuration can be the context for the next and so on), I slammed down my hands on a desk and rather dramatically declared 'I'm done, I can't wrap my head round this approach, so I'm out!'. However, I am glad I stayed, I find this a really rewarding and enlightening way to conduct research.

Study design

Steps taken at the beginning of your project will influence the data you collect, and the subsequent coding and analysis. When I started my PhD, I wanted to know ***how*** to deliver an evidence-based community stroke service within rural areas of England (Howe, 2022). Some services in rural areas were apparently doing well, delivering services in line with clinical guidelines and others were struggling. I wanted to know how these well-performing services did it. What made them so special when others were struggling?

The importance of the realist research question

How research questions are phrased is important; they shape your study design and influence your data collection. Realist evaluation offers evaluators the ability to understand ***how*** interventions work when they are implemented into organisations and not to simply determine efficacy; it is this principle which attracted me to realist evaluation. Often realist research questions are phrased as how or why statements.

My research question was:

> How can community stroke services in rural areas deliver evidence-based services in line with national clinical guidelines? What works, for whom and under what circumstances and to what extent?

A national stroke audit (Royal College of Physicians, 2015), national clinical guidelines for stroke (Intercollegiate Stroke Working Party, 2016), and a Cochrane systematic review (Langhorne & Baylan, 2017), helped shape my research question, objectives and study design. My primary supervisor and I discussed how to design the evaluation to ensure I could answer my research question. I knew we were not creating a list of barriers and facilitators; this approach jars somewhat with realist research as a barrier in one service could be a facilitator in another. My research would be of much greater benefit to the stroke community if I researched well-performing services, as they would have likely faced and overcome challenges. I quickly realised however, that community stroke services were complex multifaceted interventions, nested within complex multifaceted organisations, which is perfect for realist evaluation, as it allows you to get underneath the layers of complexity and unravel the elements of context which then trigger mechanisms to produce outcomes.

Candidate programme theories

The development of candidate programme theories is an important step in realist projects. They are used to guide programme theory refinement and inform data collection methods and tools such as interview and topic guides. An important thing to note is that no programme theory can ever explain or predict every possible outcome in every possible context (Pawson, 2013). Rival programme theories (see theory refinement below) may emerge during data collection and evaluators need to find outcome patterns, which are often referred to as demi-regularities. We acquire partial knowledge about the phenomena under evaluation which leads to a deeper appreciation and understanding. Think of programme theories as a starting point; they are meant to be tested, refined and refuted. I fell into the trap of trying to create 'perfect' candidate programme theories and spent too long on this task. They do not need to be perfect; if they were, there would be no need for you to conduct the research! I often advise novice evaluators of this common pitfall, especially when realist expertise is not present within the supervisory team. If this sounds familiar, reach out within the realist community for some advice, to help you work your way out of the programme theory maze!

Determining the 'programme' to be evaluated when there is no pre-post intervention

At one point in my PhD, my confidence hit an all-time low. I could not discern the focus of the programme I was evaluating; it felt as if everyone else had nailed this part and I was floundering. Although not all interventions need to have a pre-post scenario to be evaluated (Manzano & Pawson, 2014), a lot of published literature at the time focussed on these 'pre-post' interventions, making it really difficult to work out how my PhD fitted into the realist paradigm. I did not have a pre-post intervention; I wasn't sure that I had a 'programme' at all. I knew I needed to define an 'intervention/programme' but if you are not evaluating a newly implemented programme how do you define what your programme is? The short answer to this question, is you need to work it out!

I spent considerable time trying to determine whether the national audit of stroke services, the clinical guidelines or the components of early supported discharge (the intervention being delivered) should be the focus of my research. I spoke to anyone who would give me time and brought it up at every realist training event and seminar I attended without moving forward. I was informed many times that my research was well suited to realist evaluation, but I really struggled to articulate programme theories. I would love to tell you that I very cleverly worked it out. However, one day whilst contemplating walking away from realism, I decided that my programme/intervention was the whole service and everything in it – staff, buildings, patients – the lot. In hindsight, this is obvious, but at the time, knee-deep in detail and grappling with new terminology, I could not see the wood for the trees.

Context, mechanism and outcomes

For novice realists, articulating programme theories can be challenging, especially where intervention effectiveness is not clearly and explicitly articulated (Pawson, 2013). My difficulties were also compounded by my lack of understanding of contexts, mechanisms and outcomes. I conflated mechanisms and contexts, a common pitfall for realist researchers (Marchal et al., 2012; Dalkin et al., 2015), as 'context' and 'mechanism' are difficult concepts to grasp. What also makes it hard for novices is that 'context' is rarely defined within the realist literature (Greenhalgh & Manzano, 2021). Multiple definitions and constructs of mechanisms also exist within the realist literature (Marchal et al., 2012; Westhorp, 2018) making it harder for novices to know which is the 'right' definition and construct. The Context-Mechanism-Outcome configuration suggested by Pawson and Tilley (Pawson & Tilley, 1997) is a heuristic and may not be appropriate for your research. My advice to PhD students is: address this controversy within your thesis, decide which definition you want to use and hang your hat on it!

'If then because' statements

Dr Rebecca Hardwick encouraged me to generate **'If Then Because'** statements to help differentiate context, mechanism and outcome. **'If'** relates to context; **'Then'** is the outcome and **'Because'** is the mechanism. These **'If Then Because'** statements become the foundation for your tentative programme theories, but their generation can take some time. The **'Because'** component can be the most difficult to elucidate; mechanisms are often not articulated as such in peer-reviewed journals. I found this process frustrating. My first attempts at **'If Then Because'** statements ended with 'because they DO!!!!' Had I really appreciated I was not going to find mechanisms articulated as such within RCTs, I could have saved months of worry, and my confidence in my ability may have been higher. If I were starting now, I would either hypothesise about the mechanisms or conduct stakeholder consultation to help identify them.

Some of my early attempts at **'If Then Because'** statements were problematic, because they did not aim to answer my research question. The contexts articulated by the **If** statements needed unpacking to reveal detail, the **Because** alluded to the resources offered by the intervention but none articulated any reasoning. The **Because** part of the statement is central to realist inquiry. Once I understood what mechanisms were, it was much easier for me.

PhDs are learning journeys; a quest to *learn* how to conduct research. When I realised my candidate programme theories were not clearly articulated and that I'd conflated context and mechanism, I was worried. I could have retrospectively 'doctored' them in my thesis. However, I explained my understanding had evolved over the duration of the PhD and that I had made a common mistake. I still feel this was the right course of action; after all, it demonstrates knowledge acquisition.

Identifying the sample

Another crucial component of study design is the sample. Whom will you interview? You need to ensure your participants can provide you with the data required to refine your programme theories. Thankfully for me, via the national stroke audit, I was able to identify well-performing community stroke services, leaving me confident I would have sufficient data.

Data collection

Data sources

Data arises from multiple sources (Pawson, 2006a), think carefully about this and where appropriate factor it into your study design. In addition to realist interviews, other data sources I included were:

- **Informal meetings with service leads.** These were informal introductory theory-gleaning meetings. I collated information relating to structure, organisation and processes.
- **Observations of meetings.** Prior to interviewing, I observed at least one team meeting at each site. Observations can be useful in identifying contexts and outcomes, allowing you to probe these and tentative mechanisms in interviews.
- **Hanging around.** I used this tactic to build rapport. I engaged in opportunistic dialogue with staff at a more interpersonal level, helping me observe how things operated outside of formal meetings. For instance, one of my explanatory Context-Mechanism-Outcome configurations (CMOCs) underlying one of my programme theories was concerned with informal opportunities that staff had to talk to each other. This CMOC directly arose from my hanging around behaviour.
- **Service documents** can contain useful information about contexts and outcomes, organisational policies, national drivers, service specifications, outcome measures etc.

Ethics

Ethical approval can feel unsettling for novice researchers; find previous applications methodologically similar to yours and use them as a guide. You can ask other researchers in your department or reach out to the realist community via platforms such as RAMESES, bearing in mind there may be differences in ethics procedures between countries and institutions. Strive for a balance between specificity and flexibility to minimise the need for ethical committee amendments. For example, you may be required to stipulate how many interviews you will conduct but you are unlikely to know this upfront. One way of retaining freedom for iterative development is to state 'up to X interviews' instead of an absolute number. I had assumed that my estimation of up to 20 interviews in each site would be an overestimation. However, one of my stroke services was split into two sites (north and south). It would have been impossible to focus on the south without including the north as they were very much intertwined, so I needed the maximum limit.

Each ethical committee is different; I have submitted very different topic guides with the various studies I have participated in. Your candidate programme theories will have identified areas that you wish to evaluate, so use these programme theories to outline topics and suggested starter questions. You can, if you wish, explain that the guides will iteratively develop as knowledge is gained. Should the ethics committee require more information, they will ask for it.

Preparing for realist interviewing

When you conduct your first realist interview, you might feel nervous, overwhelmed, but also excited; after all, it is a huge milestone. Published realist evaluations rarely provide detail about how the questions were phrased. Given the influence of my psychological training, I really struggled with phrasing my questions. Thankfully, and almost like a miracle for me, Ana Manzano's 'The craft of realist interviewing in realist evaluation' (Manzano, 2016) was published shortly before I embarked upon realist interviewing. At the time it was the only practically focussed guide to conducting realist interviews. There have been more academic papers published in recent years in which realist interviewing is discussed (Gilmore, 2019; Mukumbang et al., 2020; O'Rourke et al., 2022) but it still surprises me how little is out there to help novice researchers.

Dynamics of realist interviews

A realist interview is more likely to produce rich data if you can establish a connection with your participants. Your interview style will be unique to you, and you should feel comfortable with the questions you ask. If not, this will be sensed by participants who will probably not relax. Nowadays, I have relaxed conversations or chats with participants; I'm always prepared for our conversation to take twists and turns. This can be useful for programme theory development or can take you down redundant pathways. As your interview skills progress, you become better at steering back on course. If someone tells me something new, I often enquire around this new phenomenon as I am

100% interested in what my participants say. I am regularly asked at the end of an interview if it was worth it, as participants often think their contributions are irrelevant. Reassurance from me that I absolutely think it was and seeing a smile in return from the participant is worth its weight in gold.

However, not every interview is relaxed and plain sailing; some interviews are difficult for a variety of reasons. Some people believe you have a hidden agenda and are naturally cautious, some believe they are being tested. Participants have asked me if they need to dress appropriately, i.e., wear a suit and tie, or if they should prepare anything in advance. Offering advice in pre-interview communication will help reassure participants. Following one particularly difficult interview, I sought advice from an experienced senior researcher who reassured me that not every interview progresses with ease. One hundred realist interviews later, I concur with this. Some people do not settle into the interview groove. It is important not to take it personally. Instead, reflect on the process, and see if there are things you could do differently next time.

The power dynamics at play in interviews should be addressed, since in some cultures it is considered rude to disagree with experts. (See Gilmore and Nadrine's chapter in this book on Realist data collection in less familiar settings.) If this is something you are likely to experience, you may need to adapt the phrasing of your questions and you need to consider that you may not be able to engage in the teacher-learner cycle approach. Gilmore (2019) and O'Rourke et al. (2022), have both explored cross-cultural aspects of realist interviewing, suggesting lessons in interview technique relevant for all. Power worked as an advantage for me, as the power was reversed. When I first started interviewing, I asked the most basic questions not because I was pretending to be naive but because I was naive! I was very open and transparent about that with my participants. As my knowledge evolved so did my questions. I found this approach helped me when interviewing assistants and newly qualified members of the team who always knew more than I did.

The teacher-learner approach

The general advice when conducting qualitative interviewing is to be deliberately naïve; this is where realist interviewing, and general qualitative interviewing differ. Remember, the purpose of realist interviews is to identify causal mechanisms and contexts which influence outcomes so that we can test, refine, refute or discover emerging programme theories. To do this task effectively, we are advised to employ the teacher-learner cycle method (Pawson & Tilley, 1997). Pawson used the phrase 'I'll show you my theory if you show me yours' as a way of explaining this process to people. In my early interviews, I tentatively shared my ideas (theories) with participants and asked for their opinions. Once I adopted, practiced and perfected this approach, the interviews started to flow more easily; we ended up having great conversations rich not only in context and outcomes but also in those elusive mechanisms which can be difficult to elicit.

Over the years I have found that the teacher-learner approach can un-nerve some interviewers; they are worried about confirmation bias (Vogel & Punton, 2017). (For more detailed information, see Manzano's chapter in this book on bias in realism). This is an important consideration and may have implications for some research contexts such as cross-cultural evaluations. Over the years that I have conducted interviews with NHS staff, patients and carers, I have generally found they had no problem clarifying, correcting or even laughing at my ideas (theories) if they thought I was wrong, or telling me if they thought my ideas would not work. Sometimes I ask direct questions and make statements, looking for body language cues such as nodding or shaking of heads, rolling eyes, even laughing. I use these cues to open lines of enquiry, for example, 'I can already see you are shaking your head, tell me more'. These techniques effectively give the floor to the participant, and at key points I would ask deeper probing questions.

Potential ways to phrase teacher-learner questions are:

1 My background reading tells me that A…. – what is your opinion of this?
2 One of the ideas I have is B; is that how things work?
3 A staff member in another service has told me C, do you agree with this?

Preparing for interviews: researchers with disabilities

Surviving research whilst battling with disabilities (hidden or otherwise) is a seldom articulated topic; there isn't a guide to interview hacks for disabled researchers. Research studies are designed to account for potential difficul-ties for our participants, but I have never seen anything written about allow-ances for disabled researchers. Qualitative research can take a heavy toll on researchers with disabilities. Realist interviewing is cognitively demanding and during data collection for my PhD, my health suffered. I have in recent years been very candid about my disabilities. I was seriously injured in a car accident 25 years ago, which at the time derailed my chosen career path as a clinical neuropsychologist. I have, therefore, had a long time to develop life hacks and I carried these principles into my research. Similar to conditions such as M.E., Long Covid, Fibromyalgia etc. I suffer from neurological fatigue, brain fog and can experience word finding and memory difficulties; I deal with this by being as organised and prepared as I can, and believe that the techniques I have developed can aid others with similar conditions – and can improve the confidence and preparedness of any novice researcher.

Realist interview schedules

Interview schedules can be exceptionally useful tools, but the nature of pro-gramme theory development means that standard qualitative interview sched-ules are not useful. Interview questions evolve, often during the actual interview, so you are required to think and react quickly. (See Redgate and Dalkin's chap-ter in this book on realist topic guides.) Each participant may be asked to reflect on different parts of the phenomenon under evaluation and this can be difficult to accommodate within standard qualitative interview schedules.

I was worried the long drive to my research sites would cause a flare of my long-term condition and I would forget the interview questions if I just used a topic guide. To ease my anxieties, I constructed individual interview schedules. Before each interview, I reflected on the previous interview, its accompanying schedule, meeting observations and any programme theory development which had occurred. I would tailor the interview questions to each participant. There were specific lines of enquiry I was following with certain staff groups, for example, nurses and speech and language therapists are fewer in number in community stroke services, so I was interested in the impact this had on professional development, supervision and training opportunities. Schedules for these participants had questions relating to these experiences.

These schedules were my safety net. If my words started to fail, I asked a question directly from the schedule. They gave me confidence and reassurance that no matter what my brain decided to do on the day, I was prepared! I often completed them before I left the house; they got me into the interview zone. Whilst driving, I made connections between all my data sources which were instrumental to my programme theory development. Partway through the evaluation, I realised these schedules provided a fantastic account of programme theory development. I could look back systematically and see where specific lines of enquiry emerged or questions changed to reflect the growing knowledge. Another important activity was the reflective journaling I did following each day of fieldwork, completed as soon as possible after the event. The PhD afforded me the luxury of time to engage in preparative activities. These activities increase the researcher burden and may not be feasible in all projects due to resource constraints. However, when feasible, engage with these activities, as you will reap the benefits during data analysis.

Phases of realist interviewing

One of the most important aspects of Manzano's paper that struck a chord with me was the phases of realist interview: theory gleaning, theory refinement and theory consolidation (Manzano, 2016). As you read these sections below, you may be fooled into thinking that moving from theory gleaning to theory refinement and then to theory consolidation is a linear process. However, like everything else in realist inquiry, these phases are iterative and not at all linear. As you become more experienced it is possible to go through all of the stages within one interview, or none at all if you have a particularly challenging interview.

Theory gleaning

Theory gleaning is the first phase and, if possible, you should start it before commencing interviews. Perhaps you already have some knowledge about how the programme you are researching works, and other ideas can emerge from your reading or engagement with stakeholders. In a nutshell, I think theory gleaning is about fact-finding and gaining important information. I had worked in stroke research prior to my PhD but had very little understanding about service delivery, so this first step was crucial for me. The more theory gleaning you do early on via other data collection methods such as in your literature review or other data sources mentioned earlier, the quicker you can move to other phases during your interviews.

Sampling considerations

When possible, start interviewing participants who know the most about your programme theory (Manzano & Pawson, 2014). This purposive approach to sampling is a great strategy for theory gleaning. These people possess tacit knowledge about the programme you are evaluating and provide you with information about how the programme or intervention might work (or not). At this point, you are trying to gain a broad understanding of how your phenomenon under evaluation works. Think of it as sense-making; you need to gain a good understanding of the wider context of the phenomenon you are evaluating. Identifying these key individuals may be challenging, as you may not really know who is the most knowledgeable until you interview them. In one of my sites, I interviewed the service administrator first as they happened to be available; it was a very happy coincidence. They were a gold mine of information and possessed a different perspective, which I found really useful. Administrators are often central people with knowledge across multiple areas and can be very useful for theory gleaning.

The next people to identify are those working on the frontline and actively involved with the phenomenon you are evaluating as well as the end users of the intervention. For me, this was the staff within the service. If we think of the realist mantra 'what works for whom' I wanted to ensure I represented the voices of everyone within the services. I interviewed all disciplines including assistants, service leads and administrators. I also ensured I had a broad range of staff expertise and seniority within the service to reflect differing experiences from recently qualified members of staff for example.

Articulating theory-gleaning questions

Theory-gleaning questions are exploratory. We are trying to understand what is going on, identify parts of context and outcomes and generally gather information. The types of questions asked are structured and similar across cases. I was really stressed after my first interview. I had struggled to get my participant to elicit mechanisms, and as far as I was concerned, I had failed in my mission and was going to end up with useless data! I reached out to Dr. Ana Manzano and Prof. Dalkin over their social media accounts. Thankfully, they reassured me. My advice now is, do not get worked up over eliciting mechanisms within the first few interviews. The information I gathered was related to processes and linked to my programme theories. This comprehensive information-gathering stage was useful and in subsequent interviews, I was able to elicit some mechanisms.

One useful question I asked at the end of every single interview is the 'magic wand' type questions e.g., *'If you and I were tasked with commissioning a brand-new community stroke service in a similar geographical location, what would it look like? What would we include? What would make a difference?'*. This was useful to help me determine what was working and what wasn't within their current service. Sometimes people do not feel comfortable telling you about areas they don't think work so well. This question allows them to reflect on this in a more positive way, by suggesting improvements. You can then probe (if you don't already know) why this is needed. It can also be a useful strategy to identify new theories as participants have free rein to suggest anything.

Box 6.1   Overview of theory-gleaning questions

Overview of Theory Gleaning

- Exploratory questions
- Focussed on gathering generic information relevant to programme theory development
- Semi-structured in format, but tailored to individuals you are interviewing
- Mainly identify contexts and outcomes, possibly some mechanisms

Sample Questions

1 I'd like to start by getting a little information about you. How long have you been with the team? Can you tell me a little about your role within the service?
2 What training opportunities are there for staff within the service?
3 So, what does a manager do within this service?
4 One of the things I have noticed is that administrators are so knowledgeable... how did they acquire this knowledge? Did you train them?

Theory refinement

During theory refinement, more specific information is gathered, and you increase your understanding of how things work differently for different people and how different contexts trigger different mechanisms to produce outcomes; your programme theories evolve. You may also use information gathered from other data collection sources as well as academic and grey literature, seminars, conferences or conversations with subject matter experts. These all help to influence programme theory refinement.

At this stage within my PhD, I was focussed on learning about typical and atypical occurrences, in other words, how do things normally work or not? Atypical occurrences are sometimes referred to as deviant cases. This allowed me to compare both across and within cases and understand how contexts unique to individual settings could provide vastly different outcomes by enabling or disabling mechanisms. For example, one of my programme theories focussed on care transitions. The service located within the stroke ward had the smoothest transition when compared with the other two, one located within the same hospital grounds, and one located many miles away. This functional proximity provided opportunities for cross-service collaboration and facilitated care transitions across the stroke pathway.

Theory refinement questions are less exploratory and should be designed to increase knowledge about individual contexts and mechanisms. Causal patterns and demi-regularities may emerge, though they may not be fully formulated in your head. You may uncover new or rival programme theories as I did. This new programme theory relating to how services organised their visits was identified on day one via an informal conversation, but I did not understand its significance then. However, I could chart its development through the interviews and the observations.

Box 6.2   Overview of Theory Refinement Questions

Overview of Theory Refinement

- Questions are more specific
- Causal patterns and demi-regularities are identified
- Rival or new theories may emerge

Sample Questions

1 An occupational therapist in one of the other stroke services participating in my research has told me X, how does this play out here?
2 One of my ideas is that the role of the rehabilitation assistant is important to maximise the delivery of rehabilitation. I'd like to explore how rehabilitation assistants are used in this service
3 It has been suggested that this service is interdisciplinary; some speech and language therapists have indicated they have learnt a lot more about cognition [occupational therapist role] than in previous ward-based jobs, but nurses have felt a little outside of the multidisciplinary team. What is your experience?
4 We've discussed role blurring and its benefits for service delivery, but are there any issues associated with protecting professional boundaries?

Theory consolidation

The final phase, theory consolidation, is where you fine-tune your theories. It occurs to some extent towards the end of data collection but also well beyond, into coding, analysis, synthesis and writing. Within the final interviews, you can do as much consolidation as possible. At this stage, interview questions are significantly more nuanced, probing and direct, and as a result your understanding of the phenomenon you are evaluating grows. You may decide to re-interview some people. I re-interviewed the service leads with a significant acquisition of knowledge and a deeper understanding of their service. I asked more detailed, probing questions which helped consolidate my thoughts around my programme theories. Questions, for me, were sequenced. Usually, I started with an overview of what I know about the theory. This was either confirmed or corrected by the participant. They usually understood where I was heading and often just started to talk without much prompting. The questions I asked and statements I posed during these re-interviews with the service leads were the magic wand type of questions mentioned above but we spent significantly more time exploring the how and why aspects, *'what difference would it make if that was implemented?'*, which allowed me to elicit contexts and mechanisms to further consolidate my programme theories whilst also allowing me to gain a deeper understanding of some of the shortcomings associated with delivery of community stroke services.

Box 6.3   Overview of Theory Consolidation Questions

Overview of Theory Consolidation

- Questions are more significantly more nuanced and targeted
- At the end of this process you should be able to determine: What works for whom in what circumstances and why
- Theory consolidation continues into data analysis and writing

Sample Questions

1 If we were to be on the commissioning board for a brand-new stroke service, what learning points would we take forward from it if you were to have to do it all over again?
2 What would you do or wish to have in place to be able to have the best relationship possible to facilitate those smooth discharges?

Most of my theory consolidation occurred as I wrote my findings chapters, which was an iterative and messy endeavour. I devoted a chapter to each programme theory, and after writing draft findings from each one, I conducted a focussed search of academic literature relating to each programme theory.

I prefaced each of these chapters with a short realist-inspired overview of relevant literature. Much of this literature was new to me and I completely rewrote several findings chapters as it helped me appreciate my programme theories in a new light.

Data analysis

Data analysis can be another overwhelming task largely due to the volume of data. I had several notebooks containing copious notes from meeting observations, 55 one-hour interviews (each approximately 30 pages long) and several service documents. Some researchers prefer pen and paper, others prefer computer software such as NVivo or Atlas Ti to organise data. There is no right or wrong way; the most important thing is that it makes sense to you. I used NVivo, as it was available via my institution. However, when I opened my first transcript I was completely overwhelmed. I had assumed I would code all my contexts, mechanisms and outcomes separately but given that data could be attributed to context, mechanism or outcome depending on its analytical focus I was really confused. Once again, serendipity intervened; Prof. Sonia Dalkin wrote a blog on approaches to data analysis which has since been transformed into a paper (Dalkin et al., 2021). Sonia and her colleague delivered a talk on this topic which others can use for guidance (Dalkin & McEwan, 2022).

The Dalkin method advises coding at the programme theory level (Dalkin et al., 2021). I had six programme theories, including the new theory identified during data collection. I eventually dropped one programme theory as I was over the permissible word limit in my thesis! In NVivo I created parent nodes (conceptual buckets) reflecting each theory and attributed sections of text to them. I made no formal attempt to link context, mechanism and outcomes, but this overarching approach to coding did provide deeper insights into the contexts and mechanisms influencing outcomes. Additionally, I created a miscellaneous code to capture potentially relevant data that did not fit in with existing codes. This was more to reassure me about losing relevant data, and I never used any of it. I also created memos charting my thinking and key decisions, which were useful during writing.

Next, I identified child nodes; this was an inductive process, using the data to inform the nodes. A key feature of my thinking at this stage was to determine what was driving outcomes and how they differed between sites. These child nodes predominately reflected context and the resource component of mechanisms (Dalkin et al., 2015). These sections of text contained some or all the elements of contexts, mechanisms and outcomes. Again, no formal attempt was made to identify contexts, mechanisms or outcomes, though in reality researcher hunches were being mulled over in my brain.

Once this task was complete, I exported each parent node containing the programme theory and its child nodes into MS Word. I constructed tentative CMOC tables with corresponding evidence in the form of quotes.

This process provided a holistic view and was useful in determining where similar CMOCs could be merged and highlighted how different contexts and mechanisms produced different outcomes. Subsequent tables were also constructed with data synthesised across cases and from multiple sources. These CMOC tables provided the foundations for my final programme theories and underlying CMOCs as well as the narrative explanations within my findings chapters.

Conclusions

There is so much more that I could discuss, but I hope that the information that I have provided has been useful. By way of reflection, I think my main points of advice to novice researchers are:

1 Time spent immersed in realist literature and connecting with other realist researchers is invaluable.
2 Do not be afraid to reach out and ask for help.
3 Candidate programme theories are a starting point; do not spend copious amounts of time making them 'perfect'.
4 Realist interviewing gets easier with practice.
5 Do not get overwhelmed, take it one day at a time, one task at a time and you will eventually get there.

I hope you enjoy realist research as much as I do, and I hope our paths cross in the future. Best of luck with your projects.

Acknowledgements

I would like to thank novice realist researchers, Hafsah Habib, Mary Harrison and Gurkiran Birdi for their insightful feedback on early drafts of this chapter.

7   Realist interviews in global health research

Case studies and comparative analysis with similar interview approaches

Sara Van Belle, Prashanth N Srinivas, Tom Cornu, Pragati Hebbar, Ibukun O. Abejirinde, and Bruno Marchal

Introduction

During the last fifteen years, realist evaluation (RE) has been increasingly used in the design and evaluation of global health programmes, and in research on such programmes (Marchal et al., 2018). Drivers of this uptake include (inter) national NGOs seeking alternative evaluation methods for their programmes (Radin, 2006). Another was the surge in interest in implementation research, adopted as a way to drive evidence-informed decision-making through enhanced implementation rigour and research (Van Belle et al., 2017). Addressing initial critiques that pointed to the atheoretical approach adopted by many implementation scientists, we argued earlier that theory-driven methodologies, such as RE, could be helpful in anchoring implementation science studies within existing theories and the wider body of knowledge in general (Van Belle et al., 2017). Theories on implementation processes, conditions of successful implementation, scaling up and so on could be refined by empirically testing them in implementation studies and the results of such studies could inform the implementation of future interventions.

One of the main attractions of the realist evaluation approach for global health researchers who have not been trained in social sciences has been the transparency of its methods, its potential to situate causal explanations in context and the methodological guidance and support it provides. The RAMESES project developed guidance that can be found at www.ramesesproject. org (2024) and there is a lively RAMESES email discussion list at rameses@ jiscmail.ac.uk. In recent years, much attention was directed towards methodological clarification, driven in part by increased use of the approach. RE has been combined with randomised controlled trials (Warren et al., 2022), qualitative comparative analysis (Befani et al., 2007), action research (Westhorp et al., 2016) or soft systems methodology (Dalkin et al., 2018). Detailed methodological guidance was developed regarding elicitation of the programme theory (Vincent et al., 2022). The Context-Mechanism-Outcome

DOI: 10.4324/9781003457077-8

(CMO) configuration was unpacked, with attention paid to the concepts of 'mechanism' and 'context' (Dalkin et al., 2015; Manzano, 2016; Greenhalgh & Manzano, 2021; Nielsen et al., 2022; Van Belle et al., 2023). Westhorp and Manzano have also developed guidance on realist interviewing and focus groups, relating the technique to the phases of theory gleaning, theory refining and consolidation (Westhorp & Manzano, 2017; Manzano, 2022).

In this chapter, we discuss the potential of realist interviewing to manage power dynamics between researchers and respondents, and to engage with 'context'. Power is a critical issue in any interviewing method but especially important in research and evaluation of global health programmes which are largely funded by bilateral and multilateral development agencies, while context matters a lot in the evaluation of development programmes carried out in multiple settings. First, we discuss realist interviewing in light of the current trend of knowledge co-production in applied practice fields. Then, we present real-world challenges encountered by researchers when using realist interviewing in research and evaluation of programmes in different contexts. We compare realist interviews with approaches aligned with other scientific paradigms, such as interpretivist interviewing and critical realist interviewing. We end with a discussion of key lessons learned from the case studies.

The co-production of knowledge and realist interviewing

As explained in the introductory chapter of this book, RE requires a specific approach to interviewing. Central to the realist interview is a dialogical approach where the evaluator engages in a joint sense-making process in which the theories of the evaluator regarding the intervention take centre stage. Pawson and Tilley referred to this mode of interviewing as a *teacher-learner cycle*, where the evaluator 'teaches' their programme theory to the participant, and the participant deepens the learning of the evaluator by shedding light on certain parts of the theory (Pawson & Tilley, 2004). Using the example of a maternal health programme in Nigeria, Manzano demonstrates that this dialogical approach can also be used in realist focus group discussions, where participants are selected as a sub-group or reference group in relation to their contribution to theory development. In realist focus groups, the realist evaluator is a 'deliberator' who does not seek a consensus, but facilitates creative disputation between group members (Manzano, 2022).

Several other authors have been contributing to this methodological discussion. Blamey and Mackenzie (2007) and Gilmore (2019) highlighted the question about whose theories are really being researched, pointing to the tendency of research in 'the south' often being based on concepts and theories that have been developed by 'the north' on the basis of studies on Western, Educated, Industrialised, Rich, Democratic (WEIRD) people and that may be ill-suited to settings in the south. Other authors have stressed that the teacher-learner cycle is not conceptualised by Pawson and Tilley to be emancipatory or intended to support social change (Abrams et al., 2021; Malengreaux et al., 2022). In applied practice fields, such as development, social work and environmental research, this perceived lack of emancipatory drive among realists seems to be increasingly felt as a weakness (Malengreaux et al., 2022; Mukumbang & van Wyk, 2020; Renmans et al., 2022). These concerns reflect similar debates on co-production and co-creation in the global health research and evaluation fields, where the question of stakeholder validation and power dynamics in co-production is increasingly coming to the fore (Brandsen et al., 2018; Fusco et al., 2020; Zurba et al., 2021).

Co-production of research and evaluation, and dialogical approaches in general, are not new. Participatory Action Research (PAR) and its approach to co-production of knowledge has been central to development programmes related to community organisation, mobilisation and participation (Ospina et al., 2021). Joint theorising as a way to obtain a common understanding of the issue to be addressed has been part of PAR from its origins in the 1970s. Also widely used is the Theory of Change (TOC) methodology, which was developed in the 1990s to guide the design and evaluation of community change projects. In TOC, the community organiser acts as a facilitator of a group process, which seeks to uncover a group's 'shared assumptions' on why and how a programme would work (Anderson, 2005). The resulting theory of change (or logic model) is then used to guide both the design and implementation of the programme, and its evaluation. We discuss the PAR approach and other major paradigmatic approaches to interviewing in a later section.

Experience with realist interviewing in intercultural contexts in global health development and research

In this section, we present three studies and the experiences and challenges the researchers encountered using the realist interviewing approach.

The realist implementation science lab (RIAL) in an indigenous community health intervention in South India – Realist interviewing and power dynamics

To address health inequities among the indigenous Soliga Adivasi communities in the state of Karnataka, researchers (including author P.N. Srinivas) partnered with Adivasi communities and NGOs. They aimed to set up a community-led participatory learning site, evolving out of a community-based maternal health project (Pratt et al., 2020). This inclusive and participatory approach was complemented by a realist knowledge production effort to gain a better understanding of the mechanisms underlying health inequities. Realist interviewing here was thus part of a PAR project. The study confirmed that the transformation of local power relations is a precondition for the successful implementation of community health interventions and the co-production of knowledge (Pratt et al., 2022b).

Embedding realist approaches within a long-term PAR learning and action site allowed for concomitant contributions to scholarship while co-producing locally relevant knowledge. Challenges in creating platforms where both space and voice can be claimed by the participants of the programme, in this case Adivasi communities, emerged early on (Pratt et al., 2022a). The team reframed the 'reflection' component of the action-reflection cycle of PAR as theory-building (i.e., middle-range theories explaining the historical and ongoing marginalisation of Adivasi communities). The participatory platforms created in the learning site (for instance townhall style annual meetings and focus groups of community leaders) were conceptualised as spaces to challenge and refine middle-range theories on drivers of inequities in addition to spaces for co-production. This allowed the seeding of 'academic' understanding of the explanations for inequities into community spaces, while remaining open for these 'academic' understandings to be challenged and refined. In this approach, interview and group discussion methods were seen as methods to develop and refine the understanding of downstream meso- and micro-effects of the macro-level middle-range theories that were developed in the larger participatory platforms. These downstream meso- and micro-level explanations took the form of programme theories built around specific healthcare interventions implemented through our learning site in healthcare and social institutions.

The team realised it is important to understand that the academic/researcher position was conditioned by scholarship that excluded Adivasi worldviews. Researchers hence run the risk of uncritically and (un)consciously imposing a non-Adivasi gaze onto the inquiry (Nakkeeran et al., 2021). This is evident in current public health scholarship on Adivasi health, for example, which largely problematises their geographical location ('they are living too far away…'), their distinct culture or their development achievements (or 'lack thereof'). The townhall style discussions challenged these dimensions as largely emanating from a pre-dominantly non-Adivasi scholarship. In the early years, the research team strived to integrate trained Adivasi researchers into the team. The Adivasi researchers contributed to conceptualising research as well as interrogating downstream effects of the non-Adivasi gaze and how that shapes the healthcare experience. The latter involved examining how the exclusion of Adivasi communities in the design and delivery of healthcare translates into everyday healthcare experiences by community members, during preventive health visits by community health workers, immunisation rounds or antenatal care and also in in-patient care.

The use of RE embedded within learning sites with Adivasi communities required long-term engagement to build trustful platforms for dialogue. What emerged as very important for realist interviewing was the need for an interview setting that was perceived as a dialogue space which ensured voice for Adivasi participants. Both Adivasi studies literature and the experience of the team confirm that interactions of Adivasi with outsiders were pre-dominantly conditioned by relationships of charity or missionary-style work through episodic NGO engagement, and/or by adverse interactions with the colonial and post-colonial state (e.g., violations of forest laws drawing action by officials).

In this project, the fact that the Soliga Adivasi, with whom the researchers collaborated, had worked for decades to organise themselves into a federated social movement allowed them to 'correctly' approach community consent and have gatekeepers at multiple levels; the Soliga Adivasi have organised themselves into a federated collective represented by leadership at the village, circle of villages, block and district level. However, this is not the case with many other Adivasi or other marginalised communities where legitimate gatekeeping and lack of community organisation due to historical and/or structural factors hinder the ability to engage with communities – despite the best of intentions.

Evaluating a digital health intervention in Northern Ghana - engaging community midwives in eliciting and validating realist theories

To understand how digital innovations can be used to improve the quality of antenatal care for pregnant women in low-resource settings, and its implications for health service delivery, Ibukun Abejirinde, with support from Bruno Marchal, conducted a RE of Bliss4Midwives, a diagnostic clinical decision support intervention in Northern Ghana. Reported elsewhere, and complemented by other research methods, summarily, the RE included eliciting an initial programme theory following the CMO heuristic, testing it through semi-structured interviews with midwives, patients and other implementation actors, and validating it through realist-type focus group discussions with midwives from the six health facilities involved in the intervention (Abejirinde et al., 2018b).

While the interviews with patients followed a more narrative interviewing approach, in the interviews with midwives and other frontline workers, the Pawson's teacher-learner cycle was intentionally adopted, where initial candidate theories were subtly integrated into the question guide to be refuted or confirmed by research participants. Of note is that the realist interviews onsite in Ghana were preceded by the elicitation of three candidate theories by the researcher following document analysis, a realist review and a group discussion with implementing partners of the programme in the global North. The initial candidate theories therefore informed the question guide used in the realist interviews (Abejirinde et al., 2018a).

Two conclusions can be drawn from this study. One is the importance of being aware of the stage (from theory development to refinement/validation, and to finalisation) at which different 'voices' are involved in specifying the Context-Mechanism-Outcome pathways that explain programme outcomes and how this shapes the concluding theory. That is, are all types of voices relevant to the programme and by extension, are the different levels and types of power people hold (epistemic, socio-economic and psychological) accounted for in all phases of theory evolution? Or do we intentionally (and perhaps often for practical reasons) decide whose voices shape the different 'cycles' of theory development? Perhaps the primary question is if this matters at all and what this means for the strength of the resulting theories. One can argue that the dynamic and adaptive nature of realist methodology lends itself well to the idea that the development and refinement of the explanatory causal theories that underly a global health programme will occur iteratively and will draw from diverse voices over time. In short, these different sources of knowledge may bounce off and feed into each other through multiple iterations of theory refinement.

The second conclusion is related to the earlier stated role of power and the extent to which it is shared and leads to knowledge co-production between the researcher and interviewees. In the Bliss4Midwives evaluation, interviewees were less aware that they were being positioned by the researcher to play the role of teacher during interviews. This was a decision made by the main researcher to eliminate any pressure for perfection (see Pino Gavidia & Adu, 2022) or imagined depth of expertise from the midwives regarding their contribution to the research findings. Furthermore, the socio-cultural and administrative processes of field entry had also positioned the researcher as the hierarchical expert in the room, despite her repeated objections; community partners introduced her to frontline staff as a medical doctor and researcher from the Netherlands. Whilst the researcher emphasised her African roots and values, it took weeks of relationship building, collegial conversation and demonstrations of epistemic humility to 'level out the playing field' with the midwives. This level state had not been established by the time the realist interviews were conducted. However, the theory validation exercise between the researcher and sixteen midwives, which was conducted towards the end of fieldwork and prior to a regional dissemination meeting, was structured differently – with an explicit realist style approach and a shared understanding of the teacher-learner role amongst all participants. Although participants still struggled to adopt a first-name basis with the researcher during this session, by spending time to share preliminary study findings and explain in layman terms how CMO configurations are constructed, the invitation to play the role of teacher was accepted by the midwives, who engaged heavily in the theory refinement exercise and likely felt empowered and validated by the knowledge co-production experience.

State-level policy implementation pathways of the national tobacco control programme in India – Interviewing policymakers

Pragati Hebbar and colleagues carried out a realist research study aiming at gaining a better understanding of state-level implementation pathways of the National Programme of Tobacco Control (NTCP) and the Cigarettes and Other Tobacco Products Act 2003 (COTPA). Three contrasting Indian states were identified based on nationally representative Global Adult Tobacco Survey data and in consultation with national-level tobacco control experts. In-depth interviews of 48 state- and district-level stakeholders and over 100 non-participant observations were conducted in these three states to refine the initial programme theory. Following this, two regional consultations including stakeholders from 20 Indian states were conducted for a second iteration of programme theory refinement. A total of 300 Intervention-Context-Actor-Mechanism-Outcome (ICAMO) configurations were developed from the interview data. In the next step, these were synthesised to state-specific programme theories for Kerala, West Bengal and Arunachal Pradesh. The mechanisms of collective action as norm-based human behaviour, felt accountability, individual motivation, fear and prioritisation were identified to be triggered (or not) in specific settings, leading to diverse implementation outcomes. In this study, the researchers identified gaps and policy recommendations to improve COTPA and NTCP implementation, which has important practice and research implications to further the field of implementation research (Hebbar, 2023).

Using realist interviewing with policy and implementation elites (those in-charge or at the top of the hierarchical structures) at the state- and district-level led the researchers to identify the following issues: researcher positionality, power dynamics and the insider-outsider dynamics; challenges related to applying the learning-teaching cycle in practice; expectations from realist findings, and finally, stakeholder context diversity.

The researchers experienced the issue of power imbalances during the realist interviews at different instances. While in some district and sub-district settings, the positionality of a doctoral researcher from another Indian state was accepted favourably, in some state-level settings, it did not add any advantage to rapport building or stimulating the engagement of the interviewees. Some respondents of the health departments were sceptical to engage with interviewers from 'outside' of their system, while this external positionality was relatable for stakeholders from academia and civil societies. Power imbalances were further evident during the interdepartmental focus group discussions conducted during the regional consultations. Given the focus of the study on multi-sectoral collaboration, the research team took a collective and informed decision to proceed with multi-department stakeholders in order to engage with diverse perspectives, as several departments are expected to coordinate the implementation of the policies. The facilitation of these deliberations required developing a trustful and respectful environment, while providing adequate time and opportunities for all stakeholders to contribute to the theory refinement process and overcoming language, gender and power/positional differences.

Applying the teacher-learner cycle posed further challenges in interviews where the power imbalances were not in favour of the researcher. These included stakeholders becoming defensive as they perceived such an interaction as questioning their understanding and/or actions. Some respondents who refuted parts of the programme theory were unwilling to explain why. In settings where the researcher was perceived to be in a powerful position, the researcher felt the risk that the respondent may accept most parts of the theory without countering or providing inputs to refine it, unless deliberately asked for by the researcher. With a growing interest in realist research and given the focus of the study on understanding the facilitators and barriers of policy implementation, the expectations of the stakeholders regarding the understanding of what works, for whom and how, were high. For some respondents, the interviews fuelled their expectations of identifying policy solutions to address the barriers and joint sense-making of the complexity of policy implementation shaped the course of interactions in some interviews.

Lastly, adapting the interview guide and process to stakeholders from diverse departments with contrasting contextual realities was a dynamic process. The three states had specific socio-political and economic macro-context elements that shaped policy processes, which were found to be intertwined with the meso-level departmental norms and values that ultimately shaped actors' practices as well as responses during the interviews. While this diversity added to the richness of the collected data, to make sense of this dynamic emergent nature of the context and its interactions with the mechanisms was challenging. The researchers found that recent efforts at developing ways to get a better understanding of context by Greenhalgh and Manzano (2022) were useful in the analysis process.

Dialogic approaches used in global health practice

In this section, we zoom in on other approaches to interviewing, the sheer variety of which can be overwhelming. For an overview, we refer to handbooks, for instance, Kvale and Brinkmann (2009) and Gubrium and Holstein (2014). We explore how knowledge is approached and constructed through interviewing, what knowledge product is envisaged, what each actor brings to the table in the interview, and how the interaction between interviewer and interview participant is perceived – comparing it along the way to RE. We discuss interpretive interviewing, narrative approaches to interviewing (and specifically critical narrative inquiry), and critical realist interviewing, before we return to PAR, as it is a popular methodology in global health practice and global programmes supporting social change.

Interpretive interviewing

RE is not primarily interested in the meaning people attach to programmes or events per se - only when these are part of a causal explanation (Pawson & Tilley, 1997). Yet, people's interpretations and the (lack of) shared meaning are often lurking in the shadows when subgroups in complex interventions creatively discuss and 'dispute' an event during a realist focus group (Manzano, 2022). The reading of an event is arguably related to the meaning one attributes to it. The search for causal explanation will thus often result in finding rival explanations.

In interpretive interviewing, similar to realist interviewing, interpretivists are not seeking to uncover what really happened: the interview is a meaning-making event in itself. This means that the context in which the dialogue takes place, together with the lived realities of the participants, will shape the interview 'findings'. Building on her ethnographic research with genocide perpetrators in Rwanda, Lee Ann Fuji considered the interview as inherently *relational,* a two-way sense-making event (Fuji, 2018). Data cannot simply be 'extracted' from the participant: the interview's output is determined by the interview as a communicative event – taking place at a certain time and in a given space (Fuji, 2018). Respondents will direct the course of the interview and convey meanings, values and ideas within the context of the interview as an empirical event (Scheibelhofer, 2023). Another example is the study by Santos et al. on health professionals living with tuberculosis (TB) in the Amazon region of Brazil focused on the lived realities of the respondents (Santos et al., 2020). This study adopted an interpretive phenomenological analysis, demonstrating how the experience of providers has an impact on the empathetic and sensitive care they provide for TB patients. Litorp and colleagues used in-depth interviews and focus group discussions to explore the causes of high caesarean section (C/S) rates in a university hospital in Tanzania (Litorp et al., 2015). The authors demonstrate how health professionals who operate in a culture of fear of litigation tend to divert the blame for high C/S rates (and the potential iatrogenic consequences) by citing health system issues that are outside their control (Litorp et al., 2015).

Narrative approaches to interviewing

Narrative inquiry focuses on uncovering the participant's stories by way of interviewing. In contrast with interpretive interviewing, narrative inquiry specifically zooms in on a story, consisting of elements of time, place and social interaction, by which people come to understand who they are, and how they relate to others and their lifeworld connecting lived reality to the past (Pino Gavidia & Adu, 2022). Storytelling is increasingly used in research in global health, for instance in the field of indigenous health research, but also to explore therapeutic or patient trajectories (Kaspar et al., 2023). Narrative inquiry builds on two paradigmatic approaches: interpretivist narrative inquiry and critical narrative inquiry (Pino Gavidia & Adu, 2022). We will focus on the latter.

In critical narrative inquiry, the purpose of research is to trace elements of the story back to the broader social, economic and cultural structures. Quayle and Sonn (2022) provide guidance and discuss specific ways to elicit stories from participants. The authors discuss the storytelling approach used by community psychologists with Aboriginal communities in Australia to 'give voice' to stories of structural violence in everyday life. Elders were interviewed to better understand what the communities would want future studies to focus on (Quayle & Sonn, 2022). In critical narrative inquiry, the purpose is to avoid the use and processes of dominant knowledge production further disempowers already marginalised communities through the silencing of indigenous experiences. The researchers take on the role of 'supporters' of the communities' voice (Quayle & Sonn, 2022). Moreover, the study of Gubrium provides a good illustration of how digital storytelling was used with individual follow-up interviews to uncover traumatic experiences in the sexual and reproductive health-related lived experience of Puerto Rican adolescent girls and women. Participants' engagement in the storytelling process allowed them to partially process and interrogate their experience, and fostered a sense of social support (Gubrium, 2009).

Interviewing in participatory action research

Participatory action research (PAR) is value-driven and has an explicit emancipatory agenda: it seeks to use knowledge to empower people and bring about change, stimulating critical consciousness alongside action (Baum et al., 2006). Central to PAR is the critique on the pursuit of an objective scientific truth through research. In PAR, the researcher commits to the local knowledge context of the communities. The purpose is not to test theory, but to uncover alternative lived realities or life histories. The value of research is foremost dependent on its usefulness for the community researched (Melro & Ballantyne, 2021). In PAR, knowledge is actively co-constructed by the action researchers and the communities through a 'cyclical process of fact finding, action, reflection, leading to further inquiry and action for change' (Macdonald, 2012). Interviews and focus groups with community members are mostly used at the start of the PAR cycle to obtain insight into the communities and their health issues. These inform which issues take priority, allowing for an understanding of the range of experiences and for the identification of whose voices are possibly excluded in the current community dialogues. PAR combines this with dialogic and participatory social learning approaches such as storytelling techniques, and tools such as photovoice (Burns et al., 2021).

PAR aims to bridge the chasm between 'subject' and 'object' in research, and this has an impact on how interviews and focus groups are being used. The researcher plays the role of facilitator of the process. However, processes of social change are not without challenges, as even activist researchers might have a different agenda than the communities (Pratt et al., 2020), and managing the power dynamics within communities might not be easy (Loewenson et al., 2014; Pratt et al., 2022b).

PAR has been used to act on indigenous health together with indigenous communities, for example to better understand and intervene on mental health, alcohol and drug comorbidities (Sharmil et al., 2021). Youth co-creation is a recent addition to the field of PAR, used to strengthen health promotion interventions or to enhance access to sexual and reproductive health services. Fakoya et al. (2022) describe how youth co-led the design and implementation of an intervention to enhance use of contraception in adolescents in Nigeria, Tanzania and Ethiopia, resulting in a more empathy-centred approach in implementation.

Critical realist interviewing

Brönniman (2022) recently published guidance on critical realist interviewing, building on the viewpoint of Manzano (2016) that there is a need for a realist interviewing approach to 'extract' the information that allows for theory development and refinement. Critical realism explicitly addresses power dynamics between communities or individuals and researchers by attempting to dampen its effects. The framework for realist interviewing developed by Brönniman is grounded in the work of Bhaskar and Archer, and relates to his concern for external validity and the replication of mechanisms. In his framework, the event under study is the entry-point for the interview, through which the interviewer unpacks with the interviewee the structure-agency-culture interactions behind the event. This approach requires iterative interviewing over a certain period of time to capture the interviewee's (changing) reflexive accounts regarding the potential for social change (similar to what Manzano suggested), and the structural and cultural conditions in which this happens (Brönniman, 2022). We argue that Brönniman's approach cannot be used in all interview settings. For one, it assumes a reflexivity on the part of the interviewee in relation to the structural and cultural conditions that impinge upon the event. Furthermore, Brönniman seems to align with analytical sociology, which considers social mechanisms as causal entities on their own (Harré & Moghaddam, 2016).

Critical realism has not yet been used much in global health research, perhaps because guidance for its use in global health is scant. In this book, Hastings presents a welcome 'recipe' for realist interviews in applied social science based on principles of critical realism. Also, Mukumbang and Dada report on the use of the photovoice methodology as a data collection tool for critical realist theorising (Mukumbang, 2020). The authors propose it as an alternative for focus groups and interviews when a study involves groups that have limited opportunity to express their voices. It thus can expand the range of represented voices and lived realities.

In summary, Table 7.1 illustrates the diversity of interview types and the differences in terms of the underlying paradigm, the purpose of the interview, the role of the interviewer and the interviewee and the use of theory.

Discussion

As Table 7.1 shows, few disciplines deal with power heads-on. Interviews are used as a data collection method by many disciplines, and these take different forms in function of the discipline's ontological and epistemological foundations. Interviews serve various goals, ranging from the detailed recording of the perceptions of interviewees to the empowerment of the interview participants by way of knowledge co-creation. In each approach, the role assigned to or played by the interviewee is different. Yet, in all interviews, power dynamics between researcher and interviewee are present.

Table 7.1 Diversity of interview types

Type of interview	Paradigm	Purpose	Role of the interviewer	Role of the interviewee	Use of theory during the interview
Interpretive interview	Interpretivism	To make sense of events.	Interviewer creates an opportunity in which a dialogue takes place.	Respondents direct the interview and convey meanings, values and ideas.	Usually none. Theories can provide a lens through interpretation post-interview.
Realist interview	Scientific realism	To obtain insights in CMO configurations and causal explanation at large concerning interventions.	Interviewer co-creates knowledge with the interviewee, in a dialogical approach.	Interviewee co-creates knowledge with the interviewer by reflecting on programme theories.	The programme theory is central to the interview and is critically reviewed by the interviewee.
Narrative interview	Interpretivist narrative inquiry and critical narrative inquiry	To uncover the participant's stories by way of interviewing and to trace (elements of) the story to social, economic and cultural structures.	Interviewers support the voice of people and communities.	Interviewees present their stories.	The term 'theory' is used to denote the causal explanations provided by the interviewee.
Interviewing in PAR	Constructivism and critical theory	To empower people, facilitate change and stimulate critical consciousness alongside action. PAR needs to be useful for the community involved in the research.	The researcher commits to the local knowledge context of the communities.	The interviewees offer the knowledge on which interventions can be built.	Usually none, realist (participatory) action research being an exception (Westhorp et al., 2016).
Critical realist interview	Critical realism	To develop causal explanations.	The interviewer unpacks structure-agency-culture interactions with the interviewee.	The interviewee reflects on the interaction between structure-agency-culture.	The middle-range theories are critically reviewed by the interviewee.

We argue that realist interviewing can be helpful in navigating the power differentials between interviewee and interviewer on condition that the positionality of both actors is acknowledged, and that a wide enough range of stakeholders (including representatives of marginalised groups where relevant) is included in the group of respondents. However, we also saw how issues related to power emerge when doing realist interviews. The case study presented by Prashanth N.S. showed not only that local power relations needed to be transformed so that interviewees are enabled to play an active role and the knowledge is truly co-produced. It also showed that it is essential that the interviewers acknowledge their gaze and are challenged and enabled to adopt a different perspective. The case study of Abejirinde confirmed the importance of creating a level playing field, and the substantial time which is required to build trust relationships. The case study presented by Hebbar showed how inverse power imbalances equally impede the co-production of knowledge. In all cases, power dynamics and stakeholder validation had to be actively managed.

Conclusion

Increasingly, research and evaluation of global health development programmes include participatory processes and stakeholder engagement to validate the contextual understanding of complex issues and their solutions. Yet, it is also a field where power differentials between respondent and interviewer are often amplified by the funding modalities and partnerships. We described some of the challenges encountered when doing realist interviews in research in the global South and compared realist interviewing with other interview techniques and approaches.

A key strength of realist interviewing is that it can allow the realist researcher to deepen the understanding of how context may trigger mechanisms and shape the intervention and the outcomes. Similar to the approach taken in critical narrative inquiry and critical realist interviewing, the analysis of 'context' within the CMO heuristic could be deepened if the realist interviewer pays specific attention to developing a better understanding of the interactions between structure, culture and agency. This is a much-needed next step in realist research if the aim is to check the applicability of so-called 'WEIRD' theories (Gilmore, 2019) in settings in the global south and develop programme theories that are taking into account local contexts more thoroughly.

8 Realist data collection in less familiar settings

Exploring challenges and strategies

Brynne Gilmore and Nadege Sandrine Uwamahoro

Introduction

Methodological challenges in the data collection phase of research are exacerbated in cases where researchers are unfamiliar with the research setting. Such instances are common within global health, where researchers from high-income nations often spearhead research in low- and middle-income countries. Foreign researchers are typically considered 'outsiders' because their cultural backgrounds differ from their research subjects. 'Culture' is a group's shared beliefs, values, customs and behaviours, influencing how members think, interact and express themselves. It is seen in language, religion, art and other factors that shape identities and societal norms (Singer et al., 2016). The advantages and disadvantages of the outsider vis-a-vis the insider perspective have been debated extensively by ethnographers and cross-cultural researchers (Liu & Burnett, 2022; Irvine et al., 2008). Researchers who share a language and cultural background with research participants ('insiders') may more easily establish access and trust compared to outsiders, and their knowledge of the research setting enables them to collect rich and culturally sensitive data (Merriam et al., 2001; Coloma, 2008; Falzon, 2016; Aburn et al., 2022). However, insiders may be more likely to be biased because of difficulties separating their individual experiences, feelings and ideas from those of participants (Kanuha, 2000; Abalkhail, 2021). The strengths of insiders highlight the weaknesses of 'outsiders', and their shortcomings underline the outsiders' strengths. When collaborating, an insider's cultural sensitivity complements the outsider's objectivity (Irvine et al., 2008; Liu & Burnett, 2022).

In many well-established research methodologies, discussions on challenges associated with conducting research in unfamiliar contexts are common, and researchers have ample guidance. However, conversations about conducting realist evaluations with an outsider's perspective in unfamiliar settings are emerging (Gilmore, 2019). This chapter will draw on the authors' direct experience collecting realist data, mainly through realist interviews (Manzano, 2016), as foreign researchers. It will focus on four frequently observed obstacles, which currently have little methodological guidance within

DOI: 10.4324/9781003457077-9

the realist space: power imbalance, understanding the research setting and identifying context, collecting data with the assistance of local research assistants and conducting realist interviews with participant groups that have been marginalised.

The studies and authors' experiences

The examples for this chapter come from three distinct research projects that used realist evaluation within four East African countries: Tanzania, Uganda, Kenya and Mozambique. In all cases, the authors led the realist evaluations. They were heavily involved in the realist interviews, including developing data collection plans, drafting interview guides, recruiting and training research assistants (RAs), recruiting participants, conducting interviews through the interpretation of RAs and data analysis. The authors are not from the contexts where the research was conducted, though they had varying experience levels in the research settings or similar contexts. The authors were also not fluent in the languages (except for English) spoken in the research settings, though they have conversational skills in Kiswahili and Portuguese. To our knowledge, these were the first realist evaluations undertaken within these regions/provinces. The studies were conducted in collaboration with academic researchers and implementation organisations.

One research project, with case studies in Tanzania and Uganda, involved an evaluation of a community-based maternal, newborn and child health programme implemented by non-governmental organisations (NGOs) within rural and community-based settings. Participants included community members, local healthcare workers, volunteer healthcare workers, NGO staff and relevant Ministry of Health staff. The languages used for data collection included Rukiga, Kiswahili and English. The study in Kenya evaluated a community engagement intervention implemented by an NGO to support health decision-making in Arid and Semi-Arid contexts. Participants included community members, local leaders, health staff and NGO staff. The languages used for data collection included Gabra, Borana, Maa, Kiswahili and English. In both research projects, RAs with no realist evaluation experience supported data collection and conducted realist interviews. The lead researcher/author for the two studies above is a white Canadian national who is now based in Ireland. For both studies, the author is considered an 'outsider'; however, they lived in East Africa for over five years and had previously worked in some of the research settings.

The Mozambican study is an ongoing comparative realist evaluation involving six maternity waiting homes (MWHs) in the Mozambican province of Inhambane. Maternity waiting homes are shelters located near healthcare facilities to enable timely access to skilled birth attendants and emergency obstetric care for remote and at-risk pregnant women (World Health Organization, 1996). This research seeks to test and refine nine programme theories regarding the intervention's uptake, which were developed through a realist review and synthesis of MWH literature from low-middle-income countries (Uwamahoro et al., 2022; Uwamahoro et al., 2024). Demand-side research participants include MWH users, non-users and their families. The supply-side participants involve community gatekeepers and policymakers at various health system levels, health providers, administrators and donors. Interviews were conducted in Portuguese, Xitswa and Chope by local RAs new to realist methodology. The lead researcher is of Danish nationality, born in Rwanda and raised in Zambia, with a background of living and studying in the United Kingdom. As a non-Mozambican without proficiency in Portuguese and the local languages, the author primarily occupied an outsider position. How-ever, she also had partial insider status in areas where her African background and experiences of living in countries with cultural similarities to Mozam-bique provided some connection.

Challenges of realist data collection in less familiar settings

Power imbalances

Power imbalances between researchers and participants are heavily discussed within qualitative methodologies. However, there have been limited discus-sions on power imbalances within realist evaluation (Gilmore, 2019; Ren-mans et al., 2022). In many qualitative research methods, it is acknowledged that both the researcher and the participant have power, though the power relations may not be equal. These imbalances are often, though not neces-sarily, heightened where there are social, cultural or economic differences between participants and the researcher. For instance, differences in educa-tion, access to resources as well as social or cultural norms, such as gender roles, can influence power dynamics, if not considered during designing data collection activities.

The three research studies presented in this chapter were conducted within global health and international development settings. A predicament can unfold where global health research, in its attempts to improve health and reduce inequity, may benefit from and exploit these inequities. Bena-tar and Fleischer (2007) warn about the exploitation of research partici-pants by taking advantage of power differences to meet the research goal of global health research. Any research can have large opportunity costs for participants; however, as global health research often involves populations with fewer resources or those who have been marginalised, these costs may be particularly pertinent. The potential for exploitation (whether intended or not) and large power imbalances require that global health researchers continually reflect upon and subsequently address these potential ethical dilemmas. Evaluation approaches in international development and global health research, including realist evaluation, are of Euro-Western origin and aim to advance the interests of Euro-Western stakeholders. However, ad-vocates for 'Made in Africa evaluation' and the decolonisation of global health argue that by addressing power imbalances and promoting the use of theories developed within Africa, realist evaluation shows potential for aligning with an Afro-centric epistemology (Mbava & Chapman, 2020; Renmans et al., 2022).

We both recognised power imbalances within our studies, which manifested in several ways and with different population groups. We believe these imbalances were brought about for several reasons, largely linked to our 'outsider' role and exacerbated through a lack of language skills on our behalf, education levels and association with the project or NGO teams. In settings new to realist methodology, such as the ones discussed in this chapter, the imbalance is further exacerbated by the lead researchers' knowledge regarding the methodology. This may be more apparent when the research lacks stakeholder involvement or participation throughout earlier research phases, including the Initial Programme Theory (IPT) development. However, we noticed bigger power differences between research assistants and participants due to variations in education, employment, place of residence (urban vs rural), association with the government, NGO or research institution and understanding of the research and its processes.

Of specific note is that power, or the consequence of the power imbalances, often became more apparent and influential during the directed theory development stages of the interview. For instance, and as discussed more thoroughly in later sections, we faced numerous challenges with refuting or refining some theories with certain participant groups. Though power imbalances may be impossible to extinguish in their entirety, we found some mitigating techniques, such as involving government stakeholders and communities throughout the research stages, including integrating an iterative feedback component and co-refinement of research theories. This also aligns with the African Evaluation principles, which recognise the imbalances in research capacity and expertise and recommend capacity building (Africa Evaluation Association, 2021). These perspectives seek to empower stakeholders through their engagement in the evaluation process. Stakeholder involvement is particularly important in realist evaluations led by researchers who are 'outsiders', where the context expertise of local stakeholders can be leveraged to ensure the quality of the data collection process and better determine the worth of the interventions under evaluation.

In the examples within this chapter, power imbalances were addressed through stakeholder engagement in varying degrees and approaches. For example, across all studies, stakeholders involved in designing the evaluation helped to anticipate problematic power imbalances between interviewers and interviewees and devised contextually sensitive mitigating strategies.

However, power is seen as a cross-cutting issue that influences the three more specific challenges of language, context and culture and unfamiliarity with the theory-driven approach. As such, particular approaches and recommendations are addressed more thoroughly in the subsequent sections.

Understanding the less familiar research setting

Realist researchers use their knowledge and 'hunches' of a programme and setting to uncover generative causation. However, what is the impact when realist research is conducted in less familiar contexts, and how can realist data collection in these situations be best leveraged to reduce any challenges?

Identifying underlying mechanisms and contexts, including socio-cultural and political situations, is frequently problematic (Lacouture et al., 2015; Shaw et al., 2018; Gilmore, 2019; Greenhalgh & Manzano, 2021; Nielsen et al., 2022). Another issue often highlighted by realist researchers is the difficulty of defining and distinguishing 'mechanisms' in relation to contexts (Marchal et al., 2012; Rycroft-Malone et al., 2012; Lemire et al., 2020). Identifying contextual elements has been seen as problematic, often because they are either not reported on (mostly within the literature) and/or participants have difficulty identifying everyday contextual conditions. Furthermore, multiple combinations of contexts and mechanisms can bring about one or several outcomes; thus, Context-Mechanism-Outcome configurations (CMOCs) are not always straightforward (De Weger et al., 2020; Van Belle et al., 2023). As programmes can have infinite CMOCs, developing meaningful configurations requires great detail and a skilled researcher. Thus, coding for and identifying CMOCs and theories requires a substantial amount of time that is often not anticipated (Tolson et al., 2007) and requires a considerable amount of teamwork, reflection and creativity – skills that are not always easily learned (Dalkin et al., 2015). Logistically, it can be challenging to determine how and when to conclude data collection, as theory can be continually refined. While the realist interview is meant to help elicit these relationships and unpack CMOCs, the researchers still require knowledge and insights into these elements.

Within this chapter's studies, the lead researchers did face challenges owing to their limited understanding of the organisational and socioeconomic context since the work was conducted in less familiar settings. People's behaviours were often shaped by a blend of traditional and religious norms, often not well-documented. Limited written information and data about contextual factors influencing implementation and intervention outcomes were available and/or accessible. In addition to the lack of documentation that helps identify context, the researchers sometimes struggled to elicit contexts and mechanisms from participants within the realist interview. Often, asking 'context-like' questions seemed obvious or redundant to the participant, with participants sometimes visibly confused or annoyed with the line of question, such as when asking general knowledge questions about community structures or processes or very general questions about people's understanding of pregnancy or childbirth. On the flip side, participants often misunderstood questions regarding mechanisms or did not articulate the 'whys' in the manner we were anticipating. While some of these might also come up in interviews in familiar settings, our lack of familiarity with the setting likely heightened these experiences.

As gaining insights into influential contexts and programme impacts is crucial when conducting realist evaluations, the researchers had to develop techniques to limit the negative effect of the limited understanding of the setting. By engaging local stakeholders in research design and implementation, we leveraged their comprehensive understanding of influential factors within the local context and the inner workings of evaluated interventions/programmes.

The Ugandan, Tanzanian and Kenyan studies employed multidisciplinary partnerships to enable insights that went beyond technical recommendations; clear communication channels were established to support the contribution of team members to the research process and allow more comprehensive analyses; procedures were taken to ensure engagement of decision-makers throughout the research process; reflexivity was built into the process which enabled the methodological challenges to be identified and addressed; and iterative cycles of data collection or finding dissemination sessions with participants were conducted to act as a 'validity check'. In addition, as discussed in more detail, the RAs were strategically utilised to help overcome this challenge.

The Mozambique study incorporated local stakeholder participation in alignment with the African Evaluation Principles (Africa Evaluation Association, 2021). Stakeholder involvement was organised by establishing a working group comprising representatives from participating communities, health facilities and provincial health authorities. These stakeholders were actively involved in deciding on programme theories to test, sampling, data collection methods, recruiting participants, anticipating issues during data collection and devising solutions and validating and nuancing preliminary findings. Equitable participation of these stakeholders was enhanced through a comprehensive introduction to realist methodology and immersion in the IPT through discussions around its applicability in the research context. Working group involvement is structured over four interactive workshops at different evaluation phases: pre-protocol development, pre-data collection, mid-data collection and analysis, with a pending workshop for the post-data collection and analysis phase.

The participation of individuals involved in programme implementation in evaluations is sometimes discouraged by scholars and evaluators due to concerns about potential confirmation and courtesy bias. These concerns may appear extra relevant for realist evaluation, given its focus on eliciting stakeholders' and participants' comments on the researcher's theory. Please see Chapter 2 for a more thorough discussion on the inclusion of stakeholders in realist evaluations. However, our concerns were alleviated when the discussion of the IPT with working group members elicited some 'aha moments', when they suddenly understood the mechanisms underlying some of their implementation outcomes or lack thereof. This unlocked opportunities for self-critical reflections on implementation. These discussions were recorded and formed part of the baseline data for the evaluation, which was instrumental in making initial refinements to the theory and research tools.

We encountered collective decision-making challenges due to differing priorities among working group members. Realist methodology experts advise focusing the evaluation of a few programme theories to enhance depth, so the evaluation commissioner and lead researcher would have liked to focus the evaluation on a subset of the nine IPTs (Punton et al., 2020). However, it was necessary to test all identified theories to accommodate the priorities of all stakeholders (Hansen & Vedung, 2010). While we got very useful insights from the pre-data collection workshop, engagement in this workshop was not as strong as in the subsequent workshops. This was due to several reasons, especially the fact that group members were yet to create rapport with each other and with the research team and they had not yet fully internalised the methodology and IPT. Workshop facilitation techniques evolved between workshops as the research coordinator gained a deeper comprehension of group dynamics. So far, the mid-data collection and analysis workshop was the most successful because preliminary findings sparked reflections and debates among working group members, revealing additional insights for theory refinement, including sensitive issues. However, the workshop also functioned as dissemination, with participants leaving the workshop with a commitment to improve care.

Interviewing different participant populations, especially those who have been marginalised

While realist evaluations often involve multiple methods, few detail or justify the methods chosen for specific participant groups. The realist interview is a fundamental tool within realist evaluation, yet its use or how to use it with different participant groups, such as children, adolescents, underserved and marginalised populations or persons with disabilities, has yet to be thoroughly explored. However, based on our studies' experience, participant groups may necessitate adjustments to tailor the realist interview to their capabilities.

In realist interviews, theory plays a central role, as it is explicitly and systematically integrated into every aspect of the interview process. Within a realist interview, the presentation of theory can serve as a conversation opener, enabling the interviewer to delve into different facets of the theory based on the participant's response. Nonetheless, because realist theories are often complex and pitched at a middle-range level of abstraction, engaging with them can place substantial demand on participants' abilities, particularly openness, critical thinking, communication and willingness to share ideas and opinions. Consequently, researchers need to consider the complexity of their IPT and devise approaches to present theories in a manner that aligns with the skills, capacities, abilities and preferences of intended participants and minimises courtesy and agreement bias. It is typically recommended to deconstruct complex theories into minor, partial theories to prevent undue burden on the participants and ensure a more productive and meaningful engagement in the interview process.

Generally, in our research contexts, participants' engagement in realist interviews was expected to pose challenges, especially for rural community members. This became evident in the first study in Uganda, which had many rural women as participants. Learning from the first several interviews in this study influenced subsequent interviews within Uganda. Tanzania, Kenya and Mozambique. A main challenge with some participant groups was a struggle with the collaborative theory refinement process. When presented with a theory, participants often hesitated to put forward their ideas or understanding, regularly agreeing with any position made by the researchers. The ability of the research team to 'dig deeper' was another challenge often faced. This meant it was difficult to get to reasons beyond the empirical or actual levels when identifying mechanisms by asking many 'why-type' questions. It also became obvious that this questioning annoyed or confused participants about why we asked many repetitive or simple questions. Refining theory solely based on interviews is not feasible, which is why data source triangulation is recommended (Manzano, 2016). However, due to limited access to alternative data sources for triangulation in the research contexts, we prioritised generating as much theory-refining data through interviews as possible.

Challenges arose mainly when the participant groups were community members, often living in more rural settings. One reason might be that they were unfamiliar with a realist interview style, especially since, as earlier mentioned, realist methods rely on Euro-Western forms of knowing and reasoning, which differ from Afro-indigenous approaches. Moreover, education systems in these countries often feature teacher-dominated and didactic teaching methods, with limited emphasis on encouraging students to question teachers, who are seen as the primary knowledgeable authority (Tabulawa, 2013). This can also be related to power imbalances discussed previously. For example, an educated, foreign researcher 'teaching' participants about his/her/their ideas and theories and then asking participants to 'teach' back by sharing their thoughts on the researcher's ideas and theories could be perceived as 'tell us where we were wrong'.

To overcome or limit the effect of some of these challenges, all of the studies used some common techniques. First, having local RAs or persons from the area who were collecting data was important. This is discussed further in the following section. Second, allowing appropriate time for informal meetings and discussions before the interview to make the participants more comfortable. Third, thoroughly introducing the interview style and give examples of how it might unfold or differ from other interview styles. However, when explaining, it is particularly important to use less intimidating language, for instance, by removing words like theory, refinement, teaching, etc. Fourth, start the interview with more open-ended, non-theory-driven questioning to open the dialogue and have reference material if the conversation stalls. These simple techniques were found to be important across the studies.

In addition, more specific tactics were used in some of the studies, which had varying degrees of success. In Uganda and Tanzania, a visual representation of the theories under testing was developed and shared with participant groups. The idea was that the participants and research team could draw and edit the visuals together. This approach was not as effective during the early stages of theory refinement when the theories were not as specific. It was more helpful when the participants were fed back results for theory validation towards the end of the study.

In the Mozambique study, the initial interview guide included more open-ended questions than theory-presenting ones. However, following advice from others, we revised the interview guide and included the presentation of partial theories as conversation openers. With input from local RAs and local project staff, efforts were made to present partial theories in a culturally sensitive manner and to vary the way in which theory was presented. In this study, we encountered difficulties interviewing women aged 18 to 24. In this age group, all participants were reticent and spoke minimally. They tended to align with the presented theories unless, in a few cases, the participants in question strongly disagreed. Consequently, we devised a strategy where we only interviewed MWH users and non-users who were above 24, but we interviewed some companions and male partners of women under 24 to indirectly gain insights about this population. We also experienced that single-gender focus groups were better at eliciting women's voices than mixed-gender groups.

Across all the studies, getting detailed responses, particularly from community members, was difficult and required the research teams to use many open-ended follow-up questions to uncover thoughts and feelings. Open-ended questions represented a risk of RAs losing track of the theory-testing agenda of the interview, especially when this is done through translation. Balancing the need for enough questions and prompts to assist novice realist data collectors while allowing research participants to shape the interview's direction posed a challenge. Including prompts of follow-up questions in the interview guide proved valuable for RAs, particularly when participants were hesitant or reserved. When participants had much to share, RAs understood the significance of asking follow-up questions based on participants' responses, aiming to delve deeper into the contexts, mechanisms and outcomes. This approach enabled us to cater to diverse participant needs while providing valuable support to RAs.

For all studies, techniques used to accommodate the interview style to participants included adjusting the language (removing terms such as 'teaching' or 'theory'), continual encouragement for more contribution and referring to topics the participants discussed in focus groups or individual interviews, specifically things that would refine or reject our theory.

In the Tanzanian, Kenyan and Ugandan studies, while these techniques did assist in fostering more input from participants, the most influential modification occurred when the participants first taught us their theory (with guidance from us based on what the discussions entailed). While this was only done in a couple of interviews, adjusting the interview technique in this way proved a valuable adaptation to adjust for power imbalances within the interview. While this is not an exhaustive list of potential challenges, it does highlight that the realist interview cannot be conducted similarly across all participant groups and that adjustments may be required to ensure the interview's success.

Realist interviewing through others: research assistants and/or translators

Limited language and cultural proficiency hinder foreign researchers from conducting interviews independently, without the help of interpreters or assistance from local researchers or data collectors. However, there is a serious lack of information or guidance on conducting realist interviews through RAs and/or interpreters. Few cross-cultural realist evaluation publications exist, and not all include reflections or information on how they worked with translators, interpreters or local data collectors, or if they did. Given the realist interview's task of theory development and how the data from these interviews undergoes retroductive analysis, including using the researcher's hunches, the conversation on what interviews through translation means for the realist evaluation needs to be ongoing.

Gilmore's (2019) considerations and recommendations are based on this chapter's Ugandan and Tanzanian examples. In this section, we will discuss these existing recommendations and incorporate further insights and lessons derived from the Mozambican study, focusing on the role of increased participation of RAs, including translators, interpreters and local data collectors.

The lead researcher conducted interviews in the Kenyan, Ugandan and Tanzanian cases with the support of an interpreter/RA (Gilmore, 2019). This happened in two ways, depending on the participant group and RA confidence. (1) When the RA was less confident or there was a particularly challenging interview, there was more 'direct' RA translation from the lead researcher to the participant. This often resulted in longer interviews due to the need for on-site translation but more focused theory refinement. (2) When the RA was more confident or the participant was more open and talkative, the RA would conduct the interview solely, updating the lead researcher only at certain key points during the interview. This resulted in a more flowing, shorter and pleasant interview, but it did run the risk of missing some key opportunities for theory refinement. In all studies, the lead researchers conducted English interviews, typically with NGOs, Ministry of Health staff and policy-makers.

In Mozambique, a few policy-level stakeholder interviews were done with interpretation support. The lead researcher's Portuguese was not good enough to conduct an interview, but it did allow her to identify instances when the interpreter omitted information and requested an interpretation of the missing details. Interpreter-supported interviews required more time, so to comply with the time limit outlined in the consent form, we prioritised certain theories for testing in each interview, guided by our initial understanding of the participant's knowledge and experience with the intervention.

Using an interpreter also limits the direct verbal and non-verbal contact between the researcher and the person being interviewed. Subtle tone or emotional expression changes may go unnoticed by the foreign researcher. Likewise, interpreting the facial expressions of interview participants correctly can be challenging. While the researcher can inquire with the interpreter after the interview, this may result in missed opportunities for valuable insights to refine theories. To address this, the study's RAs interpreted and followed up on meaningful non-verbal cues during the interview. When the RAs noticed discrepancies between participants' facial expressions and words, they rephrased the questions or sought clarification. This demonstrates the importance of involving interpreters in the research as RAs and not as ad-hoc communication facilitators.

For the Mozambique and Tanzania studies, the lead researchers could speak some Portuguese and Kiswahili, respectively, enabling them to establish a relationship with the interviewee through a casual chat before the interview. This aligns with recommendations within cross-cultural research that outsider-lead researchers must learn key phrases in the interview language, greet interviewees in their language and maintain contact during interviews (eye contact, nodding, smiling) to build trust (Bragason, 1997).

Across all studies, it became clear that RAs, including interpreters, need a deep understanding of the methodology and interview objectives to gather theory-refining data effectively, enabling them to interpret relevant information accurately. Equally, they needed to be very knowledgeable of the theories under test so that their questioning could constantly work towards theory development or refinement. This is crucial because interviewees, especially those with strong opinions, often share a wealth of information in one go. In such instances, RAs need to digest and summarise essential information, and a lack of comprehension regarding the realist evaluation may lead to omitting vital details for theory refinement.

Given the central role of context in realist evaluation, researchers must harness the insider perspectives of RAs. The data collection task should not merely be translating/interpreting or conducting interviews, respectively. Their active role in the research, especially in interview situations, means that a successful outcome depends on how they are selected and trained.

Selecting research assistants for realist evaluation studies

Conducting a realist interview is not easy. Therefore, it is especially difficult and potentially messy when done through translation and/or by individuals unfamiliar with the methodology, the theories or both. Realist evaluation RAs need to be knowledgeable of the methodology. Still, they must also understand the theories undergoing revisions throughout the interview to be able to 'on the spot' and collaboratively refine the theories with the participant based on their conversations and any generative causation being uncovered. It is also ideal if RAs understand the area/domain knowledge of the research because more effort can be spent imparting realist methodology and interviewing skills. Furthermore, like in any other qualitative research approach, RAs in realist evaluations should have the qualifications of a competent realist interviewer.

However, these were the first known realist evaluations conducted in these settings, and no researchers from the setting identified with prior knowledge of realist methodology and realist interviewing experience. Therefore, these prerequisites needed to be imparted through training. The language proficiency of RAs plays a pivotal role in producing high-quality interviews and transcripts (Vulliamy, 1990). It is even more significant in the context of realist interviews, which deal with abstract theories, thereby demanding advanced language and communication skills. Selecting qualified RAs can be challenging when dealing with more than two languages. For example, the Mozambican study blended Portuguese and Xitswa or Chope. Knowing the RAs' language proficiency guided decisions regarding allocating RAs to specific interviews and transcription tasks. Within the Kenyan study, four sites comprised three different tribes, each with its own language, so a minimum of three RAs needed to be hired and trained. Assessing candidates to confirm their interviewing and language proficiency is recommended. However, when no candidate has experience with realist interviewing, assumptions about their ability might need to be made. Alternatively, it might be necessary to hire on a trial basis until a candidate's ability to acquire realist interviewing skill has been determined.

Successful realist interviews require interviewers to create an atmosphere where participants feel comfortable to share their honest opinions, and as this is not easily teachable, it is important to factor it into RA selection criteria.

Training translators and/or research assistants to conduct realist interviews

If RAs conduct realist interviews independently, the training must cultivate a 'theory-testing mindset', enabling them to craft effective theory-testing questions during interviews (O'Rourke et al., 2022). RAs in all studies had prior qualitative interviewing experience, so the lead researchers taught RAs how and why realist interviewing differs from qualitative interviewing through a comprehensive introduction to realist methodology. The emphasis in realist evaluation on theory development and testing was highlighted. RAs were also introduced to the Initial Programme Theory (IPT), which was thoroughly explained and discussed, along with the evaluation design and the interview guide.

The training sessions provided opportunities for RAs to evaluate and provide feedback on research materials initially developed by the lead researchers. Their feedback aimed to enhance the translation of realist questions and make the information and questions more culturally relevant and meaningful. As in the study by O'Rourke et al. (2022), content that did not translate meaningfully into the language of the interview or that proved challenging to translate was reframed (e.g., the realist questions with the format: *'What is it about x that makes a difference?'* were reframed to *'what makes x good or bad?'* in the Mozambique study).

As IPTs can be complex, ensuring the RAs understand their logic and meaning is essential for the realist interview. For example, in Mozambique, the IPT was comprehensive, describing relationships across 19 contexts, 11 mechanisms and 31 outcomes. RAs requested support in unpacking the theories via prompts in the interview guide. The theories were also unpacked by including questions with partial theories pitched at a more granular level of abstraction. In addition, a column was included with suggestions for concrete follow-up questions and prompts. Similarly, interventions, programmes and services assessed using realist methodology are typically complex. Therefore, providing a comprehensive introduction to the intricacies of the subject being evaluated and relating these to the IPT is essential. This equips RAs to recognise when interviewees provide information relevant to theory refinement.

In all studies, what RAs found useful during the training was seeing and doing rather than explaining realist interviews. Their understanding significantly improved when they had the opportunity to review a realist interview transcript. This exposure helped them grasp how the IPTs were developed and emphasised the importance of being well-versed in these theories to test and apply them effectively. It was imperative to create space and time for RAs to deepen their understanding of the IPT, the intervention and the realist interview, practice their skills and receive constructive feedback.

In Mozambique, RAs were involved in the pre-data collection workshop, which involved discussions on logistics, recruitment and overall interview etiquette. In this workshop, RAs had the opportunity to pilot the interview guides and refine their interviewing skills by interviewing working group members and receiving feedback from interviewees. Following these pilot interviews, the lead researcher meticulously reviewed the transcripts and provided individual written feedback to each RA. A group reflection session was also conducted, featuring an experienced realist researcher reviewing the transcripts and offering general feedback to the RAs. Additionally, we organised a mock interview conducted by the lead researcher with interpretation support, which RAs observed. Using different collaborative approaches to impart knowledge and skills proved invaluable for RAs' development and preparation.

Ongoing supervision of research assistants throughout data collection

Because learning by doing was the most effective approach to learning, data collection commenced once RAs had grasped the basics across all projects. However, regular supervision and feedback were arranged to support their realist interviewing skills' continuous development and improvement. As Gilmore (2019) highlights, reflexivity is pivotal in ensuring high-quality realist interviews in unfamiliar contexts. Data was collected in intervals, and team reflection and feedback sessions occurred between intervals in all studies. In Mozambique, RAs wrote guided reflexive notes after each interview, which informed team reflection and feedback sessions with the lead researchers. In all studies, RAs were responsible for transcribing their research interviews, which helped them to process interviews and identify areas needing improvement. This also allowed them to incorporate tone of voice and body language into the transcript, which are valuable for realist data analysis. These components were included in parenthesis, and RAs included their interpretation of the meaning of the non-verbal cues.

RAs, like many realist researchers, often struggled to explore all theory components, with their primary challenge being identifying mechanisms. The best practice we have identified for uncovering mechanisms is instructing RAs to ask 'why' about everything the participants say. However, RAs found it challenging to ask 'why' repeatedly. Therefore, this approach was supplemented with questions about how participants felt or thought about experiences and intervention resources or the lack thereof.

A key challenge identified across all studies was RAs' perceived need to explore all theories in the interview guide, leading to shallow testing of individual theories. To address this, we advised them to focus on specific theories based on assumptions about each participant group's contributions. To further guide them the teams developed introductory open-ended questions to help RAs understand interviewees' expertise and prioritise theory exploration. They emphasised to data collectors that depth was more crucial than breadth, encouraging in-depth explorations of fewer theories during interviews. The shallow exploration of theories was also partly due to RAs' struggle to keep the conversation going. When the conversation stalled or the participants had difficulty responding to theory-driven questions, the RAs could use their knowledge of the subject to link it back to the preliminary discussions.

Another challenge is posing appropriate theory-testing follow-up questions, given the complexity of the theories under test. Interview guides with some theory testing questions are essential, but depending on the participant's response, it is difficult to have a guide which can be directly followed. As the interviewer needs to continue the theory-directed questioning, having some key prompts or 'theory-driven questioning' phrases can help the RA. Teaching data collectors to think critically and theorise during interviews is necessary but can be challenging. Ensuring sufficient time for piloting, practising and reviewing transcripts is necessary. Especially in the early phases of data collection, it is important not to rush but to allow time for transcription and review after each interview to develop these skills. It might also be helpful for RAs to be involved in a preliminary analysis, which can give them an idea of how the data would be used to refine the theory, thereby increasing their understanding of retroductive reasoning and the type of information needed to refine the theory. Overall, collaborating with RAs to tailor the interview guide to their evolving needs helped to increase their sense of control of the interview process.

Within qualitative and cross-cultural research, when conducting interviews to test theories, there arises a question regarding how much information the researcher should disclose to the interpreter or data collector beforehand. This dilemma stems from the potential for unintentional bias in interpretation and the questions posed by the interpreter or data collector due to foreknowledge (Udai & Rao, 1975; Roller & Lavrakas, 2015) However, our experience shows that training interpreters and data collectors can address this issue by seeking and noticing information that supports and challenges the theory rather than solely confirming it. The Mozambique study achieved this by emphasising the importance of seeking information that could refute or nuance the theory during training. During group feedback and reflection sessions, passages in the transcript containing potential new or rival theories that lacked adequate follow-up by RAs were discussed. RA's ability to tailor how much of the theory to share with a participant was strengthened through ongoing feedback.

Involvement of translators and/or research assistants in realist analysis

The input of interpreters and RAs is also vital to understanding the collected data when interviewing happens through translation. Discussions around decolonising global health research highlight the importance of equitable and meaningful local research involvement, including in interpreting and analysing data, among many things (Pant et al., 2022). Ideally, this involvement cultivates a sense of ownership of the research, and for our studies, we believe it made RAs more confident and independent realist interviewers and researchers. Having RAs analyse data with the wider team and collaboratively work to refine theories based on the findings is likely to improve the quality of the work. As the RAs conducted the interviews, their understanding of the data was essential. They are also more likely to understand any nuances of the data that outsiders might miss, such as culturally relevant sayings or examples. Their 'hunches' will also be informed by more relevant examples, thereby supporting more accurate theories.

Where it is impossible to include RAs or translators in the data analysis and theory refinement stages, Gilmore (2019) suggests interviewing them at certain points throughout the study. These time points might be when a specific participant group's data collection is complete or when a theory under exploration is exhausted. These interviews aim to understand the RAs' ideas and hunches on the theories based on their cultural understanding and insights accumulated during the interviews. In the Kenyan, and in the Ugandan and Tanzanian studies, the lead researcher conducted individual lengthy interviews with RAs after completing each case. In both studies, a half-day meeting was arranged, consisting of a 'debrief' on the study overall. This included asking the RAs how training, communication and logistics could be improved for future studies and asking them their overall thoughts on the study and the methodology. Then, the lead researchers conducted a theory-driven style interview with the RAs. After completing all interviews, the RAs were asked to consider all the insights gained and answer the research questions based on their thoughts about each theory. Lastly, in the Kenyan and Ugandan and Tanzanian studies, RAs and the lead researcher collaboratively refined the programme theories based on the interview and prepared case study-specific findings. The findings from these exercises were used to support the lead researcher's analysis of the other interview transcripts and to refer back to when there were inaccuracies, inconsistencies or questions regarding the interviews or emerging findings. The Mozambique study involved RAs in the analysis by seeking their comments on thoughts on findings at different stages. For example, they discussed preliminary findings with working group members and helped to elicit deeper insights for the analysis.

Overall, working through RAs, including data collectors and interpreters, is challenging in any context, and the same applies to realist interviews. However, with the growing interest in realist evaluations, the need to conduct realist interviews through translation will likely increase. Researchers are encouraged to document and detail their processes and lessons learned so that we can continue advancing this topic and share examples of good practice.

Moving forward: Recommendations for conducting realist interviews in unfamiliar settings

Numerous recommendations for conducting realist interviews in less familiar settings have been given throughout this chapter. These are not exhaustive and are drawn based on our experience across only a few East African research settings. Any new or unfamiliar setting will likely bring different challenges in terms of the realist interview or at least require different approaches to mitigate any of these challenges.

However, based on our experiences and observations, an approach that can assist realist evaluations being conducted in less familiar settings is collaborative stakeholder engagement, including the involvement of RAs in the evaluation process. However, a recent scoping review by Manzano (2024) found that in most realist evaluations, stakeholder engagement is often ambiguous or used intermittently in targeted evaluation phases, with few adopting an integrated approach. The study also found that in realist evaluations, the evaluator remains in charge and concluded that realist evaluation aims to determine the programme's value and accountability, not social justice or empowerment. Experiences from the cases informing this chapter demonstrate that the research process can be empowering without compromising the research end goal of determining the worth of an intervention or programme.

Conclusion

While there are many under-explored methodological questions in realist interviewing, this chapter focuses on the challenges of interviewing participants across unfamiliar cultures and settings. The chapter provides some guidance and recommendations based on the authors' experience conducting realist evaluations as foreign researchers in Kenya, Mozambique, Tanzania and Uganda. The authors recognise that this is just the beginning of the conversation, and more work is needed on this topic. For example, there is still a need to explore and document how realist interviewing can be adapted for data collection from groups that require special consideration, such as children or adolescents and diverse marginalised groups. Similarly, considerations for interviewing on sensitive topics or when the participant is placed in a particularly vulnerable position require further exploration.

No doubt, with the rising popularity of the realist evaluation, and thus realist interview, these conversations will begin to emerge. Researchers must choose approaches that adhere to methodological standards and procedures that are as ethical and respectful to participants as possible. Documenting and sharing learning and having open and honest discussions about the realist interview process can contribute towards improved practices across all realist projects and for all participant groups.

Acknowledgements

The MWH research discussed in this chapter stems from the bilateral Mozambique-Canada Maternal Health Project (2018), funded by Global Affairs Canada. The insights shared herein were made possible through the contributions of various individuals: Prof. Nazeem Muhajarine, the project's principal investigator; Jessie Forsyth, project director for Canada; project team members, including drivers, administrative personnel, and notably, the technical team consisting of Argentina Munguambe, Ruta Massunguine, Horácio Mandevo Chissaque and António Tanda; Fernanda Andre, a doctoral candidate within the project; our methods advisor, Brynne Gilmore; the diligent research assistants Assucena João Maite, Mariza Fortunato, Samuel Fabio and Tania Fernandes; Dadiva Mafala, our fieldwork coordinator; Dorcia Mandlate, the research coordinator from the Inhambane Provincial Health Directorate; translators, Eduarte Massingue and Walter Malambane; and, of course, the invaluable working group members and research participants.

The projects in Uganda and Tanzania were in partnership with World Vision Ireland, World Vision Uganda and World Vision Tanzania, with generous support from Irish Aid. The work would not have been possible without the support of the communities in North Rukiga, Uganda and Bahai District, Dodoma, Tanzania and the Ministries of Health and implementation staff. This includes Limi Malimi, Modest Kessy, Henry Mollel, Gilbert Ahumuza, Nazarius Mbona Tumwesigye and Gloria Nahabwe. The project in Kenya was in collaboration with Concern Worldwide Kenya, with funding from the European Union's Horizon 2020 research and innovation programme under the Marie Skłodowska-Curie grant agreement No 713279. It was made possible through a dedicated team of implementers, researchers and community members, including Yacob Yishak, Zaccheous Mutunga, Walton Omollo, Mollu Wario, Irene Ekalo, Guyo Dalacha and Kame Konchora.

9   Qualitative realist interviews using online video technology – challenges and opportunities

Emma Williams

Introduction

The COVID-19 pandemic forced greater use of online alternatives to face-to-face communication in many homes and workplaces, and straitened fieldwork options for researchers and evaluators. Although face-to-face communication is no longer blocked due to fears of contagion, there has not been a reversion to pre-COVID patterns. The growing awareness of the importance of environmental sustainability has become a deterrent to travel, especially air travel, if there are adequate alternatives. Many people have gained skills in online communication, own or have access to the devices required and are used to the convenience of being able to see and talk to others from their homes or other preferred locations at times convenient for them. Technology continues to develop; ongoing developments in generative artificial intelligence (AI) are making it increasingly likely that interviews will not just be conducted online, but may also involve an AI interviewer. Research interviews, such as those conducted for realist evaluations, are being affected by these technological and social developments, which offer both opportunities and challenges.

Distance interviews have been conducted for many years, using phone calls, text/email messages and other methods, some compared against face-to-face interviewing (Sturges & Hanrahan, 2004; Novick, 2008; Irvine, 2011; Vogl, 2013; Lobe et al., 2022). This chapter focuses on video interviewing, and the opportunities and challenges provided to realist interviewers using platforms such as Skype, Zoom, Google Meet, Microsoft Teams, FaceTime and similar products. Video interviewing can engage an increasing range of participants, including some who might be difficult to reach in person, but may exclude particular types of potential participants. Video interviews affect communication dynamics, with less visual information available than when interviewing face-to-face. Although they can substantially reduce travel costs, they require other resources that need to be considered, and they raise ethical issues that are less likely to apply in face-to-face interviewing. Group interviews and interviewing across cultures and languages raise additional issues. This chapter begins by examining overarching contextual factors that need to be considered in determining whether and how to conduct video interviews.

DOI: 10.4324/9781003457077-10

Subsequently, it explores the particularly high cognitive demands placed on realist interviewers, and suggests strategies to overcome these challenges, illustrating these with a realist research study investigating accountability to children and communities in international consortia.

Overarching contextual factors in video interviewing

Access and inclusion

No mode of communication is equally available to all potential participants. However, the increased use of technology during COVID-19 has led some groups, once considered unlikely to use video technology – such as the elderly – to develop considerable skills in online communication (Boland et al., 2022). Video interviewing may enable engagement with people who would have struggled to participate in face-to-face interviewing, and can democratise research participation (Lo Iacono et al., 2016) by enabling participation from widely dispersed locations within a country or internationally – providing that language and cultural issues are addressed. Video interviews may be suitable for participants challenged by mobility issues, whether caused by remote locations and/or lack of travel infrastructure, physical impairments or commitments that impede travelling, such as those of farmers or parents of young children. They may also benefit some neurodiverse people or those with mental health conditions such as anxiety or agoraphobia (Keen et al., 2022). These issues are not exclusive to interview participants; online interviewing opens up opportunities for fieldwork participation for realist researchers and interviewers who may have mobility challenges or face other barriers.

There are some potential participants for whom video interviews will not be suitable due to lack of access to or fears of technology. In some cases, these barriers can be overcome; Roberts et al. (2021) explained how they worked with shelters to enable homeless people's participation in video interviews through supported access to technology and Wi-Fi connections. However, even where project budgets and timelines enable this type of support, not everyone will have – or want – access to the devices and connections used for video interviews. Participants in realist studies are selected according to their potential to contribute to theory development or testing (Manzano, 2016). In instances where key contributors are unavailable online, even with support, employing multiple channels of communication becomes necessary rather than solely relying on online platforms.

Communication dynamics

Talking and listening via video differs from face-to-face communication in multiple ways. Working with shared visual materials onscreen can be challenging; Roberts et al. (2021) noted this with maps and flyers. Another obvious difference is that online sound and visual quality can range from excellent to poor, and there is the potential for the sound and/or picture to drop out entirely during the conversation. With any platform, it is advisable to have contingency plans and for the interviewer and participant(s) to have alternate ways to contact each other, such as exchanging email addresses and/or phone numbers prior to the interview.

However, even with a stable communication channel, what is seen in a video interview is only a fraction of what is observable in a face-to-face situation. Crucial context clues often get lost in translation. The absence of 'body language' deprives the interview of behavioural clues such as changes in posture or muscular tension that would be used in face-to-face communication (Itzchakov & Grau, 2022). Viewing one's own face onscreen can be distracting (Itzchakov & Grau, 2022; Seitz et al. 2022). Although faces are visible onscreen, facial communication is affected. Eye contact when facing each other through an onscreen camera is different from standard face-to-face communication (Paradisi et al., 2021) and video interviews tend to involve prolonged direct eye gazing, much more than would be natural in face-to-face conversations (Karl et al., 2022). To compensate for the loss of visual information, aural information becomes more important; to indicate active listening, there may be more sounds used than in face-to-face communication (Hall, 2024). These factors contribute to what has been referred to as 'Zoom fatigue'; those conducting video interviews are therefore advised to build in longer breaks than might be necessary with in-person interviews (Karl et al., 2022). A video interview may be tiring for a participant, but a series of them can be exhausting for an interviewer.

Another communication factor is the degree to which participants feel comfortable with video interviews, as this may affect the amount and type of information obtained; interviewers may therefore have to offer multiple platforms. Participants competent in their preferred platform can direct more attention to conversing and thinking through issues before responding. There is conflicting evidence on other factors that make participants feel comfortable and on how distance interviews affect which types of disclosure. Although participants with social phobias (Keen et al., 2022) may benefit from being able to talk in a place where they feel safe without another person in their space, Irvine (2011) noted that distance interviewing provides fewer opportunities for rapport-building activities such as small talk and offering refreshments. To compensate, some interviewers have developed online rapport-building strategies, such as each person simultaneously preparing a drink together pre-interview. Alternatively, email correspondence prior to the interview, or even working together to address technical glitches during the interview, can build rapport (Roberts et al., 2021). However, some participants may value video interviews for their efficiency as well as convenience, and welcome the lack of small talk.

Finally, video interviewing technology enables communications not available in face-to-face interview, which can be of great potential value. Written information may be provided through the chat function. Simultaneous transcription (Lobe et al., 2022) and even translation of conversations is becoming increasingly available as a feature in video communications. This facilitates the inclusion of people with cognitive and hearing impairments as well as speakers of other languages in video interviews.

Resource allocation: time and finances

Although it is important to build in adequate contingency time for technical glitches and communication outages, video interviews can save significant time and/or financial resources compared to those that require travel between interviews. However, there are other areas where online interviewing may require additional investment, such as in equipment and software applications. Additionally, investment is required in training interviewers to conduct online interviews, troubleshoot technical difficulties and handle communications when connections fail. Investing in time for product research is also required, as technology and participant preferences change rapidly; what worked best a year ago may not be the right choice for an upcoming project. Finally, in some cases, two interviewers may be necessary for online interviewing (Carr & Groot, this volume; Roberts et al., 2021). The second interviewer can attend to technology issues and other tasks such as taking notes, enabling the primary interviewer to focus on the interpersonal and cognitive demands of the interview.

Ethical issues

Video interviews can raise particular ethical challenges. Ensuring privacy when communicating online is not easy, especially as not all video interviewing platforms have equivalent security features. Four types of threats to security need to be noted: a participant recording the interview without permission; accidental intrusions by relatives, housemates, or colleagues sharing the participant's space; deliberate online intrusions such as 'Zoombombing' (Lobe et al, 2020); and monitoring of online communications by third parties, such as monitoring for terrorism-related terms or potentially to collect data for generative AI applications (Lo Iacono et al., 2016). The first two threats are best addressed by setting out privacy guidelines for participants, although the interviewer is unlikely to be able to monitor this effectively and must trust that participants will abide by verbal or written guidelines. The second two are best addressed through careful research into the security features enabled by each platform, which constantly evolve. However, many security features, such as waiting rooms and/or passwords to enter video sites, may affect participant ease of use (Lobe et al, 2020), so trade-offs also need to be considered.

Other ethical issues, such as power differentials, participant consent, participant distress, and the ability to withdraw from interviews, are influenced by the dynamics of online interviewing (Lobe et al., 2020; Boland et al., 2022), sometimes in positive ways. Information about the interview is typically sent online well before the interview date and some researchers have noted the value of back-and-forth exchanges about the interview and the topics that will be covered. There are multiple ways to get informed consent forms signed online, or to have participants verbally indicate their consent at the beginning of the interview and have it recorded. Participants in an online interview, compared to a face-to-face interview, can more easily withdraw if they feel uncomfortable. They can just switch off, with or without an explanation, rather than confront the interviewer. On the other hand, there is reduced opportunity to intervene personally if participants become distressed during the interview. Online interviewing on sensitive topics needs to be considered extremely carefully, and additional safeguards may be required, such as ensuring a person able to offer aid if needed is located near the person being interviewed, is aware of the interview and ready to offer support as needed. Not a great deal of literature exists on how online interviewing affects potential power differentials, but Boland et al. (2022) indicate that multiple online interactions can reduce power inequities over time.

Group interviews

Online group interviews and focus groups offer considerable challenges, including the potential for one or more participants to record others (Lobe et al., 2020). Also, with the exception of the person speaking, visual information is sparse within the very small images displayed onscreen when there are multiple participants, making it difficult to grasp group dynamics. Body language clues to matters such as who would like to speak, or who strongly disagrees with the viewpoint being presented, are difficult for the moderator to pick up. However, the online format offers alternatives such as a 'raise hand' button or equivalent, and the chat function has the potential to provide even richer information than face-to-face focus groups as simultaneous offerings are possible, and some participants may be willing to write views they would not have shared aloud. Ideally, at least one additional researcher would be available to help facilitate the group process, taking the lead on technical issues and monitoring chats (Roberts et al., 2021).

Online interviewing across cultures and languages

Language and culture are often interlinked, but each can present distinct issues and be impacted differently in online work. In regard to cultural issues in international projects, travel to interview sites, particularly international sites, although expensive, time-consuming and environmentally unsustainable, presents opportunities for building contextual cultural awareness. Observations of how people communicate and interact can teach the interviewer about body language, expected distances between conversing people and any age and gender-specific social norms for conversations, including protocols for turn-taking, a critical element of effective conversation (Boland et al., 2022). When travelling, researchers are often accompanied by a driver and/or organisational representative who can provide knowledge on local protocols and who also frequently perform introductions before moving away to provide privacy for the interview. In face-to-face communications where there are language variants, body language supplements spoken information and lip-reading can help to distinguish unfamiliar sounds. In online interviews, on the other hand, the interviewer typically must introduce themselves and may have had little exposure to local communication protocols. As noted above, auditory and visual communications are considerably less rich than in face-to-face interactions.

In cross-language work (or cross-language variants such as dialects, regional variations or accents within the same language), online environments exacerbate issues that occur to a lesser degree in face-to-face interviews. There is a considerable literature on the cognitive demands of listening in different types of circumstances, and researchers have developed multiple methods for measuring their impact (McLaughlin et al., 2021) such as word recall tests, or observing pupil dilation as an indicator of processing difficulty. Some of these methods have begun to be applied to studying the cognitive demands of listening to speech in other languages. Processing capacity in any individual is limited, so that speed and accuracy of cognitive tasks such as comprehending a conversation and working out what question to answer next are affected by listening to different accents or variants. Online communication, especially where sound quality is imperfect, makes processing even more difficult. Cristia et al. (2012) note that the effect of sound interference is greater when processing another language variant than when working in one's own language variant. Peelle (2018) notes that processing capacity is affected both by comprehending other language variants and by imperfect sound quality – and the effect is cumulative.

In addition, listening to variants significantly different from one's own language variant impacts working memory, a term used for the systems in the brain that temporarily store information and enable both language comprehension and reasoning (Baddeley, 1992). When speaking in one's own language variant, most linguistic processing is automatic. However, processing unfamiliar accents, vocabulary or syntax can engage parts of the brain that might otherwise focus on planning follow-up questions (Federmeier et al., 2020).

Not all types of interviews are equally affected. Structured interviews with a pre-determined script demand minimal planning for responses. 'Interpretive interviews', where the participant directs the conversation (Scheibelhofer, 2023), diminish the frequency of follow-up questions. In forensic/investigative interviewing, the aim is to interview witnesses, victims and (suspected) perpetrators of incidents, seeking through the interviews to establish what actually happened during an incident (Milne & Powell, 2011). This is often challenging, as memories tend to be incomplete and some of those being interviewed could have reasons for not saying exactly what they recall. Effective investigative interviewing requires building rapport, using open-ended questions and 'ensuring that the interviewee sees his or her role as an information generator rather than merely as a question answerer' (Vrij et al., 2014, p. 130), but also noting potential omissions and discrepancies to be explored later. Interviewers observe body language and facial expressions, as well as listen to what is said, and may need to take unobtrusive notes to manage the amount of information they are receiving (Baker et al., 2021). The cognitive demands of investigative interviews are already high, and as demonstrated by Hanway et al. (2021), combining investigative interviewing with another cognitive task impacts the interviewer's ability to process the information provided in the interview.

Investigative interviewing tasks – actively listening, comparing accounts, formulating hypotheses, and maintaining rapport – are akin to those of realist interviewers. However, the latter deals with theories behind intervention outcomes in various contexts, potentially heightening cognitive demands. The next section explores the particularly high cognitive demands in realist interviews, followed by the author's personal reflections on her experience conducting online realist interviews with participants speaking regional variants of English. Communication proved challenging at first, but after interviewing techniques were adjusted to fit the context, they resulted in rich information and very considerable collaborative programme theory refinement.

Dealing with high cognitive demands in online realist interview: the R-O-C-M-T approach

The cognitive demands of an online realist interview may be even greater than an investigative interview, and conducting interviews across different language variants, potentially in cross-cultural situations, presents a particularly high cognitive load for the realist interview. A potential adjustment in these circumstances would be to move towards a more structured realist interview, following a topic guide closely. Paradoxically, in these situations where a more structured approach might seem appealing, there are strong reasons to instead enhance the ability of participants to speak to issues not yet covered in the programme theory (Gilmore, 2019).

A useful approach to manage the particular cognitive demands of realist interviews involves a sequence of R – O – C – M – T. Pronounced as 'Rock-emptee', it stands for Role – Outcome – Context – Mechanism – Theory, representing the typical order of questions – although topics may be addressed flexibly as realist interviews are mostly semi-structured.

Asking about roles

The Role type of question is relevant to two issues. The first is identifying which areas of programme theory the rest of the interview should focus on.

As Pawson and Tilley (1997) noted, participants have unequal knowledge of different aspects of programmes, and therefore unequal insights into different elements of programme theory. The Role question covers not just their current role but also their path to the role, as the participant's previous years of experience may be key to their insights on programme theory. For example, in a realist investigation of workplace culture, a person with many years of experience in the organisation is well placed to discuss institutional history, but someone who joined very recently may be a better source of information on organisational induction procedures, or lack of them. Interview participants who joined an organisation after being a client of its services, or who until recently worked with a partner organisation, may provide different and valuable perspectives. The 'Role question' is therefore often phrased as "Can you tell me what your role is in X and how you came to be in this role?'

The second aspect addressed by the Role question relates to programme activities. It is quite common during fieldwork to discover that the activities actually being implemented diverge from what is assumed by the programme theory, which may have been developed in a distant head office. A useful follow-up question directly addresses what the participant does rather than what they are: 'So you are [official title] but I'm not sure what that means in practice – could you tell me about your major responsibilities?' or 'Can you tell me the sorts of things you would do in a day?'.

To sum up what a realist interviewer needs to keep track of in talking with a participant about Roles:

- They must be familiar with the programme theory, enough to identify which areas this participant is likely to know most about, once they understand their role.
- They must remember the activities assumed by the programme theory so that they can note discrepancies.
- They should recall which areas of theory are most important to explore at this point. (Initially, every area may seem equally important but over the course of a project – particularly in large projects with numerous interviews – some areas may appear relatively well-established, while others still require considerable exploration.)
- Besides these memory tasks, the interviewer must make decisions – whilst listening and maintaining rapport – on whether the responses to the Role question(s) necessitates adjusting the phrasing of their next questions and, if so, what those adjustments should be.

Asking about outcomes

Outcomes are the focus of the next question, typically phrased as: 'What sort of changes have you seen since X [programme or intervention that is the focus of evaluation] has been in place/altered?'. The word 'changes' is often used instead of 'outcomes', as for some participants – especially those with some responsibility for an intervention's success – the term 'outcomes' may mean 'what we intended to achieve'. The interviewer wants to elicit positive and negative outcomes, and also unanticipated outcomes. On occasion, when asked this open question, the participant may provide a response about something that is not a change due to the programme but to a broader environmental change, such as flows of migrants to a local area due to disruptions elsewhere, or a legislative change that affects service provision. The interviewer should note that response as a (macro) context to be investigated further, and then rephrase the question in a way that does not make it seem that the respondent's previous answer was wrong: 'Thank you for that, and have you seen changes that you think are due to X?'.

If time is limited and several outcomes are discussed in response to the open question, the interviewer must prioritise which outcomes to focus on. It is crucial to remember the outcomes mentioned by the participant in sufficient detail to revisit them later. This can be demanding on working memory, as a single answer to this question can exceed 600 words. The interviewer also needs to determine whether the outcomes noted by the participant align with the programme theory outcomes. Participants' vocabulary may differ significantly – a senior bureaucrat will likely not use the same words as a service recipient – but they may well be referring to the same outcome. Depending on the time and priorities for the interview, if the outcomes predicted in the programme theory have not yet been mentioned, the interviewer may ask about them at this point. Alternatively, they may decide to explore contexts and mechanisms for the outcomes noted by the participant, reserving discussion on elements predicted by the programme theory for later on. They need to make that decision based on which course of action seems to be most fruitful for refining the programme theory, while actively listening to responses and maintaining rapport with the participant.

To sum up what a realist interviewer needs to keep track of in talking with a participant about Outcomes:

- They need to remember the outcomes in the programme theory.
- They need to listen to the participant's words to identify whether they are talking about outputs (such as fulfilling programme commitments of activities or products) or genuine outcomes (such as changes in policy or human behaviour effected by the programme or intervention).
- They need to determine whether the participant is talking about the same outcomes as predicted in the programme theory, possibly using different words or whether they are describing outcomes not previously intended and/or identified.
- They need to use working memory to keep track of the outcomes identified by the participants and determine whether those outcomes seem sufficiently important to explore in this interview.
- They need to decide, based on this information, the content and order of their next questions.

Asking about contexts and mechanisms

Having identified some tentative outcomes, the interview moves to context. Depending on the nature of the intervention and the outcome(s) focus, the interviewer might ask 'Did you see that change every time (or in every location or whatever other question is appropriate) that X was implemented?'. If the programme theory predicts that participant groups differ, the interviewer might ask 'Did everyone in that programme change in the same way?'. These questions aim to identify contexts by identifying differences in outcomes, or paths to the outcomes, between the instances when the programme was implemented in different ways or experienced by different groups of participants. Again, although the interviewer may begin with an open question, follow-up questions are likely to include contexts identified in the programme theory: 'Did you notice any differences between when X ran the programme and Y ran the programme?'.

Once the participant has identified one or more such differences, such as 'the first time we ran it, X was the result, but the second time Y was the result', the interviewer may ask 'why do you think it was different that time/in the location/for that group' or – as some participants are uncomfortable with "why" questions – might ask 'what do you think made the difference?'. Although not every participant is comfortable with mechanism questions, increasingly refined identifications of exactly which contexts make a difference to whether outcomes are achieved serve much the same purpose, enabling the investigator to work out mechanisms, perhaps back at their desk aided by relevant social science theories. (The Redgate and Dalkin chapter in this book offers more examples of mechanism questions.)

To sum up what an online realist interviewer needs to keep track of in talking about contexts and mechanisms:

- They need to remember the programme theory contexts and mechanisms, and which outcomes they are hypothesised to generate.
- They need to listen to the participant's words to identify if they are speaking about a programme activity, a context or a mechanism – and whether the words they are using indicate a concept that may need to be further explored.
- They need to determine if the participant's responses are providing new contexts and mechanisms or validating, refining or discarding those already identified in the programme theory, although perhaps speaking about them in very different terms than used in the programme theory.
- They need to keep in mind how many contexts, mechanisms and outcomes they want to explore and how long it is taking them to explore each piece of theory with this participant. If the interviewer has committed to an hour interview, they need to ensure that they are tracking time and using it effectively.
- They need to decide, based on all of this information, the content and order of their next questions, or whether it is time to move towards concluding the interview.

Finally, although contextualisation is an important part of realist work, and is often the focus of fieldwork, de-contextualisation is equally important, enabling middle-range theories to be established as a product of realist investigations that can then be applied in multiple contexts. The 'theory' element of the interview – refining theory at a level which is not specific to the participant's own context – tends to be conducted with only some participants, depending both on how much time is left after the most important Context-Mechanism-Outcome discussions have finished, and also on the participant's apparent interest in discussing more abstract programme theory elements. This segment may entail examining one or more propositions, or presenting visual aids such as flowcharts, for participants and researchers who prefer visual thinking.

This type of R-O-C-M-T interview usually finishes with one or both of the two final questions in the RAMESES starter set (Westhorp & Manzano, 2017), as both have proven valuable in many interview contexts. The first asks what the participant would do to improve the intervention if they had the power to make changes, and the second: 'Is there anything else you would like to tell me just to make sure I really get it and I really understand?'. Particularly with the final question it can be useful to state that this is the last question of the interview and pause a second or two before saying it, giving a signal that the interviewer is willing to wait for a thoughtful response.

Accountability to children and communities in consortia – an example of online realist interviewing

In this section, I provide personal reflections on a video interviewing experience that presented challenges but resulted in extremely rich information once the interview strategies were adjusted to fit the interviewing context.

In 2022, a team of realist researchers at Charles Darwin University (Australia) were contracted by Save the Children Netherlands to research models of accountability to children and communities when agencies were working together in consortia. There was interest in how consortia – multi-stakeholder partnerships typically led by an international organisation that channels donor funding amongst partners to design and deliver programmes together (Reid & Fransman, 2021) – affected this type of accountability, that is, prioritising responsiveness to the needs and aims of children and other community members and taking responsibility for the impact of organisational actions on them. The research (Williams et al., 2023) was exploratory and included key informant interviews, a rapid realist literature review, a realist survey and case studies developed with realist interviews. Interviews with children and other community beneficiaries, although recognised as critically important, could not be conducted in this initial stage. Their engagement, and that of members of small local organisations within consortia, were called for at the conclusion of the initial exploratory research, but it was apparent that different research methods would be required.

As the consortia models were new and still emerging, the case study interviews were of particular value. To enable understanding of multiple distinct consortium and accountability models, participants were selected from sites within Nepal, South Sudan and Bangladesh. Video interviewing was identified as the most suitable method to engage participants from such widely spread locations at relatively low cost and within a relatively short period of time. As participants used and preferred different video platforms, three platforms were used for interviewing – Zoom, Teams and FaceTime, the last of which the interviewer learned to operate for the project. Time zones presented a slight challenge; some interviews had to be conducted during my night or in the very early hours of the morning. Participants who spoke English were selected and introduced to the project by a central person in each country, who had a high-level view of how consortia were operating in their country, and sometimes in other countries, depending on their employment history and life experience. Most of those selected were in some form of management position, minimising interview power differences, although participants' roles varied from those focused solely on accountability to others with more wide-ranging responsibilities. Many had experience with accountability arrangements in multiple settings.

The value of the interviews is best demonstrated in an appendix in the report (Williams et al., 2023, pp. 100–113), designed to provide transparency as to how Context-Mechanism-Outcome configurations evolved over the course of the project, detailing the origin of each proposition and how it was validated or refined at each stage of research. Only two of the original propositions remained unchanged throughout the project, and three hypothesised propositions were discarded. (They were not refuted, as it was possible that they might be valid in other settings.) Several new or refined propositions arose through the literature review, and considerable refinement of many propositions came through the input of members of the Save the Children committee overseeing the project. Committee members provided insight into the importance of different aspects of accountability and were strong in ensuring that the researchers carefully considered accountability to children specifically when developing propositions, as well as accountability to communities as a whole. Survey results also informed some proposition refinements but, as demonstrated in the appendix, the highest proportion of refinements and also of newly added propositions came from the online interviews. To achieve these results, challenges had to be overcome and adjustments made in interviewing techniques.

Gaining participant trust and ensuring clear communication

In reflecting upon the experience, two challenges stand out: gaining participant trust and ensuring clear communication. Participants were asked by someone they knew to engage with the interviewer, and prior to the interview they were emailed information on the project, as well as materials on informed consent. However, this did not always have the same effect as the personal introductions that could have been made if the interviews were being conducted face-to-face, including the typical pre-interview (often informal) conversations. Some participants wanted considerably more information than was provided in the materials, on occasion asking for a preliminary interview to engage with the interviewer and discuss details of the project. In many cases, considerable time was spent at the beginning of interviews explaining the project aims, before participants felt confident to proceed. As interviews lasted approximately an hour, this left less time for other discussion.

Communication presented other challenges, including occasional stormy weather and technical problems interrupting conversations. All participants were fluent in English and used it in their workplaces. However, even with good technical connections, communicating across different variants of English was sometimes challenging. For example, one of the first informants, answering the 'Role' question, noted their role as 'capacitation'. I quickly grew to appreciate this term, used in multiple countries but not in my own English variant – so much so that I have been trying to replace 'capacity building' with this term in Australia (so far without success). However, on this first mention it took me a minute or two to work out from the rest of the response what the term meant, time in which the participant continued to provide information I needed to comprehend to plan my next question while simultaneously working out the unfamiliar term.

There were multiple examples of this dynamic in many of the interviews. Interrupting every time there was a word I did not immediately recognise would not have been helpful to encouraging participants to speak freely. Instead, over time I worked out better techniques. For instance, before conducting interviews, I searched for YouTube examples of people speaking in the local variant of English so that I could accustom my ear to its rhythm and pronunciations before beginning the interview. I began to read more local organisational documents to become acquainted with as many local terms and acronyms as possible.

During interviews, over the course of the project I learned to adjust my usual way of asking questions: not relying on body language (difficult for me as I have lived and worked in settings where I lacked fluency in the local language, and used body language to compensate), slowing down my speech, using shorter questions expressed very clearly and allowing for longer pause times between utterances. These are useful techniques for any interview, so it is likely that the experience improved my skills. As I (like the interview participants) was dealing with quite a heavy cognitive load, I took more notes than usual, and the online nature of the interview helped this to be done unobtrusively. My note-taking uses a mixture of symbols including upward facing arrows for points that appear to verify elements of theory, downward facing arrows for points that appear to cast doubt on one or more elements of theory, tildes for puzzling or equivocal evidence – and of particular importance, the symbol I=, indicating a point of special importance that I need to revisit before the end of the interview. The notes took some of the burden off working memory, allowing me to focus more on comprehension, rapport and planning next steps in the interview.

The most time-consuming adjustment, and probably the most valuable, came in the post-interview period. Each participant received a package consisting of their transcript, a note on any words or phrases that were not yet understood, and a section on my understanding of what the participant's interview implied for how the programme theory should be refined. This step, involving participants not just in reviewing what they had said in the interview but inviting them to comment on my interpretation of what it meant for theory development, was not a step I had taken previously in other projects. There were two reasons I did it now. One was a desire to check on my understanding of what was said in sometimes challenging online communication circumstances. The other was that in many previous face-to-face projects I was hundreds or thousands of kilometres distant at the analysis stage, with no means to re-engage with participants, especially where there were literacy and/or language translation issues. In this project, I had the ability to re-contact participants and to correspond with them (but always stressing that any further responses were voluntary). Although not every participant responded, some did, providing valuable further insights which included noting points they felt I had misinterpreted.

The final stage in the theory development was undertaken collaboratively with a smaller number of participants including the three people who had coordinated participant selection in South Sudan, Bangladesh and Nepal. The result was the identification and public presentation of three models of accountability to children and communities in consortia suitable for different contexts: (1) a range of situations including urgent responses to sudden emergencies; (2) crises requiring coordination by multiple large organisations; and (3) situations where empowerment of local organisations is a priority. The collaborative theory-building process enabled by digital communication proved to be extremely valuable in the end, despite the challenges encountered along the way.

Conclusion and recommendations

Although video interviews present challenges in terms of excluding participants without online access and can make communication challenging in certain circumstances – such as poor connections or communicating across language variants – they present multiple opportunities including increased fieldwork speed, reduced costs, better environmental sustainability and ability to engage with groups who might struggle with face-to-face interviews, such as those with digital access but mobility difficulties, and those with hearing impairments. Rescheduling interviews, if needed, can be achieved more easily than when travel is involved, when the interviewer may be hundreds of kilometres away by the time the participant is free to try again. Video interviews also offer opportunities for engagement and collaborative theory refinement post-interview, even where participants are geographically dispersed. However, it is important for realist researchers to be mindful of the technical and cognitive demands associated with this data collection method. Some recommendations are provided below:

- In determining whether to use video technology for interviews, consider a range of factors including priorities for theory development/testing, project and team resources, communication equity and environmental sustainability.
- If video interviewing is identified as a preferred and/or viable method, as you identify which types of participants are required in your theory development and/or theory testing sampling frame, also identify who is likely to prefer and/or have access to which modes of communication. Build communication equity into your design as much as possible, including by using multiple modes of communication as required.
- When choosing which platform(s) to use for those participants for whom video interviewing is appropriate, consider factors such as the participants' skill in (which) different platforms, cost (for researchers and participants), ease of use, security and any special features important for the project such as translated transcription.
- Ideally, ensure that each interviewer has training and/or experience in online realist interviewing. Ensure that they are able to operate each of the platforms required, including identifying and resolving technical issues that may arise during the interview.
- Ensure interviewers are able to support participants who may be less familiar with video communication, such as letting them know how to turn off the self-view feature. Consider if two interviewers are needed to manage technical issues as well as communication with the participant(s) and potentially note-taking.
- Plan to conduct fewer interviews in a day, and build longer breaks between them, than would be usual for face-to-face interviewing, as video interviews can be tiring for participants but even more tiring for realist interviewers.
- Be aware that not all participants will have the same attitude to video interviews. Some may miss the rapport of a face-to-face meeting and benefit from additional time spent in building rapport. Yet others may value the efficiency of having an online interview at a time and place convenient to them, and value the immediate approach that a video interview enables.
- Embed fallback plans. Provide phone numbers and email addresses so that participants can contact and be contacted by the interviewers if the desired platform – Zoom, Teams or other – fails to operate. Be prepared, subject to participant agreement, to allocate time for rescheduling interviews, for example if a storm makes video communication unsafe or if unexpected interruptions disrupt the interview.

- Identify any potential project information gaps resulting from video interviewing, including: loss of cultural awareness and missed opportunities for personal introductions typically acquired through travel; limited body language clues due to only seeing each other's faces; or reduced verbal exchanges during the interview due to talking more slowly and leaving longer pauses between turns at speaking. Develop strategies to compensate for such gaps, such as spending time prior to interviews learning about local culture, terms, and ways of speaking.
- Use the opportunities offered by video interviewing, including the potential to communicate post-interview, and to share transcripts and initial analysis findings. While not every participant may wish or be able to participate in this way, those who do can provide substantial value to analysis and theory development/refinement.
- Maintain awareness of technical developments, and identify new advantages as they become available, such as improvements in simultaneous transcription and translation.

10 Lessons from realist evaluations in Canada

Advancing programme theory through patient-oriented research approaches

Tracey Carr and Gary Groot

Introduction

The importance of engaging patients, families and citizens in research represents a relatively recent paradigmatic shift in some countries and is gaining traction globally. While public involvement in research has been lauded for its potential to positively impact research priorities and the relevance of results, such engagement within the realist realm has received little explication (Domecq et al., 2014; Aubin et al., 2019). To describe how, why and under what circumstances partnering with patients, families or citizens can lead to more rich, relevant and rigorous programme theories, we will outline our experiences conducting realist evaluations with patient partners.

As we detail our journey engaging with patients in realist research in this chapter, we compare our experiences with a realist programme theory about how and why patients from a variety of backgrounds can be empowered in the research process (Zibrowski et al., 2021). This programme theory, derived from a rapid realist review based on 62 international studies, was published by a postdoctoral fellow whom we supervised. While the study outlines several contexts and mechanisms that could result in an empowered patient-centred lens for research, Zibrowski et al.'s programme theory had not been tested with primary realist studies. In describing the realist research that we have conducted alongside patient partners, we use the context and mechanisms from Zibrowski et al.'s programme theory in a retrospective analysis to understand how and why we had successful engagement with patient partners. We end by identifying potential refinements to the programme theory.

The chapter begins with a brief history of patient-oriented research (POR) in Canada, including a description of the POR Level of Engagement Tool, an indicator of patient engagement. In the second section, we outline key contexts and mechanisms from Zibrowski et al.'s programme theory to explain empowered patient-centred research (Zibrowski et al., 2021). In the third section, we describe how we engaged with patient partners in two realist evaluations in which the sets of patient partners had markedly different backgrounds. We reflect on how interactions aligned with elements of Zibrowski

DOI: 10.4324/9781003457077-11

et al.'s programme theory and areas where we identified potential refinements to the theory. We conclude with an emphasis on trust as the fundamental mechanism in POR realist research, and note that there are multiple dimensions of trust that are relevant to POR.

Patient-oriented research in Canada

Patient engagement in research elevates patients from data sources to co-collaborators in all aspects of the research process, beginning with priority setting and design and continuing to data collection, analysis and knowledge dissemination. POR was originally designed to recognise the moral, ethical and political imperatives to include patients in research that directly affects their healthcare experiences and clinical outcomes and has become a significant component of health research in Canada.

In September 2011, the Canadian Institutes of Health Research (CIHR), the principal health research funder, launched their Strategy for Patient-Oriented Research (SPOR) and established multiple national collaborative research networks (Government of Canada, CIHR, 2014). Such networks included innovative Clinical Trials platforms, the SPOR Canadian Data Platform, the SPOR National Training Entity and the SPOR Evidence Alliance. However, it was the creation of the Support for People and Patient-Oriented Research and Trials (SUPPORT) Units that enabled the formation of partnerships and connections between organisations that could directly support and advance POR in Canadian provinces and territories (Government of Canada, CIHR 2014).

In the Canadian province where we are located, the SUPPORT Unit is the Saskatchewan Centre for Patient-Oriented Research (SCPOR). To gauge patient engagement in research projects, SCPOR, alongside patient partners, developed a measurement tool: the Patient-Oriented Research Level of Engagement Tool (PORLET) (Saskatchewan Centre for Patient-Oriented Research (SCPOR), n.d.). The PORTLET uses a five-point scale to assess a project's alignment with CIHR's five designated criteria for POR: 'patients are partners', 'patient identified priorities', 'outcomes important to patients', 'aims to integrate knowledge into practice' and 'team is multidisciplinary'. Adapted from the International Association for Public Participation, the levels of engagement with patient partners are categorised as (1) inform, (2) consult, (3) involve, (4) collaborate and (5) empower (Saskatchewan Centre for Patient-Oriented Research (SCPOR), n.d.). In the following sections, as we test the patient engaged programme theory, we refer to the PORLET criteria to measure the quality of patient engagement in two realist evaluation case studies.

Patient-engaged programme theory

This section depicts relevant contexts and mechanisms from Zibrowski et al.'s programme theory and presents hypotheses regarding how and why they lead to patient engagement in research. To highlight specific contexts and

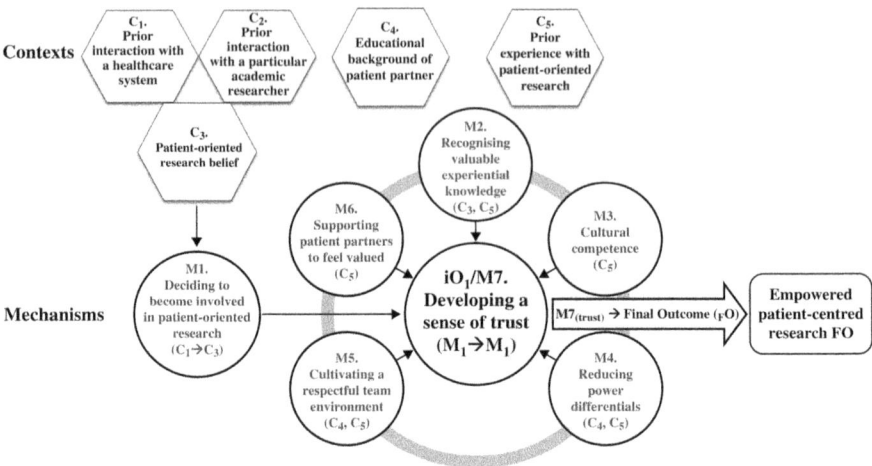

Figure 10.1 Patient-engaged programme theory (adapted from Zibrowski et al. 2021) that outlines five specific contexts and seven mechanisms that lead to empowered patient-centred research.

mechanisms as well as illustrate how and why these resonate with our experience with POR realist evaluation, we present Figure 10.1, which is adapted from Zibrowski et al. (2021).

As depicted in Figure 10.1, the theory of how and why POR is initiated begins with both the researcher's and the patient's decision to become involved (M1). This decision might be instigated by a potential patient partner's prior interaction (negative and/or positive) with a healthcare system (C1) and/or a patient partner's prior interaction with a particular academic researcher (C2). According to Zibrowski et al., decisions to become involved in POR may also be motivated by self-benefit and/or benefit to others; thus, patient and researcher could be influenced by a third context (C3) – their beliefs in POR. When patients believe they can 'pay back' their gratitude for their care or that they can improve care in the health system, they are more likely to decide to engage in POR. At the same time, researcher beliefs about POR are sometimes influenced by opportunities for funding or career advancement and disincentivised by competing time requirements (e.g., teaching, clinical duties, etc.).

As these three contexts represent the conditions under which the decision to participate in POR occurs (M1), the result can be linked to five additional mechanisms: researcher recognition of valuable patient partner experience (M2), researcher awareness of and sensitivity to the community's or patient partner's culture (M3), reducing power differentials (M4), cultivating a respectful team environment (M5) and supporting patient partners to feel valued (M6).

In Zibrowski's et al.'s programme theory, developing a sense of trust between researcher and patient partner (M7) is positioned as the central mechanism that leads to research that uses a patient-centred lens. They report trust as facilitated by several conditions, including the provision of honoraria for patient partners, consensus seeking and incorporating patient partner input, willingness by researchers to discuss their intentions for project processes and outcomes, and willingness to know patient partners and their communities. Acting as both an intermediate outcome and a mechanism, trust becomes a generative cause of a patient-centred lens and the foundation of research that represents a genuine researcher-patient partnership.

In the application of Zibrowski et al.'s programme theory to our POR realist research, we describe how these mechanisms generated trust in two evaluations (Dalkin et al., 2015). Both realist evaluations were conducted with patient partners who had prior interaction with a healthcare system (C1). At the same time, the patient partners' educational background (C4) and prior POR experience (C5) were markedly different. Despite these diverse contexts, each evaluation was an exemplar of empowered patient-centred research and could be highly rated on all criteria of the PORLET.

POR and realist research

Since our POR realist work began in 2016, we have conducted realist synthesis and evaluation by engaging multiple patient partners from various backgrounds and lived experiences (Groot et al., 2017; Waldron et al., 2020; Azizian et al., 2021; Fletcher-Hildebrand et al., 2021). Many people who seek opportunities as patient partners have similar characteristics. Patient partners are likely to be white, middle aged or older females, above average in household income and well educated (C4) (Abelson et al., 2022). Most are motivated to engage in research by past negative and/or positive interactions with the health system, which is identified in Zibrowski et al.'s programme theory as C1.

The following two cases outline our collaborations with patient partners in realist research settings and describe how we activated M2 (recognising valuable experiential knowledge), M3 (cultural competence, also known as cultural awareness or cultural responsiveness), M4 (reducing power differentials), M5 (cultivating a respectful team environment) and M6 (supporting patient partners to be valued) to amplify trust (M7) within the differing patient partner-researcher teams.

Case 1: COVID-19 vaccination in three sites in Saskatchewan: A patient-oriented realist evaluation

The first case study of POR realist research was an evaluation of the 2021 pilot phase of the COVID-19 vaccination programme in Saskatchewan and was well-suited to realist enquiry. While past vaccination programmes for other communicable diseases had been evaluated in various jurisdictions, COVID-19 vaccination on a province-wide scale was the quintessential 'black box'. Understanding how to bolster vaccine uptake was a top priority for health system and government stakeholders, and engaging with patient partners with lived experiences of the health system was essential for programme theory development, testing and validation.

The evaluation team was comprised of a master's student, three patient partners, a research assistant and the authors. As a requirement for his thesis, the master's student, who at the time held a research and quality improvement position within the health system, co-led a realist evaluation with the patient partners. Two of the three patient partners were POR 'veterans'; both had prior experience collaborating with the researchers on health system initiatives and viewed understanding vaccine delivery as an urgent priority. The third patient partner was an academic whose spouse was a resident in long-term care, a population that was among the first group selected to receive the vaccine. All patient partners had advanced levels of education, prior interactions with at least one researcher on the team and a belief that POR would result in a better understanding of how, why, for whom and under what circumstances, the vaccine delivery programme could lead to vaccination uptake (C1, C2, C3). Vaccination uptake was the outcome for the study.

Because we were working as a team for the first time and within the constraints of pandemic restrictions, the initial meeting was an informal online gathering where significant time was devoted to discussing patient partner professional and research history including family background. These informal check-ins that focussed on socially oriented team discussion continued throughout the project and were built into every online meeting agenda (*n* = 16 in total). These check-ins were instrumental in cultivating a respectful team environment (M5) and supporting the patient partners to feel valued (M6). We recognised the value of their experiential knowledge (M2) by using Mural, a collaborative visual tool (Work Better Together with Mural's Visual Work Platform | Mural, n.d.)) where patient partners could directly contribute to the development of the initial programme theories through independently adding text box descriptions. After describing the concept of Context-Mechanism-Outcome (CMO) configurations and providing a few examples that we had gleaned from a published conversation about COVID-19 vaccination, we encouraged patient partners to provide contexts and mechanisms grounded in their lived experiences.

Having patient partners as co-researchers in this project was critical to its success; their lived experiences brought an essential lens to the creation of the initial programme theories, the data analysis and final programme theory refinement. Importantly, they co-developed the interview guide with the student, then together with the student interviewed participants who had received the vaccine during the pilot phase. Guided by the initial programme theories, the student conducted an equal number of interviews with each patient partner. Patient partners collaborated in the programme theory refinement based on the interview transcripts. As patient partners were equal members of the team, they were co-authors on publications to reduce power differentials (M4) (Azizian et al., 2021).

Patient partners in this realist evaluation offered several refinements to the initial programme theories by bringing their lived experiences to the team discussions. They noted that the relationship among CMOs was complex and encouraged the notion of mechanism 'chains' that could explain the principal mechanisms of 'trust' and 'anxiety' in the initial theory. For example, the patient partner from rural Saskatchewan posited the importance of 'sense of community versus individual responsibility' as an important influence on both trust and anxiety. (Lack of) trust as a mechanism that led to the outcome of vaccine hesitancy was further explicated by patient partners to be comprised of 'trust in vaccine efficacy and safety', 'trust in healthcare institutions and medical professionals' and 'trust in leadership'. These discussions with patient partners were essential to the programme theories, and the refinements to the programme theories would not have occurred without their engagement.

By purposefully enabling the operation of mechanisms identified as important in the development of trust in patient-researcher partnerships (recognising valuable experiential knowledge, reducing power differentials, supporting patient partners to feel valued and cultivating a respectful team environment), the team developed a sense of trust (M7) which led to a successful patient-oriented realist evaluation (Azizian et al., 2021). With this group of patient partners, trust was relatively easy to develop and maintain, given the high degree of their previous experiences with POR and their preexisting knowledge of the healthcare system.

Case 2: Realist evaluation of harm reduction and residential supportive care for people with and at-risk of HIV/AIDS

The second case study involved engagement with patient partners from markedly different backgrounds than the first case study's patient partners. The programmes we evaluated were intended to meet the needs of people living with HIV/AIDS (PLHIV) through a harm reduction philosophy and the provision of patient-centred supportive care. Administered by Sanctum Care Group, a not-for-profit organisation in Saskatoon, Saskatchewan, the programmes are delivered in two homes with different populations (Sanctum Care Group, 2018). Sanctum 1.0 is a residence designed programme to assist PLHIV transition from the acute care system to independent living or to support them with their palliative care journey. Sanctum 1.5 is a home that supports pregnant women at risk of having their children taken into custody and who may have or be at risk of having HIV. The patient partners who acted as co-researchers in this case were referred to as 'resident partners'; each had completed the duration of the programme and therefore were considered programme 'graduates'.

After consultation with Sanctum Care Group stakeholders (board, staff and resident partners), we applied for and received a grant to conduct a realist evaluation. We supervised a practicum student to establish an initial programme theory regarding how, why, for whom and under what circumstances the services provided by Sanctum 1.0 worked (or not). Through a review of literature on harm reduction and housing programmes for PLHIV complemented by input from the stakeholders, we developed a realist evaluation protocol (Fletcher-Hildebrand et al., 2021).

Without meaningful partner engagement, we would not have been able to recruit programme participants. Completing the evaluations of both programmes required directly testing and validating the programme theories with programme participants. Developing trust was essential. Fostering trust with potential resident partners who were not familiar with research processes, who typically did not engage with researchers and who had lived experiences of trauma and marginalisation, necessitated researcher cultural awareness and sensitivity (M3).

Unlike the first case study, the two partners, one from Sanctum 1.0 and one from Sanctum 1.5, had no prior interaction with academic researchers (C2) nor significant beliefs about POR (C3). Instead, what led to their decision to become involved in the evaluations (M1) was positive experiences with Sanctum services (C1). As in the first case study, we found in a retrospective application of Zibrowski et al.'s programme theory that similar mechanisms (M2, M4, M5, M6) were activated that enhanced trust (M7) between the resident partners and the researchers. Because of the different contexts of the two studies (educational background of patient partners, C4, and prior experience with POR, C5), we also required a tailored approach to patient engagement. At the outset, a postdoctoral fellow who had a background in pastoral care was assigned full time to the project. He maintained regular and ongoing connections with the resident partners, which facilitated the development of a strong team. By supporting the patient partners to feel valued (M6) and cultivating a respectful team environment (M5), trust was established among team members.

Because the participants who were to be interviewed for the evaluation were considered a vulnerable population, the ethics application was deemed to be 'above minimal risk' and took a protracted period for approval. While awaiting ethics approval for the project, the resident partners and researchers met on a weekly basis, which provided ample time to cultivate a respectful team environment. Resident partners' time was prioritised, and meetings were set at their convenience. This helped to reduce power differentials (M4) between the resident partners and the researchers. Power differentials were also ameliorated by hiring resident partners as research assistants who received wages for the time they committed to all aspects of the project. Typically, in POR projects partners will receive honoraria for their time; however, by employing the resident partners they could document their contributions as recognisable work experience including the position title 'research assistant'. Not only did this acknowledge their valuable experiential knowledge (M2), but this tangible recognition of their contributions also supported them to feel valued (M6), while reducing power differentials (M4).

The CIHR SPOR modules, which were required training among those new to POR, were not particularly accessible for Sanctum resident partners, who had some high school education and limited access to technology. Therefore, both the content and the format of the modules were challenging. To overcome these limitations, the postdoctoral fellow communicated research concepts to the resident partners in lay terms and supported them in the co-development of the interview guide. This co-development with resident partners ensured the interview guide's language would be straightforward and resonate with participants. Facilitating resident partner contributions to the guide recognised their valuable experiential knowledge (M6).

Prior to gaining ethics approval, the resident partner from Sanctum 1.0 died unexpectedly. His death was very distressing for the research team who by that point in the evaluation had known each other for almost a year and had developed a sense of trust. When contemplating how to proceed, we invited the Sanctum 1.5 resident partner to take over more responsibility for research tasks on the team. Fortunately, the 1.5 resident partner was willing to take over these tasks. It was important for the team to debrief where we had the opportunity to share about the 1.0 resident partner and his valuable role on the project. With the expanded role of the Sanctum 1.5 resident partner, we continued with the evaluation.

Once we received ethics approval and could begin the interviewing process, we relied on the Sanctum 1.5 resident partner's network to recruit potential participants. In her words 'these are my people', and, because of their shared lived experiences, she could gain trust from potential participants that researchers could not develop. Her experiential knowledge was crucial (M2) for the recruitment. Shared lived experiences were essential. As a result, the rate of response was high. Potential participants were more likely to view the resident participant, someone who had graduated the programme and had similar experiences, to be a trustworthy person and someone with whom they could share information about the programme.

For data collection, we followed a process where the resident partner would contact the potential participant, schedule the interview time, then the research coordinator would arrange the technical aspects of the interview (via Zoom). After the resident partner obtained consent and briefly shared her own experiences with the programme, she asked interview questions that were intended to teach, then test, the initial programme theories in language that was relatable for the participant. While the research coordinator would be present during the interview, she did not actively participate in the interview; her video was blocked, and audio muted. Her role was to assist in the case of any technical difficulties with audio recording.

In addition to data collection, the resident partner was instrumental in the analysis of the interviews. Data analysis for the two evaluations was guided by a realist scholar who was a nursing professor. The realist scholar, the research coordinator and the resident partner met frequently throughout the analysis phase. The resident partner's lived experiences informed the analysis in a way the researchers often could not 'see'. When we refined the initial programme theories, the resident partner's perspectives were paramount to understanding how and why the programme worked. Her observations that residents' success in the programme could also be influenced by their partner's support (or lack of support) led to a unique CMO. Again, her experiential knowledge was extremely valuable (M2).

The ongoing trusting relationship (M7) between the resident partner and research coordinator was fostered by shared experiences of being moms to preschool children. As both were raising their babies, they developed a strong rapport. Their relationship continued through the knowledge transition phase of the evaluation where they co-presented the findings at two international conferences (DOHaD World Congress 2022| DOHaD Canada, n.d.; Indigenous DOHaD Gathering, 2022). The resident partner's significant role in knowledge translation, including reporting back to the stakeholder group, co-authoring publications and conference presentations illustrated her level of engagement in the research.

In this case study, awareness of and responsiveness to cultural issues was a critical mechanism (M3). In Zibrowski et al.'s original programme theory, they employed the term 'cultural competence' and underscored its significance when working with populations who have historically endured discrimination. As language in this area has evolved, terms such as 'cultural awareness' and 'cultural responsiveness' are now more often used (Government of Canada, CIHR 2005). In the context of POR, cultural awareness and responsiveness require the ability to set aside biases, recognise one's own worldview and appreciate the worldview of others. The authors had extensive experience working collaboratively with Indigenous communities and patient partners in Saskatchewan, including a realist synthesis to examine the role of trust and worldview in shared decision-making with Indigenous patients (Groot et al., 2020). We were cognisant of the historical context that had influenced the lived experiences of the resident partners. Without appreciation for this historical context and the cultural awareness and responsiveness of the researchers, trusting relationships would likely not have developed.

Discussion

In retrospect, using Zibrowski's et al.'s patient empowered programme enabled us to understand aspects of how, why, for whom and under what circumstances patients could be empowered to engage in realist research. However, comparing the literature-derived theory to our experiences in these two cases highlights new factors to consider when engaging diverse patient partners. Realist evaluations are complex, and engagement with POR invites greater complexity; marrying the two approaches brings challenges and opportunities.

The more apparent challenge with POR and realist evaluation is one that is evident in other research – the funder's requirements that limit resources and timelines. For both cases, we no longer had resources to engage patient partners in the dissemination of all knowledge translation products (including the writing of this chapter). These limits could lead researchers to primarily engage with patient partners with whom they have pre-existing relationships and with those who are 'in the majority' (Abelson et al., 2022). Potentially, POR healthcare service research and evaluation, realist or otherwise, might be conducted between patient partners and researchers who do not represent those most impacted by services. Despite these challenges, our work with patient partners produced programme theories that were valued by stakeholders.

Undoubtedly, in each of these realist evaluations, the programme theory development was augmented and elucidated by engagement with patient and resident partners. In our experience, a POR approach was essential to the process and outcome of the evaluations. We valued patients' lived experiences through recognising their unique experiences (Case 1 example: patient partner from rural setting) and treating them as equals (Case 2 example: resident partner employed as part of the team). Valuing them as equal team members was an integral part of trust building which in turn led to research with a patient engaged lens.

Conclusion

From our experience with these two case studies, the richness, rigour and relevance of final programme theories are substantial when patient partners can be engaged. Although realist research calls for stakeholder engagement in development, testing and validation of programme theory, having the opportunity to partner with patients as equal research team members in all research phases results in research processes driven by and for patients. Regardless of patient partner educational background or prior experience with POR, high levels of trust can be engendered in patient-researcher teams by activating key mechanisms. Recognising and supporting patient partners' valuable experience, reducing power differentials between patient partners and researchers and being aware of and responsive to the patient partners' culture will build trust. Trust, the fundamental mechanism in all empowered patient-centred research, can be nurtured when researchers recognise patient partners as equal team members.

11 The realist topic guide

Sam Redgate and Sonia Dalkin

Introduction

This chapter outlines how use of topic guides can assist researchers to enact realist principles within the field when collecting qualitative data. With this focus, the chapter draws on and moves between the theoretical underpinnings and practical application of realist research to inform how realist topic guides can be prepared and utilised throughout the research cycle. A topic guide (also referred to as a discussion guide, or interview schedule) in its simplest form, is a list or outline of the key issues to be explored and/or questions to be asked within an interview or focus group. These guides act as practical tools for researchers to steer discussions, keep to time and ensure key questions or areas of focus are included in the conversation, to address overall research question(s) of the study. The use of topic guides within qualitative research is not new. Indeed, one of the first social science textbooks Odum and Jocher (1929, cited in Platt, 2012) makes reference to the use of a 'schedule' within an interview approach. Such documents have become a regular feature in qualitative methodologies, as an approach to assist in providing focus and structure to interviews and focus groups. However, topic guides can vary greatly in their appearance and composition. This is predominantly dependent upon factors such as the aim of the research study, the interviewee, the underpinning philosophy of the approach taken, and to some degree, the experience and style of the researcher. Topic guides will, however, always incorporate a list of exploratory areas and/or questions to be used to aid the researcher in directing the conversation with the research participant, whether it be in an interview or group discussion. Scheibelhofer (2008) suggests that interviews can be broadly defined in two classes: interviews based on narrations, and those based on topic guides. Narration interviews are unstructured and focus on narrations and storytelling done by the interviewee, minimising structuring on the part of the researcher. Techniques which typically take this focus include the narrative interview and the ethnographic interview. (See Van Belle in this book for a detailed comparison of the realist interview with similar interview approaches.) In contrast, interviews based on topic guides require the researcher to prepare questions or themes (i.e. topic guides or

DOI: 10.4324/9781003457077-12

interview guides) and thus can be categorised as semi-structured or focused. When using a semi-structured or focused approach, the researcher designs questions to collect data about the same event with different participants. By doing so they actively use the questioning to keep on target and obtain relevant information.

Within realist interviewing there is a focus on the use of theory to drive questioning, with a suggestion that '…theory should be used explicitly and systematically throughout the interview process' (Greenhalgh et al., 2017b, p. 1). This focus lends itself to the topic guide approach, rather than interviews based on narrations, as aspects of theory can be specifically highlighted to investigate within the topic guide (Scheibelhofer, 2008). In addition, the realist approach also has links with the focused interview tradition, proposed by Merton and Kendall (1946), through its emphasis on theory development.

Within realist approaches the research process itself is iterative in nature. Initial theorising (theory gleaning and initial programme theory development) is followed by cycles of testing and refinement, prior to consolidation of theories (see Manzano, 2016 for details of theory-driven interview phases). Within this process there is a need to identify and be adaptative to patterns of information emerging from interviews and other data collection sources, and to reflect these in the questioning/topic guides moving forward. This allows interaction with, and further development of, programme theory. Due to this iterative cycle, there is a requirement for the realist topic guide to be considered differently from a non-realist topic guide (often viewed as being underpinned by constructivist principles). The realist topic guide must be sufficiently flexible to both allow the testing of a priori programme theories and for the excavation of new emerging explanatory areas. By taking this approach, generative causation can be identified and explored relating to key contextual and mechanistic aspects, and the outcomes they lead to.

Within this chapter we investigate why is it important to have realist topic guides and what this means in practice. A comparison of the realist vs. non-realist topic guide is provided alongside underpinning epistemological considerations, aided by a visual conceptualisation. This is presented with a discussion as to how these key considerations influence approaches to questioning and the topic guide development within realist studies, through outlining different question types while acknowledging the importance of being theory driven and identifying generative causation. Linking these theoretical concepts to a more tangible process, the chapter concludes with a proposed stepped process to developing realist topic guides. This is intended to assist researchers by providing advice to steer the researcher when devising a realist topic guide as opposed to being a prescriptive approach. Throughout the chapter, we adopt and refer to the theory-driven interview phases outlined by Manzano (2016) of theory gleaning, refining, and consolidation, in order to define and contextualise discussions relating to question composition and structure.

Theory development and generative causation as the focus in the realist topic guide

There is no standard topic guide format in social research methods. In its simplest form, a topic guide could be a list of topics to be covered during the discussion; at its most detailed it could contain carefully worded questions (Arthur & Nazroo, 2003). The topic guide must, however, be fit for purpose for both the researcher and in facilitating the intended outputs from the discussion. The design of the topic guide is therefore an important process, informed by the methodological approach of the study (see Table 11.1). Considerations within the topic guide should encompass subject coverage, the intended participant, language and terminology used, inclusion of follow-up questions/probes, ease of use by the researcher and flow of the discussion (Arthur & Nazroo, 2003). In addition, consideration should be given to the 'pre-interview' to contextualise the interview (Manzano, 2016), that is, to identify the extent of the participants' knowledge in relation to the components (C, M, O) to be explored in the interview, and specific relevant background influencing their responses. In realist research, there is also a need to ensure the topic guide reflects the programme theories, as it is these theories which provide the structure for the questions within the topic guide. This can be a time-consuming process and sufficient resources should be allocated to this task.

Realist research starts and ends with a theory (Vareilles et al., 2015). It aims to develop, refine, validate or falsify theories pertaining to a programme (i.e. intervention, policy or service) identifying how the programme does, or does not work, for whom and why. Thus, realist approaches focus on developing the conceptual understanding (theory development) of relational links between (1) the context interventions are situated in, (2) the mechanisms generated as a response to the intervention delivery in the context, and (3) the outcomes of interest (Dalkin et al., 2015; Pawson, 1996). These defining features of the realist approach (namely that it is theory driven and adheres to generative causation) are key to consider when generating realist topic guides.

Theory-driven basis of realist topic guides

In introducing the interview to the interviewee in a realist approach, it is the role of the researcher to introduce the teacher–learner cycle concept (see Pawson, 1996 and Pawson & Tilley, 1997 for a more detailed discussion on this approach). This involves communicating expectations of the researcher and participant during the interview. This approach includes sharing theories with the participant for them to comment on, with a view that their comments will assist in refining the programme theory (Manzano, 2016). In placing the programme theory before the participant, the researcher 'teaches' the participant about it; the participant having learned the theory, then 'teaches' the researcher about particular elements of the theory (Lacouture et al., 2015).

In adopting this teacher–learner approach to the interview, the realist researcher abandons the traditional neutral territory to engage with respondents (Manzano, 2016). It is important to highlight that this is not necessarily done as a formal word-for-word citation of the programme theory; instead, the researcher should use their discretion to present the programme theory in the most appropriate terms and format for the participant. It is possible for researchers to be explicit and describe in detail the approach of the teacher–learner cycle. However, it is more common for researchers to be informal and implicit in the approach and terminology used. For example, they may state that they will be presenting the participant with 'ideas' about an intervention/policy/service (i.e. the researcher teaching the participant their theory, or elements of their theory), and that they would like the participant to respond with their thoughts and experiences to the information presented (i.e. the participant teaching the researcher about their theory). This approach is different to interviews used in other philosophical paradigms (e.g. constructivism, grounded theory or symbolic interactionism) where the focus will often be to explore the participants' views on the topic under investigation and to capitalise on lived experience (Charmaz & Belgrave, 2012; Greenhalgh et al., 2017b).

In non-realist interviews questions are generally grouped and structured around the research aim(s). In a realist approach, they will focus on understanding, developing and refining the realist components and configurations of context, mechanism and outcome in relation to initial or developing programme theory. (See section below on 'Underpinning epistemological considerations for realist topic guide structure and development' for further discussion on this.) Therefore, questions are generally grouped by programme theory (example questions are provided in Tables 11.2 and 11.3), or in the case of theory gleaning exercises, grouped by component, that is, context, mechanism or outcome. It is, however, feasible to structure the topic guide into explanatory areas with a number of programme theories being explored within each area.

Generative causation within realist topic guides

Within theory development and refinement, question composition in the realist topic guide should be structured in a way that facilitates generative explanation and development of Context-Mechanism-Outcome (CMO) linkages. To this end, Manzano (2016) states that questioning should be focused on propositions. Taking this approach allows for the interviewer to express their view or judgement as part of the question. In doing so, questions aligning with the programme theory being tested can more easily be asked. For example, if your programme theory stated:

> Engaging in group work allows participants the opportunity to discuss their experiences of implementing new coaching strategies (context) which allows them to learn from one another and deepens their

practical understanding of and confidence in the topics learnt (mechanism), leading to increased application of the learning in real world situations (outcome).

You might ask:

It seems that group work allowed you to work through more practical applications of the strategies you had learned on the course – could you talk to me about your experience of this?

This questioning uses the teacher-learner cycle by putting forward the researcher's theory on the link between the context of group work and the mechanism it facilitates in order to deepen practical understanding through the participant's response. Subsequent follow-up questions can then be used to facilitate deeper explanation on the links between context and mechanism and context-mechanism-outcome. This allows the interview to evolve into more of a discursive format whereby the complexities of the programme theory can be thought through together between the researcher and interviewee (Greenhalgh et al., 2017b). In addition, by focusing the structure of the topic guide on propositions, theory can be interwoven within the interview. The structuring of questions is explored in the next section where we look at epistemological considerations within the topic guide.

Realist vs. non-realist topic guide structure and content

Topic guides can be used as a tool to assist researchers in enacting realist principles (as summarised briefly above) within qualitative data collection. To highlight how this can be undertaken, Table 11.1 categorises key features within sections of the topic guide. The table is intended to highlight potential similarities and differences between scientific realist and non-realist approaches to structuring the topic guide. It is acknowledged that there are many forms of non-realist approaches to topic guides which will use such guides differently, but these have been grouped for explanatory purposes. In addition, a simplified generic approach to what is contained in a topic guide has been used to illustrate these differences; however, it is noted that every topic guide will be structured to reflect the specific research aims and methodological approach of the study. Table 11.1 therefore provides a high-level overview of realist vs. non-realist topic guide structure and content as opposed to a checklist of what to include in either type of interview.

Table 11.2 has been included to provide an illustrative example of a topic guide. It is an extract from a topic guide used to guide initial programme theory development through interviews with academics delivering a Post Graduate Diploma (PGDip) in Coach Development.

Table 11.1 Realist vs. non-realist topic guide structure and content

Topic guide section	Non-Realist, i.e. more traditional constructivist approaches	Realist approach
Pre-interview	• Identify specific relevant background of interviewee which may influence their responses and require target/group specific questions (i.e. if interviewing practitioners and participants, you may have two sets of questions, one for each group).	• Identify the extent of the participant's knowledge in relation to the components (C, M, O) to be explored in the interview and specific relevant background influencing their responses. • Identification of programme theories relevant to the interviewee. This may result in different question sets (or topic guides) being used for different participant groups. • See also Manzano (2016) Guiding principle 1: Before the interview.
Introduction to the researcher and research project	• Researcher to introduce themselves • Provision of an introduction/overview of the research • Obtain informed consent • Opportunity to answer any participant questions	
Introduction to the interview	• Promoting the participant to draw on lived experience in responding to questions, e.g. stating *'There are no right or wrong answers, we are interested in your views and opinions on subject matter.'*	• Introduce the teacher–learner cycle concept. This will be more or less formal depending on the participant • Encourage the participant to elaborate or disagree with points presented to them and provide examples throughout, that is, asking *'We've been doing some work to understand the [programme name]. In this interview we'd like to work with you to understand whether our work reflects your experience, and if so or if not, how?'* • See also Manzano (2016) Guiding principle 2: Ask questions like a realist.

(Continued)

Table 11.1 (Continued)

Topic guide section	Non-Realist, i.e. more traditional constructivist approaches	Realist approach
Introductory and background knowledge	• Enable participant to feel comfortable/establish rapport • Identify the remit of the participants knowledge in relation to the interview topic(s) and specific relevant background influencing their responses	• Enable the participant to feel comfortable/establish rapport • Further identify (building on pre-interview work) the extent of the participant's knowledge in relation to programme theories to be explored in the interview and specific relevant background influencing their responses
Topic guide question grouping structure	• Group research questions into themes, relating to the research aim(s)	• Group research questions in to key realist components (C,M,O) or initial/developing programme theories (see Figure 11.1)
Question composition	• Questions are open ended or semi-structured	• Although some questions may be general, most questions are theory-driven, utilising teacher–learner concepts and aim to explore key components (C,M,O) or generative configurations (CMOCs) in depth (see Figure 11.1)
Use of follow-up questions	• Follow-up questions are not written in advance. They are constructed and used within the interview to avoid problems of understanding (Roulston, 2024)	• Follow-up questions which further investigate the programme theories, may be anticipated ahead of the interview and written into the topic guide. Also, follow-up questions of clarification to avoid problems of understanding might also be asked, particularly after the participant has explained their 'theory' as part of the teacher–learner cycle, and to elicit further ontological depth
Closing	• Thank the participant for their input and time • Explain the next steps for the research including what the interview data will be used for • Direct participant to contact details for any follow-up/communication	

Table 11.2 Illustrative example of a topic guide

Background

Redgate et al. (2022) evaluated a 'reality grounded' learning initiative; Post Graduate Diploma (PGDip) in Coach Development. The PGDip aimed to provide focused learning relating to the reality of the professional role and context of the Coach Developer, targeting the professional judgements and decision-making of experienced football Coach Developers.

In the evaluation, interviews were conducted with academics delivering the learning initiative as well as with the football Coach Developers participating in the course. The academics were perceived to have detailed knowledge of the initiative from being involved in its design, as well as delivering the course. The football Coach Developers had detailed coach development knowledge and experience, as well as relevant experience of participating in the course.

Interview section focus	Questions	Question aim
Introduction	• Just to set the scene, can you give us a quick overview of the main goals of the PGDip? What are the key aims and objectives of the course? • What changes have you noticed so far in Coach Developers? What changes would you want to see in participants by the end of the course? • Within the module documentation there is reference to 'who/what/how' a lot, how is this approach used in practice and what outcomes are expected from it? • Having spoken to [Football Association lead] regarding the course, he described the football coaching landscape as quite complex and political. Have you found this to be the case, and if so, has this affected delivery of the PGDip and the outcomes produced? • What challenges and opportunities has this landscape presented for teaching?	Understanding more about the context of the course and key mechanisms within the course related to outcomes Context development
Behaviour change	With any teaching, the aim is to influence the learning, however, do you have any techniques in place to identify if the learning from the PGDip has been put into practice and influenced behaviour change?	Identifying links to outcomes

(Continued)

Table 11.2 (Continued)

Interview section focus	Questions	Question aim
Group work	• How have you encouraged/ facilitated a community of Coach Developers? • To what extent do you think this has been successful? • What effect has the bringing together of Coach Developers from a range of backgrounds (context) had on the learning environment (mechanism)? • What effect do you feel having a group work focus has had on Coach Developers on the PGDip? • What are you doing in terms of group work? Why are you doing it? And how are you doing it? • How does learning from each other (mechanism) work within the group work elements of the PGDip (context)?	Context development/ identification of mechanisms and outcomes Identifying links between context and mechanism Context development/ identification of mechanisms Identifying links between context and mechanism
General	What effect do you think having a professional qualification at the end of the PGDip will have on the coaches? The literature talks a lot about cycles of knowledge construction - have you used this in the PGDip and if so, how?	Link to outcomes Identification of mechanisms

Underpinning epistemological considerations for realist topic guide structure and development

In realist evaluation, a wide range of participants are required to thoroughly interrogate programme theories. Participants should therefore be purposively selected based on their experience and engagement with the programme, to provide the most relevant data in the interview. This will ensure they are able to meaningfully contribute to theory development. Pawson and Tilley (1997) describe this as a participant's 'CMO- investigation potential'. These participants will have the ability to answer a wide range of questions about the programme under study. In order to ask relevant questions and adhere to realist principles, we suggest two types of questions that should be in the researcher's toolkit when developing topic guides, detailed in Figure 11.1.

Realist interviewing, as detailed earlier in the chapter, involves an openness on the part of the researcher to share their ideas and assumptions on how

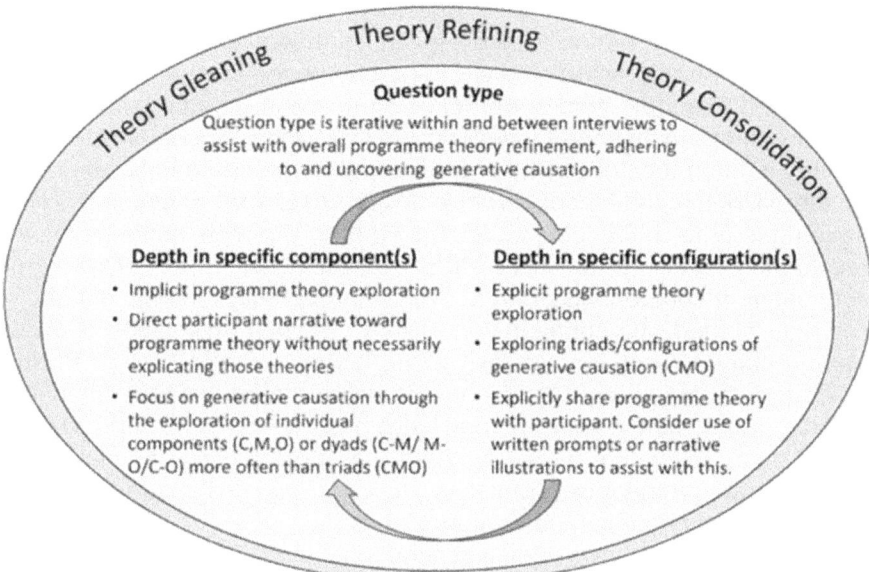

Figure 11.1 Underpinning epistemological considerations for topic guide development.

a programme works to allow the participant to assist with building and refining programme theory (Manzano, 2016; Mukumbang et al., 2020). We propose that this sharing of theory can be done either implicitly or explicitly and include full or component parts of programme theories. We categorise this as 'depth in specific component(s)' and 'depth in specific configuration(s)', in Figure 11.1. Deciding which question type approach to take within the topic guide will be dependent on a number of factors including: the phase of the interview (theory gleaning, refining or consolidation), the questions being asked, the participants engagement with the programme and the researcher themselves (described in more detail below within, Step 1: What is already 'known' and what is 'not known'?). It should also be noted that theories should not be refined solely through a single interview, but rather by combining and triangulating other 'nuggets of evidence' (Mirzoev et al., 2020) such as other interviews, and/or data collection methods, or at a minimum with the literature examining that specific theory in the same or similar programmes. In doing so, data generated through the interview can be added to, or contrasted with other evidence to enhance explanatory potential.

Choosing the right type of question(s)

As per Figure 11.1, we note that there are different approaches to question type (depth in specific component(s) and depth in specific configuration(s)) that can be used in a realist interview and therefore should be reflected in the topic guide. The placement of these question types can be considered based on Manzano's (2016) notion of theory gleaning, theory refinement and theory consolidation phases. For example, during the theory-gleaning phase, it can be expected that topic guides will focus on depth in specific component(s) based questions, in an effort to identify core C, M and Os pertaining to a programme, with an idea of potential dyad (and possible triad) linkages. Taking this approach, the participant narrative is directed toward programme theory through questions in the topic guide, but without explicitly outlining the full programme theories. In this sense, it is the researcher's role to explore in-depth different components of the C, M, Os through questioning, but also to keep sight of the CMO configuration (CMOC) through exploration of dyads, to ensure the interview remains realist (see Tables 11.2 and 11.3 for illustrative examples). However, it does not always have to be this way. Interviews may start from a more advanced knowledge base, for example, if preparatory work, such as a literature review/synthesis, has already been undertaken and initial programme theories postulated. Here you may instead look to focus more on depth in configuration(s) approaches.

In non-realist interviews often a general topic guide is written prior to obtaining ethical approval (if required). However, when using a realist interview it is often only possible to give to the committee an indication of the questions that will be asked at the point of application approval, noting that further work will take place to develop the initial programme theories once the study commences, and consequently topic guides will change. As the research progresses through to theory refinement, typically we would expect topic guides to be re-drafted to reflect the theories being refined. These topic guides will normally include a shift to more depth in specific configuration(s) approaches, whereby emerging CMO configurations are explored. This is achieved through the explicit presentation of programme theories to the participant to begin the teacher-learner cycle. This is often achieved through use of written prompts such as an explicit written statement of the programme theory, or through illustrations, which could be narrative (e.g. vignettes, pen portraits to connect theory components to experiences (Clibbens et al., 2023), etc.) or pictorial (e.g. diagrammatic visuals of the programme theory, cartoons, photos, etc.) alongside a verbal explanation of the theory. Terminology used should be adapted to best suit the participant in aiding their understanding and to ask for participants to comment with their views.

Finally, as the interviews move to theory consolidation, we would expect topic guides to focus more on depth in configuration by means of confirming and consolidating final programme theories. However, this is not to say depth in component(s) type questions cannot be used at this point. Indeed, there may still be a particular aspect of the context, mechanism, and/or outcome which warrants a more detailed investigation via a depth in component route of questioning. As with all realist research we see here the idea of iteration, moving focus as a result of ongoing analysis, both within and between interviews and question types to assist with ongoing theory refinement.

Table 11.3 Iteration between question types and focus throughout the research process

Background (see Table 11.2)	Interview aim	Type of question(s) used
Interview phase		
Theory gleaning	Interviews with academic staff delivering the PGDip to explore and refine insights and theory gained from initial scoping work undertaken by the research team	**Depth in specific component(s)** • Focus on individual components to understand (1) the context surrounding the construction and delivery of the PGDip, and (2) mechanisms viewed to be central to delivery of the PGDip. • For example, exploring an identified key context of developing a coaching community through group work; *'The documentary review showed inclusion of group work in the PGDip. Why was group work used and what did it do over and above didactic teaching and/or independent study? Could this have been related to the need to develop a coaching community?'*
Theory refinement	Interviews with Coach Developers to refine programme theories pertaining to participation on the PGDip.	**Depth in specific component(s)** • Questions asked to further refine the component and to identify causal links between Context and Outcomes. • For example, exploring a Context (social dynamics of group work) in the interview with an aim of identifying how it is linked to Outcomes (impact on peer learning); *'I understand that in circumstances where you felt comfortable with the other members of the group, that allowed you to talk through experiences and practical application of the learning with other Coach Developers - what impact has this had on your learning from the course and outside of the course? Do you think this would have been different had you not felt comfortable in that group?'*

(Continued)

Table 11.3 (Continued)

Interview phase	Interview aim	Type of question(s) used
		Depth in specific configuration(s)
		• Programme theories presented to Coach Developers verbally to comment on.
		• For example, exploring a theory on peer support, where Context is social dynamics in group work, Mechanism is group work learning approach (resource) and learning attitudes (reasoning), and Outcome is Coach Developer community; *'From observing some of the sessions, it seems that the group work you are participating in has meant that you have to talk and discuss your thoughts and approaches to coaching with some of the other Coach Developers and from this, new relationships have been built. Can you tell me a bit more about this?*
Theory consolidation	Interviews with Coach Developers and academic staff delivering the PGDip to consolidate programme theories previously identified.	**Depth in specific component**
		• Specific questions used to consolidate/finalise causal links between components with Coach Developers.
		• For example, again exploring the theory on group work and coaching communities, where Context is social dynamics in group work, Mechanism is group work learning approach (resource) and learning attitudes (reasoning), and Outcome is Coach Developer community. But at this stage looking to consolidate what the outcome of Coach Developer community entails, that is, further exploration of the outcome; *'From observing some of the sessions and previous discussions with Coach Developers, it seems that the group work you are participating in has meant that you have to talk and discuss your thoughts and approaches with some of the other Coach Developers. From this, I understand new relationships have been built as a community of coach developers. Can you tell me about these relationships?* Prompt on: *What do these relationships mean to you? What impact they have on your involvement with the course? What impact do they have on your working practices more generally?*

(Continued)

Table 11.3 (Continued)

Interview phase	Interview aim	Type of question(s) used
		Depth in specific configuration(s)

- Programme theories presented to academics verbally to comment on.
- Same format as the example provided above with a view that only minor changes will be made at this point as data to refine and support the theory has been developed over several interviews and by other means including a literature scope, observations and documentary analysis. For example, again exploring the theory on peer support where Context is social dynamics in group work, Mechanism is group work learning approach (resource) and learning attitudes (reasoning), and Outcome is Coach Developer community. But at this stage seeking support for further amendment of the theory, *From observing some of the sessions and previous discussions with Coach Developers and academics delivering on the course, the group work aspect of the course appears to have a significant impact on the Coach Developers application-based knowledge and skills. Through participating in group work, Coach Developers have become more comfortable with one another, and engage in peer learning discussions with their fellow coaches. This is seen to influence their attitudes towards Coach Development and has forged a Coach Development community. Does this statement align with your views from delivering the course and if so, or if not, how?*

It is important to note that topic guides may include questions on both depth in configuration(s) and depth in component(s). A researcher may, for example, begin by exploring depth in specific component(s) in an interview and then move towards depth in configuration(s) within the same interview. A worked example of how this iteration between question types can be used throughout the research process is provided in Table 11.3.

Depth in specific component(s) and depth in specific configuration(s) questions are not standalone question types. We propose that these question types will be iterative both within and between interviews as to assist with overall programme theory refinement, adhering to and uncovering generative causation. Furthermore, these two question types blend with one another, especially within the flexibility required in a realist interview. If a participant moves towards explanation of a configuration when asked a depth in component question, we encourage the researcher to allow this excavation of CMO configuration. As with all realist research, this is a messy and complex process, which will look different dependent on the individual study and interview.

Using the constructs in Figure 11.1 and acknowledging the iterative nature within and between interviews, topic guides help to focus questioning in the realist interview, using depth in specific component(s) and depth in specific configuration style questions. They can be used as a tool to assist the researcher in maintaining theoretical awareness while establishing generative causation between components (C, M, O) within the interview.

Designing realist topic guides

In this section, we provide advice in the form of a stepped approach intended to steer the researcher in developing a realist topic guide (see Figure 11.2). Although steps are presented sequentially below, in practice the process is likely to be more iterative, and there will be movement between, and repetition of some of the steps. This iteration is in response to emerging data from the research. The realist topic guide has a requirement to ensure that it is structured in such a way that can facilitate dialogue that identifies and explores key CMO components and their links, with an aim to 'inspire/validate/ falsify/modify' (Pawson, 1996, p. 295) programme theories. Information presented below in Figure 11.2 is linked to Figure 11.1 to assist in bridging the gap between this conceptual endeavour and a more tangible process.

Step 1: What is already 'known' and what is 'not known'?

A useful topic guide that facilitates the participant to share their relevant knowledge is grounded in carefully crafted programme theories. Although questions will be focused on the programme theories, the programme theories are not themselves the interview questions. Following the development of initial programme theories, it is important for the researcher to consider

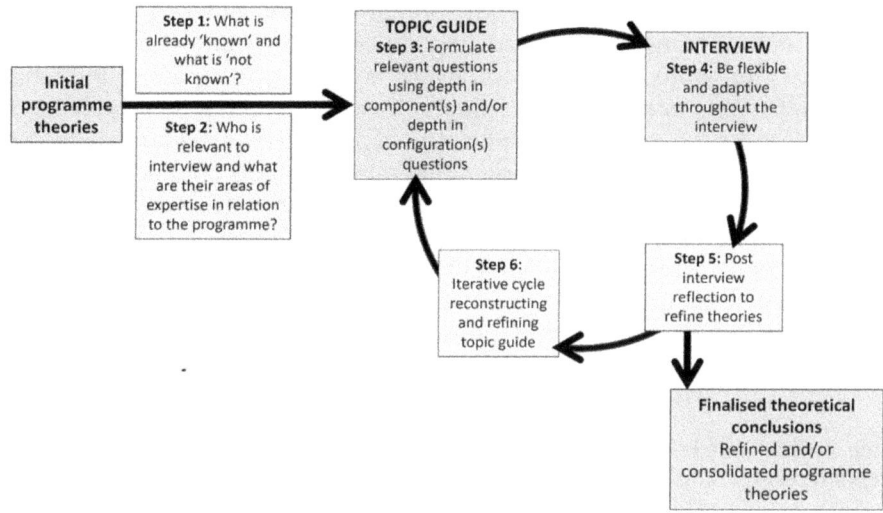

Figure 11.2 Stepped approach to developing the realist topic guide.

what is now 'known' versus what are the 'known unknowns', that is, what requires further investigation to focus the questioning in the topic guide while acknowledging there will also be 'unknown unknowns', that is, things that we do not know we don't know (Pawson et al., 2011). This focus may include depth in component(s) and/or depth in configuration(s) approaches to questioning (see Figure 11.1).

By 'known' we do not insinuate that this is a 'done deal', but rather there is something tangible which we can then explore further. We may for example 'know' that social dynamics in group work is a key context but need further exploration of how this fits within a configuration, thus prompting a depth in configuration type question.

On a practical level, the designing of topic guides can provide space for reflection and focus on existing programme theory(ies), by identifying gaps in knowledge which require exploration. The notion of what is 'not known' is extremely important; it is often the case at this point in the research cycle that causal links are tentative or that we have confidence in one or two components (e.g. O and M) but need to know more about what their bedfellow is (e.g. C). As highlighted previously, these two approaches are not mutually exclusive, and it is expected that there is iteration in question type both within and between interviews.

Step 2: Who is relevant to interview and what are their areas of expertise in relation to the programme?

Participants in realist studies are selected in relation to their potential to contribute to discussions on causation, to build and refine theory about what worked for whom, how, in what circumstances, and why, rather than being a representative of a broad population under study (Coorey et al., 2020). It is therefore important to consider who the participant is and what they may be able to contribute to theory development, that is, what parts of the programme theory they might be able to provide relevant knowledge on (see Table 11.1). It is important to note here that you do not need to ask all participants the same question(s), and even the same 'type' of participant (e.g. those receiving the intervention) may need to be asked different questions, as their experience and relevant knowledge may not be the same as their fellow participant. As the interview progresses, questions will become even further tailored in response to the information provided by the participant.

Step 3: Formulate relevant questions using depth in component(s) and/or depth n configuration(s) questions

When designing the topic guide, it is important to identify how the answers to the questions will be used, not by simply asking *'what are the evaluation questions?'*, but instead *'for what will the answers be used?'* (Westhorp, 2014). Using the constructs within Figure 11.1, we can use depth in component(s) questions to provide focus on exploring individual or dyadic components of theory. On the other hand, we can use depth in specific configuration questions to provide a more nuanced account of postulated generative causation between components. Taking this approach allows for questions to be structured in such a way that they can assist in theory gleaning, refining and consolidating. It is important at this step to phrase your questions like a realist with the focus on theory development and uncovering generative causation while keeping in mind the 'type' (depth in component(s) or depth in configuration(s)) of question you think you need. Questions should focus on the programme theory while exploring the '...how, where, when and why programmes are and are not effective' (Greenhalgh et al., 2017b). See Table 11.3 for examples of types of question.

Step 4: Be flexible and adaptive throughout the interview

There is a need for flexibility and adaptiveness throughout the realist interview. A lot of this flexibility will need to be 'in the moment' during the interview in response to emerging data from the participant, enacting the teacher-learner cycle. This therefore demands a thorough knowledge of the programme theories under investigation, or at least the ones being presented to the interview participant (see Step 2), prior to entering the field. Having this knowledge allows you as the interviewer to be agile and respond to the expertise of the participant in the interview. This can be facilitated using follow-up questions posed within the teacher-learner cycle which can help to encourage participants to elaborate and provide further detail on points made. In addition, it allows for flexibility should the 'unknown unknowns' emerge, that is, components that you had not previously considered or theorised about.

Step 5: Post-interview reflection to refine theories

After the interview, there is a need to be reflective. Ask yourself what went well, which questions yielded good responses, what did not work, and try to understand why this was. Was it the way the question was phrased, for example, or was it because the participant did not have the relevant knowledge to answer it? This reflective process allows you to consider whether any changes are needed in the topic guide in relation to explanations or phrasing to better facilitate your participants in providing relevant information to progress theory gleaning, refinement or consolidation. However, it is important to remember that sometimes one participant may find a question difficult to answer and another may find the same question easier, due to relevant personal experience. Therefore, although a question did not work well, you might not have to radically change it prior to the next interview.

Step 6: Iterative cycle reconstructing and refining topic guides

The topic guide in realist research is iterative, not only in relation to the type of question used, but in reflection of the refinement of theory as data collection progresses. This iteration should develop and transform as the researchers' thinking does. This is a key concept of realist topic guides. As the researcher gets 'wiser' (Kvale, 1996, p. 100), the topic guide should be amended to incorporate the new dimensions uncovered in the previous interviews along with any other data collection methods in the study.

Ideally the topic guide should be reflected upon after each interview in order to identify if any amendments in light of new knowledge are required. However, in practice this is very difficult to do, for example if there are multiple researchers using the same topic guide, or if there is little time between interviews. Therefore, a pragmatic approach to whether the topic guide needs to be updated to reflect new learning should be taken. This reflection can take many shapes and forms and could include (but is not limited to):

i A question could need to be taken out or given less priority within the topic guide because you feel you have sufficient evidence.
ii A question needs to move from a depth in component(s) question, to a depth in configuration(s) type question (or vice versa).
iii A new area or programme theory that had not previously been considered needs to be further explored (an unknown unknown) and requires the addition of new questions. These may be single standalone questions, but

sometimes a new section/area of interest including several questions in the topic guide may be required.

iv A focus may be put on questions that explore programme theories for which there is currently scarce data (instead of those that participants have explored in depth in previous interviews).

v If there is a change in the circumstances surrounding the intervention (e.g. a new policy introduced or the intervention attracts a lot of press attention) then additional questions may need to be added.

If working in a large research group with more than one person collecting data it is essential that a deliberative analytic approach (Carr et al., 2017) is used in meetings when doing data analysis, but also when updating the topic guide to ensure collective learning is reflected (see also the chapter in this book by Michaelis on managing quality in realist evaluations with extensive qualitative data).

Conclusion

This chapter has highlighted the need for the realist topic guide to be focused on theory development and uncovering generative causation, to be in line with the underpinning principles of realist research. In taking this focus, we suggest that questions within topic guides can be grouped by programme theory and will contain patterns of 'depth in specific component(s)' and 'depth in specific configuration(s)' questions within them. In defining these two types of question, we can start to interrogate how questions can be structured within the topic guide to inform theory development in relation to individual, dyadic or triadic theory configurations. This approach, combined with the stepped process of developing a topic guide highlighted within the chapter, bridges the gap between linking the theoretical concepts of realist methodology and a more tangible process, offering a framework to steer researchers when devising a realist topic guide. The information presented in this chapter presents one way of developing a realist topic guide and we invite others to build upon these ideas to further elucidate the process of generating realist topic guides, facilitating learning across the realist community.

12 Developing a recipe for realist interviewing using critical realist ingredients

Catherine Hastings

Introduction

Critical realism is a collection of philosophical or meta-theoretical ideas to guide thinking about the nature of the world, our knowledge of it, and our values. In this chapter, the focus will be on how critical realism can be applied to develop social science research methodologies with a focus on the interview method. Given that realist evaluation is a methodology associated primarily with scientific realism (Pawson & Tilley, 1997), the chapter will discuss the core similarities and differences between the two sets of realist ideas.

It can be challenging to define critical realism, as many scholars work on and within philosophical positions that seek a properly post-positivist social science. However, there are overlapping ideas on ontology, causation, structure, persons and forms of explanation (Archer et al., 2016). In this chapter, I refer to the distinctive characteristics of critical realism as expounded by Roy Bhaskar (2016) and also elaborated in the work of Archer (2000, 2003), Porpora (2015), Sayer (2000, 2011), Collier (1994) and Danermark et al. (2019). To cite Bhaskar, I will refer primarily to Bhaskar's (2016) final (posthumous) book, *Enlightened Common Sense: The Philosophy of Critical Realism*. It provides a condensed yet detailed summary of his philosophical ideas and, via its referencing, serves as a gateway to his earlier original works.

After describing the core features of scientific realism, I will explore the most significant differences between the two realist approaches. The chapter will provide a summary introduction to a critical realist logic for research and the philosophical ideas that justify such an approach. I will introduce five areas of critical realist thinking that support causal explanation through interview data by differentiating structure and agency and taking the values, motivations and emotions of people seriously. Finally, I will provide an example of their application in structuring interview guides, datasets and analysis.

Scientific realism

Although realist evaluation is understood to be situated in the scientific realist philosophy, Pawson and Tilley (1997) also claim to be influenced by authors such as Bhaskar (2008), Archer (1995) and Sayer (1992)—all vital contributors

DOI: 10.4324/9781003457077-13

in the attempts to leap from scientific realist explanation to critical realist social explanation. Sometimes, scientific realism and critical realism are described as two 'prominent forms of realism' differing in how the core ideas of realism are 'accented' (Mukumbang et al., 2023, p. 505, 508). At other times, critical realism is described as a form of scientific realism, where scientific realism is the catchall term for a range of realist positions (Joseph, 2007). There are sophisticated versions of scientific realism expressed as a philosophy of (natural) science and subsequent attempts to apply its principles to social science. This has resulted in numerous interpretations and definitions that sometimes contradict each other (Garrett, 2018).

In basic terms, scientific realism is any philosophy of science that 'emphasises the physical existence of things, in contrast to theories that dispense with things or objects in favour of ideas' (Garrett, 2018, p. 71). It is generally considered that the first principle of scientific realism is a metaphysical belief in the independent existence of reality—a 'mind-independent reality'—in contrast to the assumptions of idealist, hermeneutic, most constructivist and most poststructuralist philosophical views (Joseph, 2007). The nature and structure of the world are something that is objectively real and exists rather than being the product of our cognition or imagination (Mukumbang et al., 2023). The second principle relates to the 'semantic notion'—the relationship between theories and the world. Scientific theories try to capture the truth of the nature of reality (e.g. scientific objects, events, processes, properties, and relations). Scientific realism holds that scientific theories are 'truth-bearers' and are true or false depending on whether the theory correctly describes reality, that is, 'true or false *in virtue of reality*' (Ruyant, 2021). The final principle is the 'epistemic notion' of scientific realism, which is described differently by different realists. This notion often suggests that the best and most plausible scientific theories represent an approximation of reality (truth), starting from a common sense or abductive position. The claims are considered true, rather than only 'useful', because there are reasons (evidence) to believe the theory. However, scientific theories are only truth-approximating, and over time, they can be developed or discarded as part of the progressive nature of science (Garrett, 2018; Mukumbang et al., 2023). As scientific realism argues the reality of 'unobservable and underlying structures, processes, generative mechanisms and causal relations' (Joseph, 2007, p. 346), it is necessary to develop theories of reality using a retroductive logic of inference.

There are many overlapping ontological understandings when comparing scientific and critical realism. For example, they 'share similar understandings relating to the existence of a mind-independent reality, the existence of the unseen, upward and downward causation, stratified reality, emergence, the embrace of multiple methodologies, and the importance of theory in science' (Mukumbang et al., 2023, p. 508). The version of 'practical' (Pawson, 2013, p. 2) scientific realism, operationalised as a methodology in realist evaluation (and synthesis), is grounded in the idea that observed regularities (or demi-regularities) are caused by generative mechanisms, with their operations always contingent on contexts (Pawson & Tilley, 1997).

The two most significant differences between scientific realism—as expressed in realist evaluation writings by Pawson and Tilley (1997)—and critical realism, concern ideas about structure and agency and the role of values and normativity in social science (Porter, 2015; Alderson, 2021; Hinds & Dickson, 2021; Mukumbang et al., 2023). First, according to critical realist ontology, it is necessary to clearly distinguish the mechanisms of social structures emergent from human agency to achieve explanatory theories that more closely approximate reality. A fuller introduction to critical realist conceptions of structure and agency follows as part of the discussion on developing critical realist interview questions.

Second, critical realism has an axiology which develops principles on 'how to think about the ultimate objectives and moral implications of knowledge building' (Brunson et al., 2023, p. 4). At a minimum, these ideas challenge the possibility of a Humean 'fact/value' distinction and the pretence of objectivity in science, arguing that facts are influenced by values and values by facts (Gorski, 2013). This aspect of critical realism, particularly as articulated by Bhaskar, is strongly rejected by Pawson (2013) who exhorts realist evaluation practitioners to beware of such ideas. However, as will be discussed in more detail later in this chapter, these observations also help to focus attention on the role of motivations, concerns and ethics in human agency and argue that reasons must be analysed as causes (Sayer, 2011) and understood to influence the reflexive 'internal conversation' through which human agents mediate the causal powers of structures (Archer, 2003).

In addition, critical realism's axiology also outlines a commitment to the emancipatory potential of social science, with critique and evaluation serving as integral elements of research and applications of knowledge. Researchers' judgements 'influence the selection of issues, the emphasis placed on different factors, and the descriptions they attach to them' (Porter, 2015, p. 77), meaning that evaluators should reflect on and make their values explicit (Sayer, 1997). Some critical realists follow Bhaskar's moral realist perspective that values are real entities available for discovery through social science, not simply subjective individual preferences or a reflection of social norms (Bhaskar, 2016). Other critical realists employ a more pragmatic or Habermassian perspective grounded in an ethic of deliberation with value proposals accepted through consensus (Archer et al., 2016; Brunson et al., 2023). Regardless, critical realism emphasises the obligation for researchers to promote social justice and human flourishing (Sayer, 2000; Gorski, 2013). Compared to scientific realism, these ideas provide a rationale for research (including evaluation) that explicitly engages with values and ideology, the political, and what motivates people in the search for what is the 'truth' about reality.

Critical realism

In this chapter, I focus on the ramifications of adopting a critical realist ontological conception of a stratified, contingent and emergent social reality (Bhaskar, 2016) in evaluation, on the basis that these dynamics are necessarily the focus of explanatory critical realist social science in all its forms (Danermark et al., 2019). First, there is stratification between structures (or the objects of the social world) according to their nature and their generative mechanisms—with the fundamental question: what makes the object what it is and not something else? Second, there is a distinction between structures and their mechanisms and the events they produce (observed, unobserved or unobservable). Third, critical realist approaches stress the importance of mapping the ontology of the area of research interest. They understand reality as layered (stratified) and endeavour to explain how structures and mechanisms account for events within and between layers—including creating new and emergent structures at a higher ontological level. Ontologically 'deep' causal explanation requires research that integrates analysis of structures (objects in the real), mechanisms and outcomes at all relevant levels to answer the research question, incorporating the use of study designs and methods most appropriate to each level (Danermark, 2019). Depending on the object being studied, explanations may include physical, biological, psychological, psycho-social, socio-economic, cultural and normative kinds of mechanisms, contexts and effects developed using empirical and theoretical knowledge from each relevant discipline or area of knowledge.

Some of the critical questions that a philosophy of social science may seek to answer are:

- Do structures in society exist externally to the individuals on whom they exert powers (holism), or do the actions of individuals sum to create social structures (individualism)?
- Is a value-neutral social science possible or even desirable? (Little, 1991)

Critical realism develops ways of thinking about these questions, which provide some reconciliation of traditionally contradictory or problematic positions. As discussed above, realist evaluation (and synthesis) have been critiqued for 'conflating' structure and agency and underestimated the role of values in evaluation research (e.g. Porter, 2015; Hinds & Dickson, 2021; Mukumbang et al., 2023). Therefore, within the overarching theme of the implications of a critical realist stratified, contingent and emergent ontology for interviewing in realist evaluation, there will be a specific focus in this chapter on ideas about structure and agency, and the role of values.

Realist interviewing inspired by critical realism

To show how critical realism can be applied to inspire, structure and scaffold a form of realist evaluative research, it is necessary to introduce the conceptual ideas from which the more practical advice will develop. These will include concepts justifying a critical realist logic for social science research, guidance for how methods may be developed within a critical realist-inspired methodology and an introduction to five conceptual ideas within critical realist thinking—Bhaskar's *transformational model of social activity* and *four-planar social being*, Archer's *morphogenetic/morphostatic model* and the *internal conversation*, and the explanation for why reasons must be analysed as causes.

A critical realist logic for scientific research

Bhaskar elaborates a model for doing critical realist empirical inquiry (Bhaskar, 2016). It is a model of theoretical explanation which becomes the logic for scientific enquiry. Bhaskar's logic looks simple and common sense, and in a way, it is. However, doing research in this way does present a challenge—as does doing any research based on realist principles.

Bhaskar describes science as a creative activity in which one moves from a description of events (and other phenomena) to theoretical causal explanations in terms of the structures and mechanisms that produce them. The DREI(C) model of theoretical explanation is the simplest version of Bhaskar's description of a research logic based on critical realist principles (Bhaskar, 2016. p. 7, 30–31, 79–80). The acronym stands for the stages of:

- **D**escription of some phenomena or pattern of events
- **R**etroduction of many possible explanatory causal explanations by 'the imagining of possible mechanisms that, if they were real, would account for the phenomenon or pattern in question' (2016, p. 30)
- **E**limination of competing explanations by discounting those that do not apply in this case, leading to
- **I**dentification of the generative mechanism at work (followed by **C**orrection of earlier findings in the light of this identification)

Moving through this cycle and identifying the structure or generative mechanism causing the pattern or phenomenon that is the object of study becomes the impetus for a new cycle of discovery and theoretical explanation. Retroductive inference is used again to explain this newly identified level of a stratified reality, with the process continuing as far as is helpful to explain the events or things that are the object of scientific study.

The justification for this logic of scientific enquiry can be found in the core tenets of critical realism. I will focus on how Bhaskar describes the *domains of reality* and three core pillars of critical realist thought (combining *ontological realism, epistemic relativism* and *judgemental rationality*). Taken together, these concepts mean that a critical realist-inspired approach to a methodology for evaluation makes a search for theorised generative mechanisms its goal, weaving together existing knowledge and new analysis of context-specific empirical data.

Bhaskar's transcendental argument asks, 'What must the world be like for experimentation to be possible?' (Bhaskar, 2008). He establishes a stratified depth to reality in three domains: the empirical, actual and real. The domain of the *empirical* is what we experience in the world, our 'facts' mediated by theoretical concepts; the domain of the *actual* refers to events that happen in the world, whether experienced or not; and the domain of the *real* is that which can produce events in the world such as structures, powers, generative mechanisms, causal potentials and liabilities. This means that what is observable in the empirical domain is not direct evidence of causality, regardless of the structure of the data or the data analysis method. Causal explanation is instead a theoretical description of the real domain based on the indications, hints, patterns and signals observable in the empirical domain (Bhaskar, 2016; Danermark et al., 2019).

Consequently, critical realism develops the basic structure of the transcendental realist account of scientific activity. Science is, at the same time, *transitive*—a social process reflecting our changing knowledge of things—studying the *intransitive* or independently existing and acting objects of reality (Bhaskar, 2016, p. 24).

Likewise, *ontological realism* is the belief that there is a world existing independently (in the natural world) and relatively independently (in the social world) of what we know or think we know about it. *Epistemic relativism* recognises that our knowledge of the world is obtained through facts and theories, paradigms and models, methods and techniques of inquiry, which are a fallible, socially constructed, historically specific, changing, theoretical and extending knowledge of the world. Finally, *judgemental rationality* describes the possibility of adjudicating which accounts about the world are better or worse, that is, making claims to knowledge and claims about false beliefs. This involves judging between different, competing and contested epistemic accounts of reality based on elements of normativity, rationality, coherence, consistency and choice, in a cognitive process that recognises ontological realism and epistemic relativism, and also meta-epistemic reflexivity and ethical (moral, social and political) responsibility. The consequence of ontological realism and epistemic relativism is the *necessity* of judgemental rationality—whilst acknowledging the difficulty of separating facts from values and values from facts (Sayer, 2000; Archer et al., 2016; Bhaskar, 2009, 2016; Quraishi et al., 2022).

In summary, the essential approach of critical realist empirical social science is to collect data which encourages, supports and justifies retroductive inference and the move from description of events and observations to theorised causal explanation across all relevant strata of reality. In realist evaluation interviews are designed to test hypotheses that are 'elicited, developed, refined and tested' (Manzano, 2016, p. 352). According to Bhaskar's logic for social science inquiry, critical realist research would typically be more exploratory in its first phases, starting with the object of interest and looking to reveal empirical events and theorise structures and mechanisms (Brönnimann,

2022). Although, this logic does not preclude the use of interviews to test theories and assumptions, in general, interviews are more broadly a tool for investigating the reflexivity of human agents and a resource for understanding aspects of the layered or structured social reality (Smith & Elger, 2014).

Interview method development within a critical realist paradigm

There is no one approach to developing interview guides and collecting interview data within critical realism, just as there is no single critical realist methodology for social science or evaluative research. Critical realism is a philosophy or meta-theory, not a methodology recommending a specific approach to interview. As Bhaskar says, 'it is the nature of the object that determines how it should be studied (together with the current state of the research process)' (2016, p. 11). In the context of evaluation, the approach to interviewing will be guided by the scope and purpose of the evaluation, nature of the evaluand, and what is possible given the research team's expertise and knowledge. In any evaluation, the approach to interviewing will be influenced by the philosophical principles of the researcher and those of the authors of, for example, realist evaluation's methodological frameworks (Smith & Elger, 2014; Manzano, 2016).

Although there is no prescribed critical realist approach, there are many conceptual frameworks within the philosophy that may be utilised to develop evaluative research, depending on context. They can assist an evaluative researcher in collecting rich data, enabling retroduction to structures and mechanisms in a stratified, contingent and complex causal reality to both generate and test theoretical ideas. This section of the chapter will discuss some useful frameworks and show examples of how they have been applied. However, first, we must remind ourselves of how interview data fits into any empirical research project, of which realist evaluation is one example.

All research requires the integration of solutions to a substantial range of meta-questions which connect the philosophical underpinnings of a project to its practical methodological approach. Explicit (or implicit) interrelated knowledge claims across all project elements combine to develop a 'conceptual architecture' for the research (Nichol et al., 2023). A representation of the relationships of meta-questions within research projects is illustrated in Figure 12.1. It demonstrates the linkages between assumptions contained in philosophical principles, the theories and conceptual frameworks that help us explain what is happening in the world, and how a methodology enables the social research practice to answer a specific set of research questions. Thinking about the interconnected parts of a research design systematically and their influence on each other, along with the consistency (or not) of their embedded assumptions, will help prompt the meta-questions that, when answered, will develop the components of a linked-up project structure. This is a recursive and iterative process that will look different from one evaluative or social research project to the next (although similar types of evaluations in

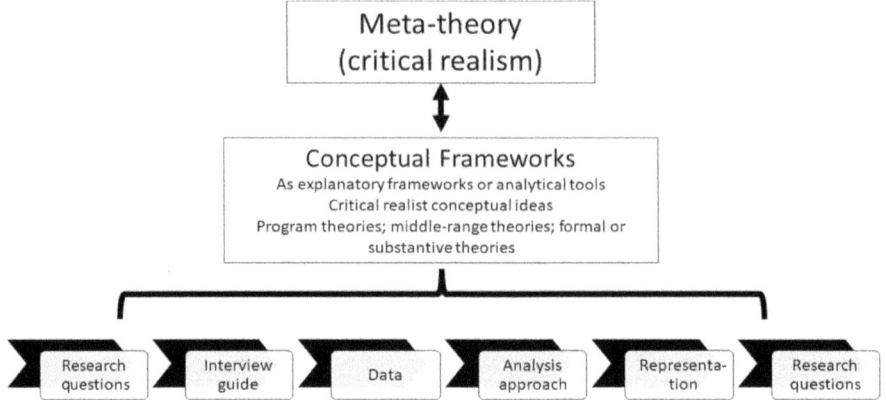

Figure 12.1 Method design within an internally consistent methodology.

similar contexts may start to develop recognisable patterns of approaches). At its core, this is a process that will bring meta-theory, theories, research practicalities and the objectives of the research into alignment to build scaffolding to support and sustain the project.

In considering the practicalities of doing interview research, the overarching meta-questions could be articulated as follows:

- What interview questions do I need to ask (and of whom) to generate the richness and range of data that I expect will provide evidence for retroductive causal analysis in the context of this evaluation, given the nature of what is being studied?
- What theoretical and conceptual material can be used to develop such an interview guide and provide inspirational frameworks for analysing the data it produces?

Critical realist ingredients for developing realist interviewing

In evaluation research, it is common to ask questions such as: how are things expected to work, how are they currently working, how have things worked in the past, how do we understand them to have changed in response to a stimulus (or intervention) and why? These are causal questions. How they are answered will be deeply influenced by the philosophies of science in which the evaluation methodology is grounded. Hence, the importance of the breakthroughs associated with realist evaluation approaches. The aim of this chapter is not to suggest an substitute to the approaches or logics to realist interviewing suggested by others (Pawson, 1996; Manzano, 2016). Rather, as discussed above, I argue that critical realism offers conceptual 'fodder' to further enrich realist evaluation approaches within a stratified, emergent, complex and contingent critical realist conception of causality. The concepts I will work with are clustered around critical realist models for (1) understanding the relationship of social structures and human agency over time and (2) thinking about facts, values, motivations, ethics and why people act how they do (or are able to).

Transformational model of social activity

Two crucial features characterise Bhaskar's conception of the relationship between structure and agency: (1) a laminated or stratified understanding of reality and (2) emergence. It is summarised in his *transformational model of social activity (TMSA)* (2016, p. 51–52). First, social structures or forms enable or constrain human agency and the activity of human agency reproduces or transforms social structures. Over time, social structure pre-exists the human agency that transforms it and post-dates the actions through which it is changed. Second, social structures and human agency 'constitute *radically different kinds of things*' (2016, p. 52) due to emergence. The properties of the *emergent* phenomena are irreducible to those of their constituents, with their specific structures, forces, powers and mechanisms, even though the new higher-level entity is dependent on those below and could not exist without them. Therefore, objects at the social strata level are emergent from lower strata, such as the level of the psychological or biological. Social structures are emergent from human agency. According to critical realism, ignoring emergent properties leads to an inadequate explanation of social phenomena (Sayer, 2000) compared to reductionist approaches, with the whole being functionally a sum of its simpler, constituent, interacting parts (Garrett, 2018).

The morphogenetic/morphostatic model

Archer's morphogenetic (change)/morphostatic (stays the same) model shares fundamental similarities with Bhaskar's approach, conceptualising the temporal relationship through which structure and agency emerge, intertwine and redefine one another (Archer, 2003). Archer describes her work as an explanatory framework facilitating social researchers to explain the social world (Archer, 2011). Her explication of the model suggests the questions a researcher may ask to explain the difference in social systems over time and how to break up the flow of events into analytical phases. When Archer outlines the phases of structural conditioning, social interaction, and structural elaboration (or change), she suggests analytical prompts such as: What are the components of what I am studying? How have they changed? Who was responsible? What interactions brought it about? What was wanted or not wanted because of what is there? Who did what, with or against whom, and with what outcome? Who had the resources? (2011, p. 62–66). It is thus very practical. Archer also theorises culture systems as a form of social structure, explaining their causal powers and interactions with human agency in an equally helpful way.

Four-planar social being

Finally, in this introduction to a critical realist view of structure and agency, there is the very helpful elaboration of the TMSA in Bhaskar's conception of the *four-planar social being*. This is the idea that 'all social activity and all social being occurs simultaneously on the four dimensions of:

a material transactions with nature;
b social interactions between people;
c social structure; and
d the stratification of the embodied personality' (Bhaskar, 2016, p. 53).

That is, all actions by agents and their being as social objects can be understood by paying attention simultaneously across all these four dimensions. Taken together, the conception of a laminated social being 'explodes' the relations across the stratified structured reality that describes a person at a point in time and as these relations are transformed over time. *Material transactions with nature* can refer to the physical world, environment, spaces and material 'things' with which a person interacts. *Social interactions between people* capture interpersonal interactions between individuals. Interactions with *social structures* describe the already mentioned enablement or constraint of human agency over time and the reproduction or transformation of social structures by the activity of agents. Finally, the *stratification of the embodied personality* refers to those features of our internal psychological makeup that make each of us distinctly individual — our motivations, beliefs, personality attributes, psychological state, subjectivity, reflexivity and intentionality mediating our agency as actors in social life. Each dimension of the four-planar social being suggests the possibility of different kinds of generative mechanisms implicated by the outcomes we observe in the social world.

The internal conversation

Archer also contributes to conceptualising the human agent as being both partly transformed by their sociality and having the capacity partly to transform their society by theorising a stratified model of agency (Archer, 2003, 2011). Without examining the attributes of this model here in detail, Archer distinguishes between *persons* (accounted for by the emergence of self-consciousness, personal identity, and social identity) who are also *actors* (incumbent of a role) and *agents* (occupying a position on society's distributions of scarce resources). She advances the concept of the *internal conversation* to describe how agents reflexively deliberate on the social circumstances they confront. Relevant to evaluation and understanding how, why, for whom and in what contexts interventions bring about changes (or not), Archer writes, 'fundamentally, we cannot account for any outcome unless we understand the agent's project in relation to her social context. And we cannot understand her project without entering into her reflexive deliberations about her personal concerns in conjunction with

the objective social context that she confronts' (2003, p. 131). Reflexive deliberations mediate structure and agency — representing the 'subjective element
which is always in interplay with the causal powers of objective social forms'
(2003, p. 130). Archer describes how agents strategise (fallibly) about how to
best achieve their objectives, which they determine themselves, but in circumstances not of their choosing.

Reasons must be causes

Therefore, to investigate a stratified, emergent and conjunctive causal reality in
the context of a realist evaluation, Archer's writing implies the necessity of attempting to grasp the concerns, motivations and beliefs of, for example, participants and others involved in the programme. Bhaskar argues that 'reasons must
be causes' (Bhaskar, 2009, p. 135), meaning reasons why people act (or not) are
real and have causal powers. In the book *Why Things Matter to People,* Sayer
shows how people's 'relation to the world is one of concern' (2011, p. 1). People are evaluative beings, with their concerns susceptible to evidence and argument, what kind of a person they are and what happens to them—in the past and
the present. The ethical and normative dimensions of life motivate people. These
concerns must be analysed in relation to the social and cultural structures that
shape but do not fully determine agential actions. Likewise, personhood can be
understood to be emergent from 'fully real' human capacities—for good or not
for good—emergent from the human body and brain (as they operate in the material and social environment), the causal powers of which 'endow humans with
the ability to bring about changes in material or mental phenomena, to produce
or influence objects and events in the world' (Smith, 2010, p. 42).

Using critical realism

As already discussed, there is no one critical realist interview method. However, the philosophy, including those aspects profiled in this chapter, provides
some guidance for what to pay attention to when considering the possibilities
of interview data. In general, the interview guide must facilitate data collection suitable for realist analysis (description and retroduction) according to the
research objectives and the (evaluative) questions the research seeks to answer.

The logic of critical realist research suggests two phases of theoretical
analysis which can be adapted and applied to projects seeking a theoretical
causal explanation for observed outcomes (Danermark et al., 2019; Hastings,
2021). First is a **structural analysis** in which the 'field' or scope of the inquiry
is 'mapped' using *conceptual abstraction* from the empirical evidence to the
features of a phenomenon. It is a cognitive process through which what is
already known about a phenomenon is reinterpreted to give an improved understanding of observable events, the connections, relations, and properties
of the social object. At this stage of analysis, it can be helpful to ask the sorts
of questions suggested by Sayer (Sayer, 1992, p. 91), including: 'What does

the existence of this object (in this form) presuppose? Can it exist on its own as such? If not, what else must be present [or absent]? What is it about the object that causes it to do such and such?'.

Second is a **causal analysis** which employs *retroduction* to imagine a model of a mechanism that, if it exists, would account for the phenomenon (outcome) in question. Usually, explaining something in a complex social context would involve developing a model accounting for the interaction of generative mechanisms associated with multiple social objects or structures within a stratified social ontology. In critical realism, this process is understood to be aided by *abduction*—a redescription or recontextualisation of what is observed using existing theoretical or conceptual language as an aid to evoking mechanisms (Danermark et al., 2019). For example, an observed behaviour could be described as 'racist'. What in our theoretical understanding of racism suggests how that observed behaviour may act on others or the mechanisms by which it was generated? Further refinement of the theorised operation of mechanisms can be developed using *retrodiction*, that is, by considering the possible interactions and conjunctions of mechanisms that could bring about the outcome of interest (Elder-Vass, 2015). For critical realists, what is essential is holding 'together' in causal analysis a recognition of social systems as open systems, ideas of complexity, lamination, emergence, context, contingency (mechanisms can moderate, reinforce or counteract each other), and what conditions are necessary versus sufficient for an outcome (Bhaskar, 2016; Byrne, 2004). In addition, critical realism asks that we identify what is absent or what has been absented (or excluded) for the phenomenon to be what it has become (Norrie, 2010).

In empirical research, these structural and causal analysis procedures occur in response to the evidence of patterns, hints and shapes discovered through data analysis. The inferential or theoretical processes involved are aided by existing empirical and theoretical research and ideas. *So, how can interviews develop the appropriate data to promote structural and causal analysis in service of the research objectives of the project?*

Interviews are typically understood as useful for generating data that captures, for example, what an interview participant knows about something; what they have seen, heard or experienced; how they understand the circumstances and opportunities available to them (or not); how they understand or interpret their experiences of the world or the experiences of others; their processes around decision making; their feelings, motivations, concerns, values, attitudes and opinions; what they are like as individuals (their attributes); or their response to the dynamics of complex situations. However, in a critical realist (versus more constructivist or interpretivist) approach, the participants' reflections, experiences and motivations, in themselves, are not the research subjects. Instead, critical realist interviews 'focus on people's relational actions with causal effects on each other in an objective reality' (Brönnimann, 2022 p. 16). What is crucial is to discover the social conditions under which these ideas, feelings, motives and experiences were shaped and what behaviour they may trigger. Fundamentally, what can interview participants tell us about the ontological landscape of the object of the research, including about the reasons, values and experiences that have causal powers? Depending on the focus of the research question and the resultant mapping of the ontological landscape of the subject under investigation, interviews can provide forms of evidence across all relevant parts of a stratified social ontology.

Critical realist conceptual frameworks inspire the process of translating research questions into interview guide questions that speak to ontological depth. Thinking in terms of a stratified and emergent ontology in the design of questions, particularly using critical realist conceptions of the relationship between structure and agency, strengthens the potential for compelling causal explanation by enriching the dataset from which the theories will develop. Rich data will increase the likelihood that all relevant structures or social objects are identified and incorporated into the mapping process of structural analysis. Rich data will provide the fuel for retroduction in causal analysis. Rich data and ontologically 'deep' conceptual analytical frameworks will bring explanatory theory closer to describing the real in all its complexity.

Considering a school context with an intervention theoretically working through behavioural change in teachers as an example, critical realist thinking about structure and agency, using the frameworks described above, would encourage questions to capture the teacher's interactions with:

- the material environment of the school—nature of spaces and their position in relation to each other, quality and accessibility of materials, levels of comfort (temperature, safety or crowding), distance of school from residence
- other persons in their environment—their interpersonal interactions with other teachers, parents, students, their own family, other workers and volunteers in the school environment. What are the relationships, and what is the nature of each relationship (power, trust, influence, regularity, quality, differences and similarities), and what influences do they have?
- social structures—what are the administrative and teaching systems, workplace cultures, ideologies, pedagogical influences, education policies or structured power imbalances that have the causal power to constrain or enable the actions of teachers? What are teachers' actions in response, despite of, or in conflict with these structures? How are their activities reproducing or transforming these structures? How have systems or cultures changed over time? What actions or events brought about change (or not)? What else was needed or absent? What helped or hindered why, where, when or where? What resulted? How are interview participants positioned relative to the resources available (enabling their capacity to choose their roles and maximise agency)?
- their stratified embodied personality—what is their sense of self in the personal or work context, what capacities, concerns, feelings, reasons for acting (or not), ethical positions, motivations, hopes, and mental states could be influencing how they act (or not) in a given situation? Whose perspectives are needed to cover a 'saturated' or encompassing sense of the ontological landscape?

In this hypothetical case, the conceptual ideas are being used to generate avenues of inquiry, ensure facets of the ontological landscape (particularly in the relationship between social structure and human agency) are not overlooked, and collect data that evidences mechanisms by suggesting how things work, why they do, for whom and in what contexts within a complex, stratified and contingent realist social reality. They are prompting general research questions which can be edited down in number and made specific to the research to be appropriately framed as questions in the interview guide. In other words:

- What are the relevant social and cultural structures, and how are they constraining or enabling human agency? How are human agents acting to reproduce or transform these structures over time?
- What is the nature or structure of each of the relevant social objects in relationship to the object of study? How are they emergent from the interaction of other mechanisms to have specific structures, forces, powers and mechanisms?
- What is it about a social being's material transactions with nature, social interactions with other people, interactions with social structures and the stratification of their embodied personality that may help explain the subject of the research, in this circumstance?
- How can we understand the reflexive deliberations and concerns of agents in their social context and the implications of both on how they act?
- How has the evaluative capacity of people, their ethical and normative frames, their exposure to evidence and argument and their individual combination of personal attributes and capacities influenced their thinking and produced their agential influence on things in the world?

In the context of evaluation, there are many positions in this conception of stratified reality in which an intervention could be 'interfering' and using critical realist concepts can help to identify them more thoroughly.

Interviewees are selected according to their 'differentiated patterns of respondent expertise' (Smith & Elger, 2014, p. 110). The logics of sampling articulated by Manzano (2016) also provide helpful guidance on a realist rather than 'constructivist' or 'positivist' approach. She highlights that saturation is not the goal, as even single reports or 'fragments' may be the key to explanation; that purposeful sampling is used to focus on the contexts that matter within the realist process of theory-testing; and that the aim is to collect as much rich data as possible given the constraints of the project. She also advocates for research designs that enable repeat interviews 'to explore and further develop evaluator's theories as he/she is becoming more knowledgeable about the programme' (p. 349). Therefore, sampling methodologies and sample size will be a pragmatic response to the data needs of the project, following the iterative analysis processes which direct us to seek clarification or more information in certain directions. However, within a complex, contingent and stratified critical realist social ontology, it is probable that interviewees may not always have all the answers, as the role of social or cultural structures maybe hidden, unrecognised and unacknowledged. Other data sources will be necessary to fill gaps and suggest other ways of interpreting or explaining a phenomenon.

Finally, a word on critical realist thinking about values in theory building and evaluation. Multiple explanatory theories are possible with any set of available evidence. Our theories are, according to realist ontology, fundamentally underdetermined by evidence, meaning that other criteria must be used to choose between available explanations. These criteria will often be based on epistemic and ontological values or philosophies; and the corresponding assumptions that a researcher makes about human personhood and capacities when seeking to interpret social science data (Gorski, 2013). Critical realism argues that facts and values 'are not so easily or neatly insulated from one another' (2013, p. 543) as is often assumed by social scientists. Values influence facts and facts influence values. The implication of this is that the values and ethics of the researcher in an evaluation will influence the basis of how they construct a project, generate data, see patterns in the data, retroduce to mechanisms and evaluate rival theories. How the statements of interview participants are interpreted will also depend on if their ethics, motivations and beliefs about a problem and intervention are allowed to influence an evaluation's design, assessment criteria and evaluative judgements.

A framework for phrasing more appropriate critical realist research questions

Brönnimann (2022, p. 2) introduces his paper on critical realist interviewing with the statement that his framework's 'aim is to develop interview questions that are more coherent with the underlying realist philosophy to support retroductive analysis methods'. The framework combines Bhaskar's ontological conception of the *three domains of reality* with Archer's *morphogenetic sequence* (both of which are described above). It also draws on the critical realist methodological principles developed by Wynn and Williams (2012), suggesting a sequence of actions for collecting and analysing empirical data. These can be summarised as involving exploration, retroduction, validation (or invalidation) of theorised mechanisms through a return to the dataset or collection of additional data (e.g. additional or repeat interviews), and the use of triangulation of other methods and data types to build evidence. Brönnimann argues that 'in combination, these concepts provide structure to direct the development of questions, that can explicate events as well as social structures and agency' (2022, p. 2) by generating data supporting retroductive analysis.

The resultant nine-cell framework shows that different objects, events or observations are in focus in the (1) real, (2) actual and (3) empirical domains. At the same time, distinct processes will be the focus at each stage of the morphogenetic cycle, being (1) conditioning by structures, (2) interactions with agents and (3) resulting morphogenesis or morphostasis. The paper shows how each cell of the framework indicates the types of questions that need to be asked to generate data with ontological depth and available for retroduction to the mechanisms of social structures and agency. Brönnimann stresses the importance of developing quality interview data through paradigm-conforming transcription, analysis, compositing of findings and subsequent publication. Therefore, the philosophical perspective must 'logically inform' the data collection and analysis methods. The framework he offers provides one such logic through structured guidance for developing interview questions. His question examples show how the framework can inspire applied and evaluative questions about the adoption of, in this case, a new business process.

Conclusion

Critical realism is a philosophy of science offering a version of realist social ontology, epistemology and axiology to support realist evaluation, and in the case illustrated in this chapter, in the design of interview methods. It offers useful ways of conceptualising the interaction of structure and agency over time and the values and motivations of agents and the researchers that study them. This chapter argues that taking seriously each of these aspects of reality will allow for better theoretical truth approximations in realist evaluation research.

13 Theorising through the lens

Introducing a realist photovoice technique

Ferdinand C Mukumbang and Sara Dada

Making a case for a realist photovoice technique

Photovoice is a participatory research method using participant photographic dialogue to encourage reflections on relevant social issues while empowering the participants to take control of the situation. The photovoice technique is claimed to improve the participation of vulnerable groups and empower them, thus emancipating them (Budig et al., 2018). Its ability to facilitate an authentic and meaningful collaboration to co-create/co-produce knowledge in healthcare makes it attractive to researchers (Halvorsrud et al., 2019). Like the teacher-learner realist interview approach, participatory research emphasises an 'educational aspect of social investigation' and translates participants' lived experience and everyday knowledge, supporting its potential compatibility with realist principles (Westhorp et al., 2016).

We recently applied the photovoice technique in critical realist-informed research to explore its potential to uncover generative mechanisms and emancipatory potential (Mukumbang & van Wyk, 2020). It enhanced the connection between the empirical data and theoretical analysis as the information shared by the participants emanated from their volition per the research objective(s) (Mukumbang & van Wyk, 2020). To this end, the photovoice technique favours retroductive theorising, a retrospective approach to unearthing the generative (social) mechanisms and structures responsible for the outcomes observed when an intervention, programme, or policy is implemented in a particular setting (Mukumbang, 2023; Mukumbang et al., 2023).

In this chapter, we introduce a realist photovoice technique which provides practical applications and guiding principles for using photovoice in realist evaluations and possibly other realist-informed inquiries. We unpack the photovoice technique as a potential tool in the toolbox of realist researchers and explore its potential contribution to enhancing programme theory co-elicitation between the researchers and stakeholders. In the following sections, we will underpin the photovoice methods in realist principles and illustrate how these methods can constitute a valuable data collection tool to enhance retroductive theorising and emancipate the stakeholder groups involved. Furthermore, we will demonstrate how the realist photovoice

DOI: 10.4324/9781003457077-14

technique addresses power inequities during researcher-participant engagements by giving participants ownership over the research process. Finally, we consider when and why to use the realist photovoice technique and when it might not be appropriate.

The photovoice technique

Photovoice integrates images and words to encourage the exploration of people's experiences, perceptions, and meaning-making processes. Wang and Burris (1997) first proposed photovoice as a process through which participants own and share their narratives by capturing photographs that depict their lived experiences (Figure 13.1). As co-researchers, participants are asked to reflect on their experiences or feelings relating to the research question and select photos to instigate this discussion, with this selection process meaning they take on a significant role in driving data analysis. This technique has been applied at both the individual and group levels. In these discussions, researchers may consider adapting existing frameworks or developing their guiding questions (Wang & Burris, 1997).

The photovoice technique values local participants' experience and knowledge and gives power to participants as co-researchers to control

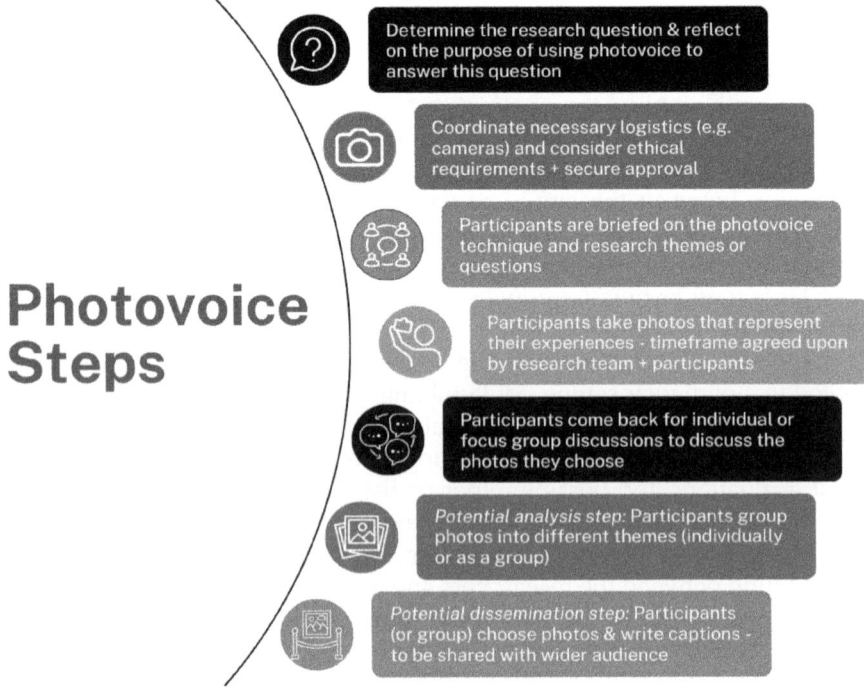

Figure 13.1 General steps followed in implementing photovoice.

and voice their narratives and can encourage collaborative learning across community members, researchers, and decision-makers (Hergenrather et al., 2009). Creative participatory activities help build trust and disrupt the researcher-participant relationship's 'traditional power structures' (Mannay, 2010). Visual activities such as photovoice can allow individuals to participate more freely, without concern for literacy or language barriers influencing the interview dynamic (International HIV/AIDS Alliance, 2006). Wang and Burris (1997) described how photovoice empowers participants and communities to define and represent their realities; as a result, they may put forward ideas that challenge the expectations and narratives of the researcher, contributing to the mitigation of power imbalances in research. Photovoice also allows communities to engage and discuss issues collectively when used in a group or at the community level (Catalani & Minkler, 2010). Previous photovoice participants have appreciated the platform, suggesting it provides a safe space to reflect and communicate creatively (Sutton-Brown, 2014). By actively addressing the power dynamics in hierarchical and heterogeneous research settings, incorporating photovoice approaches has the potential not only to improve participation in realist research but to facilitate the process of generating insightful knowledge with meaningful implications for practice (Jagosh et al., 2015; Vaughn & Jacquez, 2020).

However, there are also potential challenges to consider in conducting photovoice, such as the ethical implications of privacy and taking and sharing photographs, especially those depicting people (Woodgate et al., 2017; Teti & van Wyk, 2020). Additionally, researchers must consider the logistical and practical components of implementing photovoice, from the availability of cameras and film to communicating or explaining the 'ask' of what participants should do (Catalani & Minkler, 2010). Finally, while photovoice is lauded for addressing power imbalances in data collection, little is known about how photovoice can be used to engage participants in co-designing and defining the direction of the research. Researchers must, therefore, remain cognisant and intentional in ensuring participant-driven storytelling and acknowledge the other ways power imbalances may still be present throughout the research process (Wang and Burris, 1997). While applying the photovoice technique, how we define 'participation' and achieve capacity building through participants' engagement is explored less.

The photovoice technique, power dynamics, and emancipation in realist evaluation

Participatory research encompasses research designs, methods, and frameworks that use systematic inquiry in direct collaboration with those affected by an issue being studied for action or change (Vaughn & Jacquez, 2020). The photovoice technique is frequently adopted in collaborative evaluation and empowerment evaluation approaches. Although realist evaluation has not traditionally been considered part of collaborative evaluation and empowerment evaluation approaches, participatory research methods such as photovoice align with the realist paradigm and have been adopted within realist evaluation designs (Harris, 2020; Renmans et al., 2022). Participatory research methods value genuine and meaningful participation in the research process, and their methods are predominantly applied when some of the stakeholder groups involve vulnerable and at-risk groups.

Realist evaluation is a theory-driven approach that guides the implementation of complex interventions through iterative theory development, testing, and refinement. Participatory evaluation involving the active participation of relevant local stakeholder groups or representatives is gaining traction in realist-informed evaluation (Griffiths et al., 2022). Adopting the photovoice technique in realist evaluations enhances stakeholder participation in theory formulation. Bhaskar (2008), in his critique of the conventional evaluation methods, revealed that the science of evaluation should start by recognising that the fate of social [interventions and] policies lie in the choices of choice makers. This assertion is supported by Pawson and Tilley's (1997) conceptualisation of mechanisms as resources plus actors' reasoning, which also puts the actors at the centre of realist evaluation.

Participatory research methods, such as photovoice, encourage active involvement and co-production of knowledge to empower stakeholders (Budig et al., 2018). Nevertheless, these methods are conspicuously less considered in realist-informed inquiries. While Pawson and Tilley (1997) paid less attention to using participatory research methods in realist evaluation to consider power dynamics, Bhaskar (2009) was concerned with power dynamics issues and considered emancipation an essential aspect of research conducted using realist-informed methods. He suggested that emancipation speaks to the world becoming meaningful to the stakeholder in question, where their thoughts, understanding, and values are no longer seen as subjective classifications of the mind but constituting their reality (Bhaskar, 2009). Although this meta-reality is individualist, it can lead to collective action oriented toward emancipation to achieve social justice (Dean et al., 2006), an explicit goal of the photovoice methodology.

Regarding emancipation, therefore, critical realist approaches strive to contribute to changing the world for the better through the creation of structures that are wanted, needed, or generally emancipatory (Wilson & Greenhill, 2004). This is achieved by unveiling how things are necessary to demonstrate the place of human acts in the 'reproduction of social structures and relations that stand in the way of emancipation' (Ackroyd & Fleetwood, 2003, p 23). Through retroductive theorising, uncovering underlying mechanisms and structures that explain an observation or a phenomenon (Jagosh, 2020), such as inequity in healthcare service delivery, realist-informed research approaches enable reflections on alternative structures where genuine and equitable healthcare service delivery can be considered.

Layered ontology

Bhaskar's (2008) book *A Realist Theory of Science* lays out the foundation of the realist 'deep' ontology. He proposed that the world is stratified into three domains: the domain of the *'empirical,'* which entails our observations of events that occur in the domain of the *'actual,'* which are caused by underlying mechanisms and structures that are part of the domain of the *'real.'* Realists' position is that the object of science should be unearthing these mechanisms and structures, which are usually hidden.

Photos and other visual tools have been used to uncover social mechanisms that can explain a social phenomenon. By taking pictures and sharing their significance with others, the researcher can unveil the individual's thought process and emotional state to understand their decision-making vis-à-vis the observed behaviour. These emotions and thought processes are found in the 'real', which have caused the events (situated at the *actual*) the individual is recounting or describing using the images and the images and discussions (situated in the *empirical*).

Intransitive and transitive parts

Causal entities such as gravitational forces are usually unseen and are considered intransitive entities —human actions cannot change them. They represent laws and properties of the world independent of our knowledge of (and efforts to understand) them. Through research activities, we can formulate theories and develop models to postulate their existence. These models and theories, like programme theories developed through realist evaluation, are considered transitive entities—amenable to alteration by human action. An individual's worldview is related to their social role. Individuals can play multiple roles at any time, and the types of roles can vary across time and place (Dean et al., 2006). While playing different roles, individuals may be involved in various relationships, each exerting peculiar causal tendencies (Dean et al., 2006). The meaning-making opportunities that the photovoice technique offers using images allow individuals to represent their different roles and the meanings they attribute to them to capture their social situations. These different roles can be observed when individuals enter designated social positions to engage (or not) in social practices (de Souza, 2013). For example, Lennon-Dearing and Price (2018) used photovoice to explore the realities of women living with HIV, which allowed them to systematically unpack their roles as mothers, patients, substance abusers, criminals, and lovers, thus identifying the relevant generative mechanisms for the outcome or observation of interest.

The photovoice technique allows participants who live and experience a phenomenon to take centre stage rather than being foregrounded through the researchers' viewpoints (Glaw et al., 2017). Because the study participants are central to setting the study's agenda, most photovoice practitioners consider them as co-investigators (Woodgate et al., 2017). The philosophical implication is acknowledging that participants' experiences produce knowledge of themselves. Within this context, various stages of meaning-making are associated with the photovoice technique; the participants' narratives and reflections during the image discussion sessions are analysed by the researchers to understand the meaning attached to them. Therefore, different layers of meaning can be unearthed as the photovoice components evoke deep emotions, memories, and ideas through multiple interpretive and subjective moments. These interpretive and subjective representations constitute the transitive, as they can change over time as the emotions and perspectives of the co-investigators change.

Emergence and open systems

Emergence occurs when a whole (an outcome) possesses one or more emergent properties (Elder-Vass, 2010). Unobservable entities are structured, and these structures are nested within other structures, for example, family dynamics nested within cultural or religious practices. These entities are usually unobservable, and their operations depend on situational conditions created by complex interactions with other things (Brönnimann, 2022). The occurrence of novel qualities from the interactions of these existing entities is described as emergence. The emerging outcomes are not the sum of the parts of the interacting entities. Thus, they cannot be reduced to the entities that combined to form them. For instance, perceived HIV stigma can be attributed to a combination of cultural norms and an individual's interpretation of the cultural norms, but cultural norms alone cannot cause perceived stigma. The photovoice technique can capture these emergent behaviours by recording multiple moments and aspects of the phenomenon under consideration.

The notions of open and closed systems further capture the concept of emergence. Realists contend that the world is an 'open system' with a constellation of structures, mechanisms, and other entities responsible for the observed demi-regularities. Bhaskar (2016) explained that human capacity and agency are omnipresent and unceasing in their capacity to alter their environment. Within the open system, structures and other entities can potentially influence demi-regularities or outcomes. Interventions are implemented in systems that involve multiple factors associated with the intervention, the context and the people involved. These factors can influence each other in creating creative and unexpected but influential effects on results (Allana & Clark, 2018). The role of the photovoice technique is to work with agents considered part of the open system to unpack those contextual and structural issues that influence their attitudes and actions.

Aligning the photovoice technique to realist principles

The principles underpinning realist evaluation constitute an amalgam of scientific and critical realism philosophies of science (Mukumbang et al., 2023). Following the notion that the adopted methodology and epistemological foundations should inform the data collection and analysis processes (Nichol et al., 2023), we situate photovoice, a participatory research method developed from an interpretivist point of view, in realist evaluation. The premise of our argument here follows that interpretivism and critical realism recognise the importance of ideas, experiences, narratives, and discourses in understanding social phenomena. However, realist-informed research employs these forms of expression to explore causal explanations (McEvoy & Richards, 2006). The understanding is, therefore, that while the data collection technique developed from an interpretivist perspective might be useful, it must be adapted to align with methodological realist principles to harness its full potential in realist evaluation. Therefore, we extend this argument to introduce a realist photovoice technique. To achieve this, we discuss how realist principles should guide adopting photovoice techniques in realist evaluation.

Situating photovoice within realist evaluation study design

Realist evaluation is generally conducted in three phases: theory gleaning, theory testing (refining), and theory consolidation (Manzano, 2016; Mukumbang et al., 2020). The theory-gleaning phase, as the name suggests, is exploratory. Usually, it entails developing an initial programme theory or conceptual framework about the underlying mechanisms of the intervention, policy, or programme (Sobh & Perry, 2006). Different sources of information can inform the development of the initial programme theory. The existing information through systematised reviews, document analysis, and interviews with relevant stakeholders can inform the initial theory construction (Mukumbang et al., 2018). The realist photovoice technique can also be employed to elicit relevant information from the targeted population to inspire the development of the initial programme theory.

The theory testing phase also takes an eclectic methodological approach. This phase usually follows an explanatory theory-building approach designed as case study research (single or multiple cases). It involves formal data collection and analysis methods to validate, falsify, and modify the initial programme theory. The photovoice technique can be a suitable data collection tool used in isolation or combined with other data collection methods. We had previously successfully used photovoice as a single approach to unpack the dynamics around antiretroviral medication adherence among adolescents living with HIV (Mukumbang & van Wyk, 2020).

The theory consolidation phase is the second-level refining and fine-tuning of the initial programme theory. It represents the final stage of retroductive theorising and may entail the application of retrodiction when conducting cross-case analyses and comparing in-case theories from selected cases to obtain a more refined theory. Photovoice exhibits could be harnessed as a potential avenue for theory consolidation and higher-level abstractions, especially when implemented on a participant basis – bringing together different types of participants or case studies, if applicable.

Pawson and Tilley (1997) identified context, mechanisms, and outcomes as the three central constructs to explaining how and why programmes work or not, with the notion that an outcome (O) is generated by a mechanism (M) being triggered in a particular context (C). Realist programme theories are primarily formulated using the Context-Mechanism-Outcome configuration (CMOC). The goal of data analysis in realist photovoice is to identify CMOCs within the conversations instigated by the photos in tandem with the transcripts. Gilmore et al. (2019) emphasise identifying linked CMOCs within the transcript excerpts; this informed our development and inclusion of the CMOCs and the presented photos in the case study described in this chapter. However, it is noteworthy that Jackson and Kolla (2012) suggest identifying linked dyads (mechanism-outcome, context-mechanism, context-outcome) and triads (context-mechanism-outcome) during analysis, which may be a preferred approach in some cases.

A realist photovoice technique: Experiences from Zambia

The realist photovoice technique was recently used in a realist evaluation focused on the community engagement conducted by Safe Motherhood Action Group (SMAG) volunteers in the Eastern Province of Zambia (Dada et al., 2024). This multi-method study conducted focus group discussions with community members and in-depth interviews with SMAGs, local leaders, health facility staff, and pregnant women. In this case study, data was collected through observations, interviews and focus groups with different stakeholders, and the realist photovoice technique was used to test programme theories (Table 13.1) initially developed in a realist review (Dada et al., 2023). The realist photovoice technique was conducted with the pregnant women (PW) participant population to test these programme theories and uncover their feelings, perspectives, and experiences with the community engagement intervention, messages, and decisions to seek antenatal care.

Before deciding on, planning, and conducting data collection through the realist photovoice technique, the considerations (expressed as reflective questions) in Table 13.2 were examined.

Two prompts, described in reflective question 5, were chosen to uncover the generative mechanisms to explain SMAGs' influence on antenatal care attendance in the first trimester of pregnancy. In addition to determining what participants should capture in the photos, the researchers also had to coordinate the logistics of the photography equipment. Previous photovoice experiences have used disposable or non-disposable film cameras, digital cameras, and smartphones (Hergenrather et al., 2009). Based on experiential knowledge of the community and available resources, inexpensive digital cameras were chosen over disposable film cameras and provided to participants. While many in the communities could access cell phones, smartphones with built-in cameras were uncommon. The digital cameras were simple to use and durable, with rechargeable lithium batteries, eliminating the need for

Table 13.1 Theories tested through realist evaluation using realist photovoice (Dada et al., 2023)

Programme theories (PTs) tested in realist evaluation in Zambia	
PT 1: Community is actively involved (co-creation)	When communities are actively involved throughout the identification, design, and implementation of messaging delivered by the SMAGs, the communication is more relevant, acceptable, and trusted. Community members and SMAGs play an active role in co-creating the communication messaging by informing what information should be communicated, identifying challenges or misunderstandings, and raising overall awareness of the project and early antenatal care through tailored messaging. This increases ownership and enables longer-term sustainability.
PT 2: Messaging and programme are acceptable	When the project acknowledges and considers local practices/norms and power structures in communication messaging and processes, and these approaches and programme goals are tailored appropriately to the community, then the project and its messages will likely be acceptable to and shared further by the community.
PT 3: Communication sources are trusted	When messaging aligned with community members' values and experiences is delivered through familiar or agreed-upon communication avenues/structures by respected and influential SMAGs, the communication for the community engagement programme is trusted.
PT 4: Community has a reciprocal relationship with the programme	When the actors involved in maternal and newborn health programmes and delivery (including local leaders, SMAGs, and health providers) develop a positive relationship with community members and directly act on feedback from the community to inform the programme and messaging, community members feel heard and valued as equals.
PT 5: Community sees value or benefit from the programme	When a community experiences or perceives benefit from the project through the shared messaging, knowledge gained, or services provided, they are inclined to support/participate and disseminate messages further. This enables the longer-term sustainability or continued functioning of the maternal and newborn health programme.

extra batteries, and included a micro-USB charging cable and lanyard. The researchers included a 32 GB micro-SD memory card in each camera (as well as a micro-SD to SD adapter). These were fully charged before they were distributed to participants, allowing for eight hours of use, and participants were encouraged to turn off the camera when it was not in use to preserve the battery. When participants returned for the follow-up conversations, the researchers inserted the micro-SD card into a USB memory card reader on a laptop. The participant and researchers could see the photos on the laptop screen, and the participant pointed to which photos they wanted to share.

As was appropriate in the community, participants in the realist evaluation received a nominal financial amount for their transportation costs. Because photovoice participants were met twice, they received half the amount in

Table 13.2 Reflective questions in planning for and conducting a realist photovoice
technique

Reflective question	Zambia case study example
1 Why do I want to use Photovoice?	The researcher (as an outsider) wanted to address potential power imbalances with participants to encourage open discussion based on previous experience observing this group's interview hesitation.
2 What role would photovoice play in my realist evaluation?	The realist photovoice technique aimed to test programme theories developed in a realist review; however, photovoice prompts could also cause new theories to emerge.
3 What perspective am I trying to capture?	The researchers want to understand the influence of community engagement on pregnant women's decision-making about care-seeking:
	a What factors influence or prompt pregnant women to seek antenatal care early?
	b How do community engagement activities affect this?
	c What is pregnant women's perception of/experience with this community engagement?
4 Who can provide this perspective?	Pregnant women: this is often a less enfranchised group, and the researcher is trying to uncover the generative causation in their decision-making processes to seek care.
5 What photovoice 'prompts' can provide this perspective?	Participants take photos representing feelings at two different time points:
	a How they felt about care-seeking 'before' interacting with a SMAG.
	b How they felt about care-seeking or the SMAG 'after' they met.
6 How will participants take photos, and what supporting materials do they need?	a Decide whether to use digital cameras, film cameras or smartphones.
	b We developed verbal and pictorial instructions in English and local dialects.
	c Included a photo release form specifying the use and dissemination of photos in ethics applications.

the first instruction meeting, and the other half at the end of the follow-up
conversation. Photovoice participants kept the cameras at the end of their
participation in the research. To address ethical implications for the photovoice activities, consent and photo release forms were signed by participants
to ensure dissemination of the photos in research and policy publications.

Realist photovoice prompts, instructions on how to use the cameras, and
general information about the project for the consent process were provided
in English and Nyanja, the local language, to participants when the cameras
were given (Figures 13.2 and 13.3). When the researchers explained the photovoice activity in the initial meeting, they provided an example of a photograph
that could be taken, and tested for participants' comprehension of the activity
by having an initial discussion as a group about what they would consider

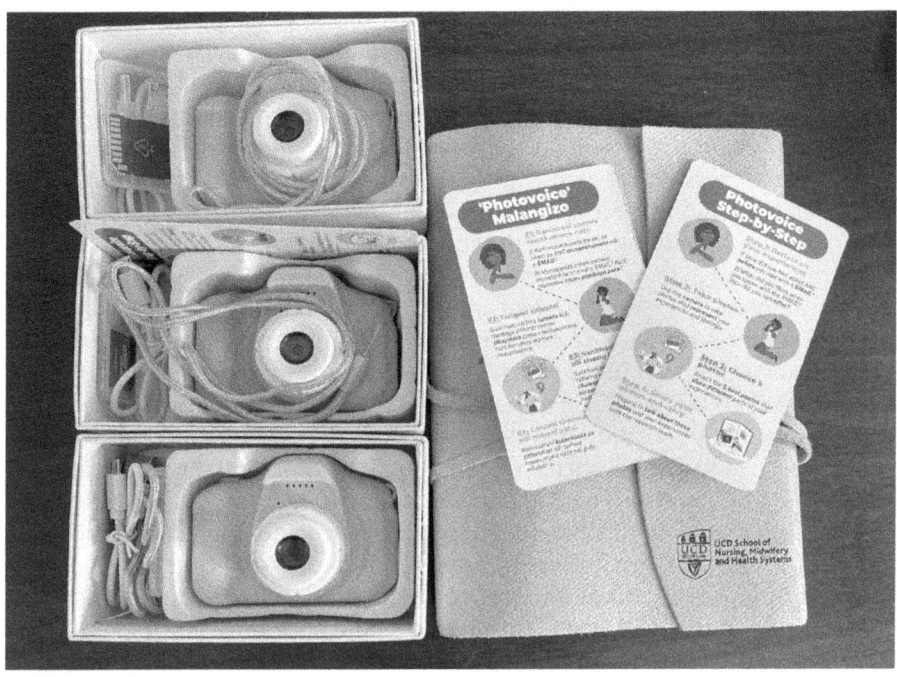

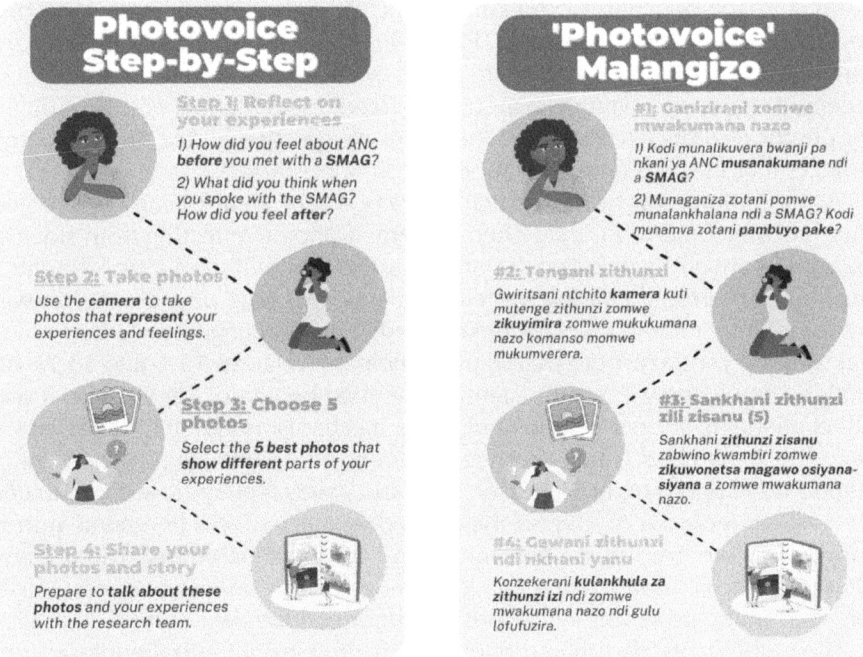

Figures 13.2 and 13.3 Equipment and support materials given to participants.

photographing to answer the prompts. If comfortable, participants were encouraged to reflect on their experiences and feelings and discuss the activity with their family and friends before taking photos. The researchers and participants then agreed on the time and place for the follow-up conversation. According to the project timeline, these occurred four to six days after initial introductions.

The researchers conducted a pilot interview with a participant who was introduced to photovoice and given approximately five days to take photos before the scheduled follow-up conversation. After this first conversation transcript was reviewed, adjustments were made to the process before finalising recruitment. For example, researchers incorporated informal discussions with participants on what photographs they might take, to test their comprehension and understanding of the two prompts (how they feel before and after interacting with an SMAG). Furthermore, the researchers informed potential participants that they could exit the study without consequences, such as being denied health care services. Consequently, two potential participants declined to participate, and researchers were able to recruit other participants.

The participants generally seemed to understand and apply the photovoice prompts. While participants brought several distinct images that could potentially be interpreted differently, they often described the pictures in similar ways. For example, Figures 13.4 and 13.5 illustrate how participants generally 'felt good' after meeting the SMAGs, mainly because they acquired knowledge from them. Although the researchers used follow-up questions to clarify, unpacking what this meant specifically or how the photos were distinguished was often challenging. However, the purpose of photovoice is for participants to decide what to share and to what extent; therefore, researchers accepted vague or repetitive responses. Indeed, the participants' use of different photos to represent the same feeling or perspective on the SMAGs could indicate that this was an important or dominant feeling.

While the prompts asked participants to capture their feelings before and after meeting the SMAG, they often presented photos reflecting both sides of the same concept (e.g. a bench without a cushion and then a bench with a cushion to represent gaining something new). This type of presentation was predominantly related to a lack of knowledge and gaining knowledge, which was also the central aspect shared by participants (Figures 13.6 and 13.7). Although knowledge was a consistently described benefit of the SMAGs, it was still challenging to uncover the underlying mechanisms that may have been at play. The researchers asked probing questions about why gaining new information was important, how it made the participants feel, or how it influenced their future decisions to unravel the generative mechanisms behind acquiring knowledge (the 'resource'). This finding remained valuable because the emphasis on information sharing and knowledge acquisition was not previously reflected in the programme theories that informed the data collection tools.

The participants also shared photos, providing insight into the interactions and demeanours of the SMAGs when they met with them. These examples, demonstrated in Figures 13.8 and 13.9, were often less literal than some of

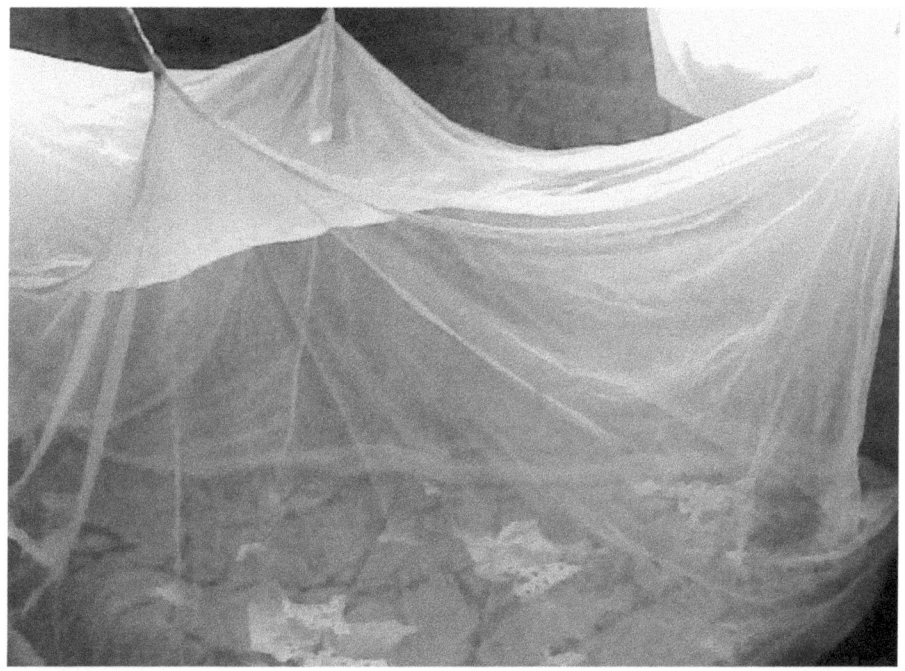

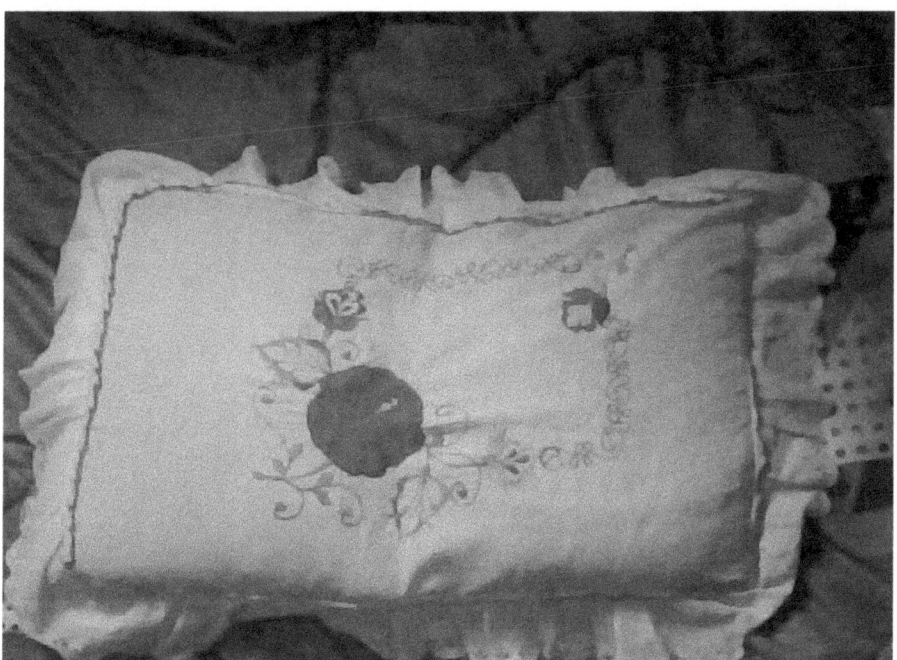

Figures 13.4 and 13.5 Photovoice examples about 'feeling good'.

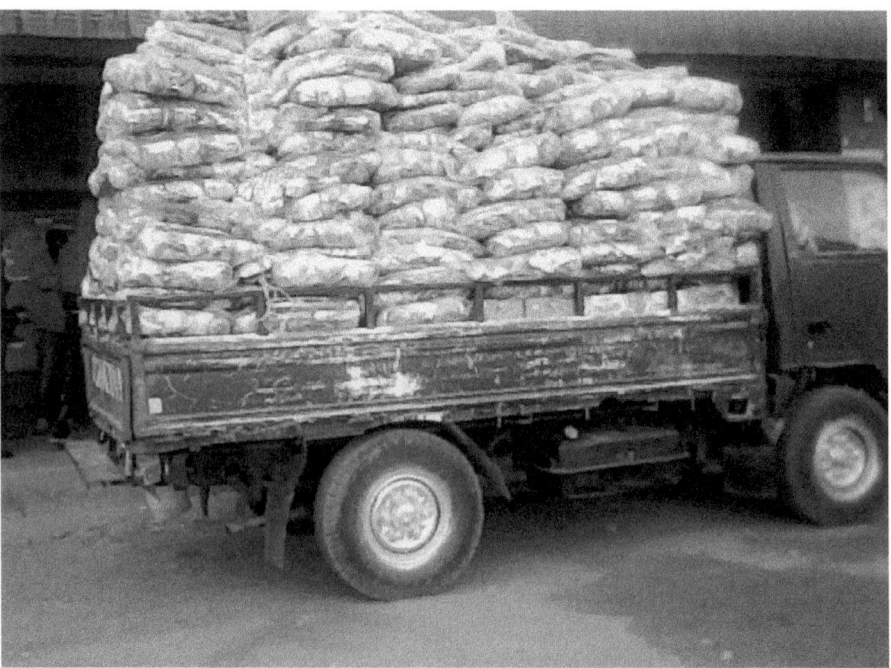

Figures 13.6 and 13.7 Photovoice examples relating to before/after learning information.

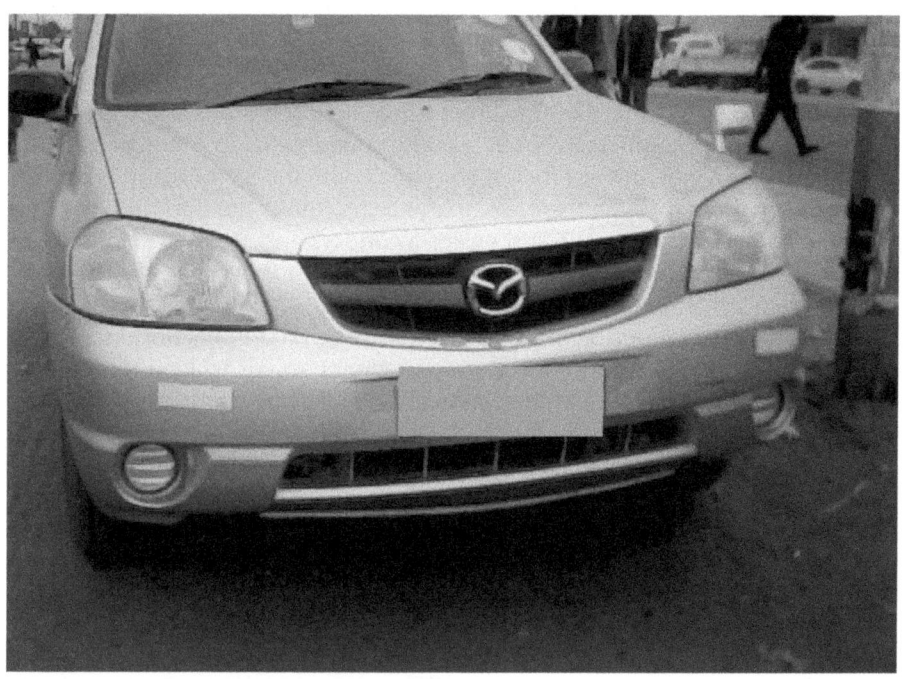

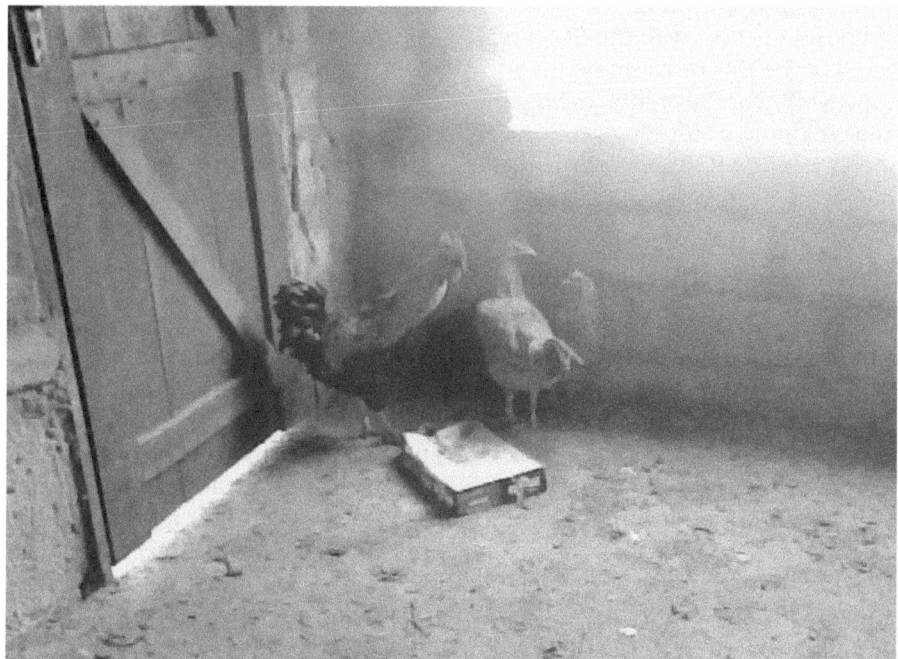

Figures 13.8 and 13.9 Photovoice examples of interactions with SMAGs.

the other photos shared and could be considered more reflective of the pro-gramme theories being tested and refined in this study. For example, one par-ticipant shared a photo of a car, expressing that it would carry any passengers no matter who they were. This idea represents how the SMAGs served any of their community members without passing judgement. Another participant described the jovial nature of their interactions with the SMAGs and how they learned from them through their use of humour to make the information more relatable to their experiences and easier to understand. The participant cap-tured this in a photo of chickens playing to represent how the SMAGs 'play' with them as pregnant women.

The prompts used during the realist photovoice data collection in Zambia were intentionally broad to encourage participant voices to lead the conver-sations. Researchers were familiar enough with the programme theories be-ing tested in the realist evaluation that they could follow up or probe these concepts when participants shared a photo or experience related to one of them. In Figure 13.9, the photovoice conversations provided insight into a programme theory that had been challenging to discuss with other interview participants. Throughout data collection, when asking about how the SMAGs communicated with the community and pregnant women (relating to PT 2 on acceptable messaging), participants often described the information (e.g. danger signs in pregnancy) rather than how the information was shared. In this realist photovoice conversation with a pregnant woman, she organically brought up this dynamic of 'how the chickens are playing' as a representation of her interaction with the SMAGs. This representation allowed the research-ers to probe this programme theory about what type and how messaging was conveyed. Our illustration of how the realist photovoice technique contributes to developing or revising programme theories is typified in Table 13.3, which shows how CMOCs, informed by the realist photovoice data and other case study data, were analysed, and synthesised to inform a new programme theory.

Challenges and reflections when conducting realist photovoice

Photovoice enables participants to communicate their experiences to pro-vide explanatory value while maintaining control over which experiences they disclose, and how they are represented by choosing the direction of the discussion through which photos they share (Amenyah et al., 2021). As with many experiences in data collection and research, the realist photovoice technique was not conducted without challenges. After adjusting the pho-tovoice introduction process following the lessons learned from the pilot, we received some thought-provoking photographs from the participants. They were metaphoric — using animals and cars to represent their experi-ences with SMAGs in ways the researchers did not always expect. Some participants struggled to articulate why they took some of their photos when sharing their stories, and the onus was handed to the researchers interpret their symbolic meaning.

Table 13.3 Refining and developing programme theories with realist photovoice data

---

Programme Theory: Sharing valuable and relevant information to the community contributes to a positive relationship between the SMAGs and the community, especially pregnant women, as this new knowledge provides value and benefit to the community

---

CMOC1: Knowledge is caring.
In a community with limited institutional knowledge around maternal health issues (Context), when the SMAGs share maternal health information/knowledge (Mechanism – Resource), pregnant women feel that the SMAGs care about them (Mechanism – Reasoning), which contributes to a positive relationship between the SMAGs and the pregnant women (Outcome).
Data sources: Realist photovoice – PW1, PW2, PW4, PW5; Focus Group Discussion
Thought process: This CMOC relates to SMAGs sharing information and knowledge with the community/pregnant women, thus influencing their relationship positively because they feel like they care or are trying to help.

CMOC2: Knowledge makes me feel good.
In a community where pregnant women are not aware of maternal health practices (Context), SMAGs providing useful information about maternal health care (Mechanism – Resource) are positively received (Outcome) because women perceive value in learning about how to take care of their health (Mechanism – Reasoning).
Data sources: Realist photovoice – PW3, PW4, PW5
Thought process: This idea of 'feeling good' is associated with the information provided—partially because they learned how to address any ailments or illnesses they were experiencing during pregnancy.

Notes on how these CMOCs contribute to theory refinement:
These CMOCs, in addition to CMOCs from other data sources, contributed to refining theory. The realist photovoice data emphasised the role/importance of information and knowledge in the dynamic relationship between SMAGs and the community, particularly pregnant women. This emphasis was not previously reflected in any programme theories in the enquiry, so this new programme theory has been formulated.

Participants, especially programme end users, seldom explicitly present generative mechanisms during realist interviews. This challenge remained true for the realist photovoice in the Zambia case study. For example, participants shared photos that represented *'feeling good'* after meeting the SMAGs. Although the photos would differ and likely hold distinct meanings to the participants, their verbal reflections and explanations would return to *'I felt good because they gave me information.'* When asked why they felt good or how that made them feel good, the responses relayed ideas like *'I didn't have the information before, but after meeting the SMAGs, I did, so I felt good.'* Researchers responded to this by asking questions in new and different ways, including giving examples of their own experiences or describing what they had observed in the community. Additionally, it is essential to remember that not every question and answer has to be about a specific programme theory, and the information gleaned from an interview can still provide valuable insights even when it does not go as planned (Gilmore et al., 2019; Manzano, 2022). Although it was difficult to determine the different implications of feeling good, this emphasis on perceiving information acquisition as a benefit was still a valuable learning in this case study.

When participants were less verbally expressive about their photos, researchers incorporated more 'traditional' realist interview questions relating to the programme theories to ensure participants could still reflect on the programme theory ideas. For example, the researchers presented the programme theory on trusted communication sources (PT 3) to one participant during a photovoice conversation: *'Similar to what you have told us about your 'granny SMAG,' there is this idea that when the community respects a SMAG, people will trust them and their messages. What do you think of that?'* This approach was incorporated at the end of the discussion or throughout the conversation as participants shared a photo or idea that was tangential to the programme theory areas. The following excerpt with a different participant demonstrates this:

Participant: *The patients need to trust the SMAGs, and the SMAGs need to trust the patients.*
Interviewer: *That's very interesting because there is this idea that when a SMAG is known in the community, people will trust them and the information they share. So, what do you think of that?*
Participant: *I don't agree with the idea because even someone from a different area can come to your community and educate you on something you don't know that even that person doesn't know.*

Another challenge that is not unique to the realist photovoice experience is ensuring the willingness and interest of participants to participate in the project. First, the researchers addressed this by gauging how enthusiastic participants were to participate during the introductory meetings. Like other qualitative interview experiences, it can be challenging to encourage participants to be expressive. Photovoice was incorporated in this case study to meaningfully engage with the participants and empower them to express their stories comfortably. In practice, some participants were still reluctant and potentially influenced by the researcher-participant dynamic. For example, a participant conversant in English was jovial and talkative when the researchers interacted with her around the facility or in the community. She participated enthusiastically and took notes throughout the introductory meeting and on her photos to share during the interview. Once the audio recorder was turned on, she became demure and responded to questions only in Nyanja. To address this challenge, the researchers continued to spend time in the facility and the community to develop positive relationships with potential study participants. The initial realist photovoice conversations were also conducted in Nyanja with simultaneous English translation. To improve the rapport and conversational dynamic in these interactions, the researchers transitioned to having the local research assistant lead the interviews directly in Nyanja without any simultaneous translation into English to make participants feel comfortable.

Using translators to enable communication between the researchers and the co-investigators is a common practice in both photovoice and realist studies. Challenges with using translators in realist evaluation studies have been noted, especially regarding its implications for investigating and developing CMOCs (Gilmore, 2019). As illustrated by the Zambia case study, language played a significant role in the dynamic between researcher and co-investigators. The impact of language was particularly apparent when participants were asked to tell a story around the photo to elucidate its meaning. In many cases, we observed that co-investigators were less expressive, potentially due to differences in language structure. We noticed that Nyanja could be a complex language, using long phrases when written; this might have influenced word choice and the flow of conversation, especially when a participant was shy. In cases where researchers use realist photovoice in a group setting, it is also essential to consider the group dynamic and ensure the participation of potentially lesser-heard voices. Group settings offer what Manzano (2022) describes as 'group intelligence' (or 'group reasoning'), which can be realised when each participant is allowed to reflect on photos shared by other group members (Mukumbang & van Wyk, 2020).

Another important consideration when planning the realist photovoice technique is the logistics, such as the type of camera provided to the co-investigators. In a previous realist-informed photovoice study, we provided Samsung cell phones because the price of disposable cameras and printing film almost matched that of the phones, which produced better photo quality (Mukumbang & van Wyk, 2020). While there were concerns that the co-investigators could be robbed of their cell phones during the study period, the investigators thought these devices could be helpful for the individuals beyond the study scope. Another benefit of providing the phones to the co-investigators described by the study coordinator, a medical doctor at the clinic, was the opportunity to create treatment support WhatsApp forums. We could also opt for smartphones because South Africa had a steady electricity supply to ascertain that the phones would be charged. In comparison, basic digital cameras were chosen in the Zambian case study because of their simplicity and cost, whereas smartphones would have been less appropriate in this setting. In other resource-limited countries, the availability of electricity and/or film should be considered for the type of device used in a photovoice study.

Relatedly, researchers must consider the perception of giving participants a camera; this introduces a dynamic of gift-giving and requires participants' engagement in a research project through activity outside the direct researcher-participant interaction. In the case study, a participant expressed that her husband was sceptical about where she received the camera and initial transportation compensation and became upset. When the participant shared this experience with the researchers, the approach outlined in the ethics application for cases where psychosocial support was followed: highlighting potential support mechanisms available, asking the participant what she wanted from us, and ensuring she led the next steps. In this situation, the participant suggested the researchers meet with the family to introduce the project and case study directly to them and hand over the camera and transportation compensation in front of the group, which was received well. Providing compensation to participants, whether monetary or other benefits such as the cameras, has ethical implications that should be considered to ensure the process is appropriate and not perceived as transactional (Ng et al., 2023). As with other research activities involving compensations, the value and implication of the gift should be reflected, including when and for which participants it is appropriate and safe. Based on these learnings and experiences, Figure 13.10 provides guidelines and recommendations for planning and implementing the realist photovoice technique.

Photovoice activities in research provide an excellent opportunity for dissemination through the co-development and co-curation of content with the participants (Liebenberg, 2018). Previous photovoice projects have used the photos of participants in photo essays, booklets, and exhibitions to contribute to research dissemination and knowledge translation (Lennon-Dearing & Price, 2018). For instance, Lennon-Dearing and Hirschi (2019) found that sharing photographs and stories with the public via community exhibits empowered women living with HIV, where they combined a sense of personal

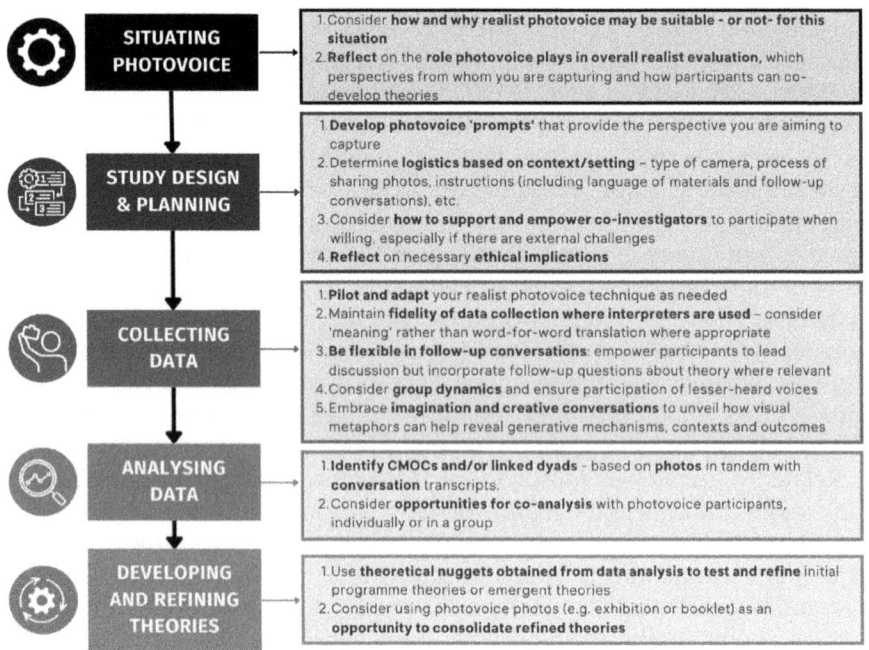

Figure 13.10 Guidelines and recommendations for a realist photovoice technique.

control with the ability to influence their environment and affect the behaviour of others actively. This activity can enhance the theory consolidation process. Realist photovoice discussions could play an essential role in translating the findings to policymakers and programme implementers in creative and digestible ways.

Future research directions and the use of the realist photovoice technique may entail considering its impact on data collection versus conducting only a 'traditional' realist interview. However, it is essential to note the challenges in conducting a thorough assessment of the contribution of photovoice to realist data collection because the experience of implementing photovoice depends on the individual participants, their interpretations of the prompts, their willingness to participate in the project, and their articulation of their narratives.

Conclusions

We argue that while there is room for adopting existing qualitative data collection methods which are well-developed within other paradigms, such as photovoice, to lines of realist inquiry, we should also delink these methods from their ontological backgrounds and adapt them to conform with realist ontological and epistemological principles. Thus, our realist photovoice allows for the creative imagination of information sharing during a realist inquiry's theory gleaning and testing phases. This chapter introduces a realist photovoice technique by providing lessons learned from experience, practical applications, and guiding principles for using photovoice in realist evaluation and possibly other realist-informed inquiries.

Bibliography

Abalkhail, M., Stead, V., Elliott, C., & Mavin, S. (Eds.). (2021). Being 'native': Insider research in qualitative studies of gender and management. *Handbook of research methods on gender and management*, 130–160. Edward Elgar Publishing, https://doi.org/10.4337/9781788977937.00017

Abejirinde, I., Ilozumba, O., Marchal, B., Zweekhorst, M. & Dieleman, M. (2018a). Mobile health and the performance of maternal health care workers in low- and middle-income countries: A realist review. *International Journal of Care Coordination, 21*. https://doi.org/10.1177/2053434518779491

Abejirinde, I. O., Zweekhorst, M., Bardaji, A., Abugnaba-Abanga, R., Apenti-badek, N., De Brouwere, V., Van Roosmalen, J. & Marchal, B. (2018b). Unveiling the black box of diagnostic and clinical decision support systems for antenatal care: Realist evaluation. *JMIR Mhealth Uhealth, 6*, e11468. https://doi.org/10.2196/11468

Abelson, J., Canfield, C., Leslie, M., Levasseur, M. A., Rowland, P., Tripp, L., Vanstone, M., Panday, J., Cameron, D., Forest, P.-G., Sussman, D., & Wilson, G. (2022). Understanding patient partnership in health systems: Lessons from the Canadian patient partner survey. *BMJ Open, 12*(9), e061465. https://doi.org/10.1136/bmjopen-2022-061465

Abrams, R., Park, S., Wong, G., Rastogi, J., Boylan, A, Tierney, S., Petrova, M., Dawson, S., & Roberts, N. (2021). Lost in reviews: Looking for the involvement of stakeholders, patients, public and other non-researcher contributions in realist reviews *Research Synthesis Methods, 12*, 239–247. https://doi.org/10.1002/jrsm.1459

Aburn, G. E., Gott, M., & Hoare, K. (2022). Experiences of an insider researcher–interviewing your own colleagues. *Nurse Researcher, 30*(3). https://doi.org/10.7748/nr.2021.e1794

Ackroyd, S., & Fleetwood, S. (2003). Realism in contemporary organisation and management studies. *Realist Perspectives on Management and Organisations*, 3–25. https://doi.org/10.4324/9780203164433-9

Africa Evaluation Association. (2021). *The African evaluation principles*. https://afrea.org/AEP/new/The-African-Evaluation-Principles.pdf

Alderson, P. (2021). *Critical realism for health and illness research: A practical introduction*. Policy Press.

Allana, S., & Clark, A. (2018). Applying meta-theory to qualitative and mixed-methods research: A discussion of critical realism and heart failure disease management interventions research. *International Journal of Qualitative Methods, 17*(1), 1–9. https://doi.org/10.1177/1609406918790042

Allard, T., Stewart, A., & Manning, M. (2019). The virtues of rubbish research: A novel way of measuring the impact of crime prevention interventions in public spaces. In

G. Farrell and A. Sidebottom (Eds) *Realistic evaluation for crime science: Essays in honour of Nick Tilley* (pp. 77–99). Routledge.

Amenyah, S. D., Murphy, J., & Fenge, L. A. (2021). Evaluation of a health-related intervention to reduce overweight, obesity and increase employment in France and the United Kingdom: A mixed-methods realist evaluation protocol. *BMC Public Health*, *21*(1). https://doi.org/10.1186/S12889-021-10523-3

Anderson, A. (2005). *The community builder's approach to theory of change. A practical guide to theory development.* The Aspen Institute Roundtable on Community Change.

Archer, M. (1995). *Realist social theory: The morphogenetic approach.* Cambridge University Press.

Archer, M. (2000). *Being human.* Cambridge University Press.

Archer, M. (2003). *Structure, agency and the internal conversation.* Cambridge University Press.

Archer, M. (2011). Morphogenesis: Realism's explanatory framework. In A. Maccarini, E. Morandi, & R. Prandini (Eds.), *Sociological realism* (pp. 59–94). Routledge.

Archer, M., Decoteau, C., Gorski, P. S., Little, D., Porpora, D., Rutzou, T., Smith, C., Steinmetz, G., & Vandenberghe, F. (2016). What is critical realism? *Perspectives*, *38*(2), 4–9.

Arthur, S & Nazroo, J (2003). Designing fieldwork strategies and materials. In Richie, J & Lewis, J (ed.) *Qualitative research practice, a guide for social science students and researchers* (pp.109–137), SAGE.

Astbury, B., & Leeuw, F. L. (2010). Unpacking black boxes: Mechanisms and theory building in evaluation. *American Journal of Evaluation, 31*(3), 363–381. https://doi.org/10.1177/1098214010371972

Atkinson, M. (1968). On the sociology of suicide. *The Sociological Review, 16*, 83–92.

Aubin, D., Hebert, M., & Eurich, D. (2019). The importance of measuring the impact of patient-oriented research. *Canadian Medical Association Journal, 191*(31), E860–E864. https://doi.org/10.1503/cmaj.190237

Azizian, A. R., Carr, T., Muhajarine, N., Verrall, T., Hartness, C., Vanstone, J., Yasinian, M., Skrapek, C., Andreas, B., Farthing, G., & Groot, G. (2021). Developing a patient-oriented realist evaluation for COVID-19 vaccine implementation in Saskatchewan: A methodologic framework. *Canadian Medical Association Open Access Journal*, *9*(4), E1034–E1039. https://doi.org/10.9778/cmajo.20210041

Baddeley, A. (1992). Working memory. *Science, 255*(5044), 556–559. https://doi.org/10.1126/science.1736359

Baker, M., Fessinger, M., McWilliams, K., & Williams, S. (2021). The use of note-taking during forensic interviews: Perceptions and practical recommendations for interviewers. *Developmental Child Welfare, 3*(1), 20–35. https://doi.org/10.1177/25161032211002187

Bankhead, C.R., Spencer E.A., & Nunan, D. (2019) Information bias. In: *Sackett Catalogue of biases.* https://catalogofbias.org/biases/information-bias/

Bareinboim, E., Tian, J., & Pearl, J. (2022). Recovering from selection bias in causal and statistical inference. In P. Glymour & R. Scheines (Eds.), *Probabilistic and causal inference: The works of Judea Pearl* (pp. 433–450). Wiley

Barrett, D., & Heale, R. (2020). What are Delphi studies? *Evidence-Based Nursing, 23*(3), 68–69. DOI: http://dx.doi.org/10.1136/ebnurs-2020-103303

Battersby, M. (2016) Enhancing rationality: Heuristics, biases, and the critical thinking project (2016). OSSA Conference Archive. 2. https://scholar.uwindsor.ca/ossaarchive/OSSA11/keynotes/2

Baugh Littlejohns, L., Hill, C., & Neudorf, C. (2021). Diverse approaches to creating and using causal loop diagrams in public health research: Recommendations from a scoping review. *Public Health Reviews, 14*(42), 1604352. https://doi.org/10.3389/phrs.2021.1604352

Baum, F., Macdougall, C. & Smith, D. (2006). Participatory action research. *Journal of Epidemiology & Community Health, 60*, 854–7. https://doi.org/10.1136/jech.2004.028662

Beach, D. (2017) Process tracing methods in social science, *Oxford Research encyclopaedia of politics* https://oxfordre.com/politics/display/10.1093/acrefore/9780190228637.001.0001/acrefore-9780190228637-e-176

Becker, H. S. (1967). Whose side are we on? *Social Problems, 14* (3), 239–247.

Befani, B., Ledermann, S., & Sager, F. (2007). Realistic evaluation and QCA: Conceptual parallels and an empirical application. *Evaluation, 13*(2), 171–192. https://doi.org/10.1177/1356389007075222

Befani, B., & Stedman-Bryce, G. (2017). Process tracing and Bayesian updating for impact evaluation. *Evaluation, 23*(1), 42–60. DOI: https://doi.org/10.1177/1356389016654584

Benatar, S. R., & Fleischer, T. E. (2007). Ethical issues in research in low-income countries. *The International Journal of Tuberculosis and Lung Disease, 11*(6), 617–623.

Bennett, A., Fairfield, T., & Soifer, D. H. (2019). Comparative methods and process tracing. *American Political Science Association Organized Section for Qualitative and Multi-Method Research, Qualitative Transparency Deliberations, Working Group Final Reports, Report III.1.* http://dx.doi.org/10.2139/ssrn.3333405

Beran, T. N., & Violato, C. (2010). Structural equation modeling in medical research: A primer. *BMC Research Notes 3*, 267. https://doi.org/10.1186/1756-0500-3-267

Bergen, N., & Labonté, R., (2020). "Everything is perfect, and we have no problems": Detecting and limiting social desirability bias in qualitative research. *Qualitative Health Research 30*(5): 783–792. https://doi.org/10.1177/1049732319889354

Better Evaluation. (2024). *Describe the theory of change.* https://www.betterevaluation.org/frameworks-guides/managers-guide-evaluation/scope-evaluation/describe-theory-change

Bhaskar, R. (2008). A realist theory of science. In *Medical History* (Vol. 25, Issue 1). https://doi.org/10.2307/2184170

Bhaskar, R. (2009). *Scientific realism and human emancipation* (2nd ed.). Routledge.

Bhaskar, R. (2016). Enlightened common sense: The philosophy of critical realism. In Mervyn Hartwig (Ed.), *Journal of critical realism* (Issue 4). Routledge.

Birt, L., West, J., Poland, F., Wong, G., Handley, M., Litherland, R., Hackmann, C., Moniz-Cook, E., Wolverson, E., Teague, B., Mills, R., Sams, K., Duddy, C., & Fox, C. (2023). Protocol for a realist evaluation of Recovery College dementia courses: Understanding coproduction through ethnography. *BMJ Open, 13*(12), e078248. https://doi.org/10.1136/bmjopen-2023-078248

Blamey, A. & Mackenzie, M. (2007). Theories of change and realistic evaluation. Peas in a pod or apples and oranges? *Evaluation, 13* (4) 439–455. https://doi.org/10.1177/1356389007082129

Boland, J., Banks, S., Krabbe, R., Lawrence, S., Murray, T., Henning, T., & Vandenberg, M. (2022). A COVID-19-era rapid review: Using zoom and skype for qualitative group research. *Public Health Research & Practice, 32*(2). https://www.phrp.com.au/wp-content/uploads/2021/07/PHRP31232112.pdf

Boudon, R. (2014). What is context? KZfSS Kölner Zeitschrift für. Soziologie und Sozialpsychologie, 66(1), 17–45. https://doi.org/10.1007/s11577-014-0269-2

Bouyousfi, S.E. & Sabar, M. (2022). Realistic evaluation and the process-tracing method: A combined approach to scrutinizing causal mechanisms. *Canadian Journal of Program Evaluation, 37*(1), 83–103. https://doi.org/10.3138/cjpe.71050

Bragason, E. H. (1997). Interviewing through interpreters. *Newsletter–Centre for Qualitative Research, 23.*

Brandsen, T., Steen, T. & Verschuere, B. 2018. *Co-production and co-creation. Engaging citizens in public services.* Routledge.

Brault, N. (2021). Une brève histoire du concept de biais en épidémiologie. Epidemiology and Public Health. *Revue d'Epidémiologie et de Santé Publique 69*(4): 215–223. https://doi.org/10.1016/j.respe.2021.04.134

Brönnimann, A. (2022). How to phrase critical realist interview questions in applied social science research. *Journal of Critical Realism, 21*(1), 1–24. https://doi.org/10.1080/14767430.2021.1966719

Brousselle, A., & Champagne, F. (2011). Program theory evaluation: Logic analysis. *Evaluation & Program Planning, 34*(1), 69–78. https://doi.org/10.1016/j.evalprogplan.2010.04.001

Brunson, L., Lauzier-Jobin, F., Olson, B., & Cote, L.P. (2023). Seven key insights from critical realism and their implications for ecological think and action in community psychology. *Journal of Community Psychology, online.* https://doi.org/10.1002/jcop.23054

Bryman, A. (2012). *Social research methods,* 4th edition. Oxford University Press.

Budig, K., Diez, J., Conde, P., Sastre, M., Hernán, M., & Franco, M. (2018). Photovoice and empowerment: Evaluating the transformative potential of a participatory action research project. *BMC Public Health, 18*(1). https://doi.org/10.1186/s12889-018-5335-7

Buetow, S. (2019). Apophenia, unconscious bias and reflexivity in nursing qualitative research. *International Journal of Nursing Studies, 89,* 8–13. https://doi.org/10.1016/j.ijnurstu.2018.09.013

Burns, D., Howard, J. & Ospina, S. M. 2021. Challenges in the practice of participatory research and inquiry. In Burns, D., Howard, J., Ospina, S.M. (ed.) *The Sage handbook of participatory research and inquiry.* SAGE.

Byng, R., Norman, I., & Redfern, S. (2005). Using realistic evaluation to evaluate a practice level intervention to improve primary healthcare for patients with long term mental illness, *Evaluation, 11*(1), 69–93. https://doi.org/10.1177/1356389005053198

Byrne, D. (2002). *Interpreting quantitative data.* SAGE.

Byrne, D. (2004). Complex and contingent causation – The implications of complex realism in quantitative modelling: The case of housing and health. In B. Carter & C. New (Eds.), *Making realism work: Realist social theory and empirical research* (pp. 50–66). Routledge.

Campbell, D.T. (1988) A general "selection theory", as implemented in biological evolution and in social belief-transmission-with-modification, in science. *Biology & Philosophy 3,* 171–177.

Carr, T., Quinlan, E., Robertson, S., & Gerrard, A. (2017). Adapting realist synthesis methodology: The case of workplace harassment interventions. *Research Synthesis Methods, 8*(4), 496–505. https://doi.org/10.1002/jrsm.1261

Catalani, C., & Minkler, M. (2010). Photovoice: A review of the literature in health and public health. *Health Education & Behavior, 37*(3), 424–451. https://doi.org/10.1177/1090198109342084

Charmaz, K. & Belgrave, L. (2012). Qualitative interviewing and grounded theory analysis. In Gubrium, J, Holstein, J, Marvasti, A & McKinney, K (ed.) *The Sage handbook of interview research: The complexity of the craft (2 ed).* (pp. 347–366). SAGE.

Chen, H. T. (1990). *Theory-driven evaluations.* SAGE.

Chernoff, F. (2007). Critical realism, scientific realism, and international relations theory. *Millennium, 35*(2), 399–407. https://doi.org/10.1177/03058298070350021701

Clibbens, N., Baker, J., Booth, A., Berzins, K., Ashman, M., Sharda, L., Thompson, J., Kendal, S. and Weich, S. Explanation of context, mechanisms and outcomes in adult community mental health crisis care: The MH-CREST realist evidence synthesis. Southampton (UK): National Institute for Health and Care Research; 2023 Sep. (*Health & Social Care Delivery Research,* No. 11.15.) Chapter 2, Review methodology and methods. Available from: https://www.ncbi.nlm.nih.gov/books/NBK596123/

Collier, A. (1994). *Critical realism: An introduction to Roy Bhaskar's philosophy.* Verso.

Collins, H.M. (1985). *Changing order: Replication and induction in scientific practice.* SAGE.

Coloma, R. S. (2008). Border crossing subjectivities and research: Through the prism of feminists of color. *Race Ethnicity & Education, 11*(1), 11–27. https://doi.org/10.1080/13613320701845749

Coorey, G, Peiris, D, Neubeck, L & Redfern, J (2020). A realist evaluation approach to explaining the role of context in the impact of a complex eHealth intervention for improving prevention of cardiovascular disease. *BMC Health Services Research 20*, 764. https://doi.org/10.1186/s12913-020-05597-5

Coryn, C. L., Noakes, L. A., Westine, C. D., & Schröter, D. C. (2011). A systematic review of theory-driven evaluation practice from 1990 to 2009. *American Journal of Evaluation, 32*(2), 199–226. https://doi.org/10.1177/1098214010389321

Cristia, A., Seidl, A., Vaughn, C., Schmale, R., Bradlow, A., & Floccia, C. (2012). Linguistic processing of accented speech across the lifespan. *Frontiers in Psychology, 3*, 479. https://doi.org/10.3389/fpsyg.2012.00479

Dada, S., Praveenkumar, A., Aoife, D. B., De Brunún, A., Barreix, M., Chelwa, N., Mutunga, Z., Vwalika, B., & Brynne, G. (2023). Understanding communication in community engagement for maternal and newborn health programmes in low- and middle-income countries: A realist review. *Health Policy & Planning.* https://doi.org/10.1093/HEAPOL/CZAD078

Dada, S., Praveenkumar, A., Aoife, D. B., De Brunún, A., Barreix, M., Chelwa, N., Mutunga, Z., Vwalika, B., & Brynne, G. (2024) We move together: a realist evaluation of the safe motherhood action groups in Eastern Province, Zambia [Manuscript submitted for publication]

Dalkin, S., Forster, N., Hodgson, P., Lhussier, M., & Carr, S. M. (2021). Using computer assisted qualitative data analysis software (CAQDAS; NVivo) to assist in the complex process of realist theory generation, refinement and testing. *International Journal of Social Research Methodology, 24*(1), 123–134. https://doi.org/10.1080/13645579.2020.1803528

Dalkin, S. M., Greenhalgh, J., Jones, D., Cunningham, B., & Lhussier, M. (2015). What's in a mechanism? Development of a key concept in realist evaluation. *Implementation Science, 10*(1), 49. https://doi.org/10.1186/s13012-015-0237-x

Dalkin, S., Lhussier, M., Williams, L., Burton, C. R. & Rycroft-Malone, J. (2018). Exploring the use of soft systems methodology with realist approaches: A novel way to map programme complexity and develop and refine programme theory. *Evaluation, 24*(1), 84–97. https://doi.org/10.1177/1356389017749036

Dalkin, S., & McEwan, K. (2022). *Managing messiness in the real research world using NVivo.* https://mediaspace.nottingham.ac.uk/media/Managing%20Messiness%20in%20the%20Real%20Research%20World%20Trimmed%20Recording/1_4qn10qlt

Danermark, B. (2019). Applied interdisciplinary research: A critical realist perspective. *Journal of Critical Realism, 18*(4), 368–382. https://doi.org/10.1080/14767430.2019.1644983

Danermark, B., Ekström, M., & Karlsson, J. Ch. (2019). *Explaining society: Critical realism in the social sciences.* Routledge.

Daston, L., (2005). Scientific error and the ethos of belief. *Social Research*, 1–28.

De Ries, K. E., Schaap, H., van Loon, A. M. M. J. A. P., Kral, M. M. H., & Meijer, P. C. (2022). A literature review of open-ended concept maps as a research instrument to study knowledge and learning. *Quality & Quantity, 56*, 73–107. https://doi.org/10.1007/s11135-021-01113-x

De Souza, D. E. (2013.). Elaborating the Context-Mechanism-Outcome configuration (CMOc) in realist evaluation: A critical realist perspective. *Evaluation, 19*(2), 141–154. https://doi.org/10.1177/1356389013485194

De Weger, E., Van Vooren, N., Wong, G., Dalkin, S., Marchal, B., Drewes, H., & Baan, C. (2020). What's in a realist configuration? Deciding which causal configurations to use, how, and why. *International Journal of Qualitative Methods*, *19*, 1–8. https://doi.org/10.1177/1609406920938577

Dean, K., Joseph, J., Roberts, J. M., & Wight, C. (2006). Realism, philosophy and social science. *Realism, Philosophy & Social Science*, 1–199. https://doi.org/10.1057/9780230502079

Delgado-Rodriguez, M. & Llorca, J., (2004). Bias. *Journal of Epidemiology & Community Health*, *58*(8), 635–641. https://doi.org/10.1136/jech.2003.008466

Department for International Development. (2020). FCDO Ethical Guidance for Research, Evaluation and Monitoring Activities, Last updated 23 January 2020 https://www.gov.uk/government/publications/dfid-ethical-guidance-for-research-evaluation-and-monitoring-activities

DOHaD World Congress 2022 | DOHaD Canada. (n.d.). https://dohad.utoronto.ca/dohadworldcongress2022/

Domecq, J. P., Prutsky, G., Elraiyah, T., Wang, Z., Nabhan, M., Shippee, N., Brito, J. P., Boehmer, K., Hasan, R., Firwana, B., Erwin, P., Eton, D., Sloan, J., Montori, V., Asi, N., Dabrh, A. M. A., & Murad, M. H. (2014). Patient engagement in research: A systematic review. *BMC Health Services Research*, *14*, 89. https://doi.org/10.1186/1472-6963-14-89

Douglas, J.D. (2015). *Social meanings of suicide*. Princeton University Press.

Drummond, C & Fischhoff, B. (2019) Does "putting on your thinking cap" reduce myside bias in evaluation of scientific evidence? *Thinking & Reasoning*, *25*(4), 477–505, https://doi.org/10.1080/13546783.2018.1548379

Durkheim, E. (1897/1951). *Suicide: A study in sociology*. The Free Press.

Edwards, P. K., O'Mahoney, J., & Vincent, S. (Eds.). (2014). *Studying organizations using critical realism: A practical guide*. OUP Oxford.

Elder-Vass, D. (2010). The causal power of social structures: Emergence, structures and agency. In *Structure (first)*. Cambridge University Press. https://doi.org/10.1017/CBO9780511761720

Elder-Vass, D. (2015). Developing social theory using critical realism. *Journal of Critical Realism*, *14*(1), 80–92. https://doi.org/10.1179/1476743014Z.00000000047

Emmel, N. (2013). *Sampling and choosing cases in qualitative research: A realist approach*. SAGE.

Emmel, N., Greenhalgh, J., Manzano, A., Monaghan, M., & Dalkin, S. (Eds.) (2018). *Doing realist research*. SAGE.

Fakoya, I., Cole, C., Larkin, C., Punton, M., Brown, E. & Ballonoff Suleiman, A. (2022). Enhancing human-centered design with youth-led participatory action research approaches for adolescent sexual and reproductive health programming. *Health Promotion Practice*, *23*, 25–31. https://doi.org/10.1177/15248399211003544

Falzon, M.A. (2016). *Multi-sited ethnography: Theory, praxis and locality in contemporary research*. Routledge.

Farrell, G. (2013). Five tests for a theory of the crime drop. *Crime Science*, *2*, 5. https://doi.org/10.1186/2193-7680-2-5

Farrell, G., Laycock, G. & Tilley, N. (2015). Debuts and legacies: The crime drop and the role of adolescence-limited and persistent offending. *Crime Science 4*, 16. https://doi.org/10.1186/s40163-015-0028-3

Faulds, H. (1880). On the skin-furrows of the hand. *Nature*, October 28th, 605.

Federmeier, K. D., Jongman, S. R., & Szewczyk, J. M. (2020). Examining the role of general cognitive skills in language processing: A window into complex cognition. *Current Directions in Psychological Science*, *29*(6), 575–582. https://doi.org/10.1177/0963721420964095

Fisher C., & Downes, B. (2008). Performance measurement and metric manipulation in the public sector, *Business Ethics: A European Review*, *17*, 245–258. https://doi.org/10.1111/j.1467-8608.2008.00534.x

Fletcher-Hildebrand, S., Alimezelli, H., Carr, T., Lawson, K., Ali, A., & Groot, G. (2021). Understanding the impact of a residential housing programme for people living with HIV/AIDS: A realist evaluation protocol. *BMJ Open*, *11*(4), e044522. https://doi.org/10.1136/bmjopen-2020-044522

Foreign, Commonwealth & Development Office. (2023a). *FCDO evaluation strategy.* Updated 4 September 2023, https://www.gov.uk/government/publications/fcdo-evaluation-strategy/fcdo-evaluation-strategy-2#outcome-2-high-quality-evaluation-evidence-is-produced-2

Foreign, Commonwealth & Development Office. (2023b). *UK International Climate Finance results*. 28 September 2023 https://www.gov.uk/guidance/uk-international-climate-finance-results#evaluation-reports

French, J., & Morgan, R. (2015). An experimental investigation of the indirect transfer and deposition of gunshot residue: Further studies carried out with SEM–EDX analysis. *Forensic Science International*, *247*, 14–17. https://doi.org/10.1016/j.forsciint.2014.10.023

Fuji, L. A. (2018). *Interviewing in social science research. A relational approach.* Routledge.

Fusco, F., Marsilio, M. & Guglielmetti, C. (2020). Co-production in health policy and management: A comprehensive bibliometric review. *BMC Health Services Research*, *20*, 504. https://doi.org/10.1186/s12913-020-05241-2

Galdas, P. (2017). Revisiting bias in qualitative research: Reflections on its relationship with funding and impact. *International Journal of Qualitative Methods*, *16*(1), p.1609406917748992. https://doi.org/10.1177/1609406917748992

Garfinkel, H. (1967) *Studies in ethnomethodology*. Prentice Hall.

Garrett, B. (2018). *Empirical nursing: The art of evidence-based care*. Emerald Publishing. https://doi.org/10.1108/9781787438132

Gilmore, B. (2019). Realist evaluations in low- and middle-income countries: Reflections and recommendations from the experiences of a foreign researcher. *BMJ Global Health*, *4*(5), e001638. https://doi.org/10.1136/bmjgh-2019-001638

Gilmore, B., McAuliffe, E., Power, J., & Vallières, F. (2019). Data analysis and synthesis within a realist evaluation: Toward more transparent methodological approaches. *International Journal of Qualitative Methods*, *18*, 1–11. https://doi.org/10.1177/1609406919859754

Glaser, B., & Strauss, A. (2017). *Discovery of grounded theory: Strategies for qualitative research*. Routledge.

Glaw, X., Inder, K., Kable, A., & Hazelton, M. (2017). Visual methodologies in qualitative research. *International Journal of Qualitative Methods*, *16*(1), 160940691774821. https://doi.org/10.1177/1609406917748215

Glynn, A. N. (2013). What can we learn with statistical truth serum? Design and analysis of the list experiment. *Public Opinion Quarterly*, *77*, 159–72. https://doi.org/10.1093/poq/nfs070

Goldsmith, L. J. (2021). Using framework analysis in applied qualitative research. *The Qualitative Report*, *26*(6), 2061–2076. https://doi.org/10.46743/2160-3715/2021.5011

Gorski, P. (2013). Beyond the fact/value distinction: Ethical naturalism and the social sciences. *Society*, *50*(6), 543–553. https://doi.org/10.1007/s12115-013-9709-2

Government of Canada, CIHR. (2005).Ethics of Health Research Involving First Nations, Inuit and Métis People – CIHR. https://cihr-irsc.gc.ca/e/29339.html

Government of Canada, CIHR. (2014). Strategy for Patient-Oriented Research – Patient Engagement Framework – CIHR. https://cihr-irsc.gc.ca/e/48413.html

Greenhalgh, J., & Manzano, A., (2021). Understanding 'context' in realist evaluation and synthesis. *International Journal of Social Research Methodology*, *25*(5), 583–595. https://doi.org/10.1080/13645579.2021.1918484

Greenhalgh, T., Pawson, R., Wong, G., Westhorp, G., Greenhalgh, J., Manzano, A., & Jagosh, J. (2016). *Quality standards for realist evaluation. For evaluators and peer-reviewers.* http://ramesesproject.org/media/RE_Quality_Standards_for_evaluators_and_peer_reviewers.pdf

Greenhalgh, T., Pawson, R., Wong, G., Westhorp, G., Greenhalgh, J., Manzano, A., & Jagosh, J. (2017a). *Frequently asked questions about realist evaluation.* The RAMESES II Project, https://www.ramesesproject.org/media/RAMESES_II_FAQs_about_realist_evaluation.pdf

Greenhalgh, T., Pawson, R., Wong, G., Westhorp, G., Greenhalgh, J., Manzano, A., & Jagosh, J. (2017b). *The realist interview.* The RAMESES II Project (www.ramesesproject.org). https://www.ramesesproject.org/media/RAMESES_II_Realist_interviewing.pdf

Greenhalgh, T., Pawson, R., Wong, G., Westhorp, G., Greenhalgh, J., Manzano, A., & Jagosh, J. (2017c). *Philosophies and evaluation design.* https://ramesesproject.org/media/RAMESES_II_Philosophies_and_evaluation_design.pdf

Greenhalgh, T., Pawson, R., Wong, G., Westhorp, G., Greenhalgh, J., Manzano, A., & Jagosh, J. (2017d). *Realist evaluation, realist synthesis, realist research – what's in a name?* https://www.ramesesproject.org/media/RAMESES_II_RE_RS_RR_whats_in_a_name.pdf

Greenhalgh, T., Pawson, R., Wong, G., Westhorp, G., Greenhalgh, J., Manzano, A., & Jagosh, J. (2017e). *"Theory" in realist evaluation.* The RAMESES II Project https://ramesesproject.org/media/RAMESES_II_Theory_in_realist_evaluation.pdf

Greenhalgh, T., Pawson, R., Wong, G., Westhorp, G., Greenhalgh, J., Manzano, A., & Jagosh, J. (2017f). *What is a mechanism? What is a programme mechanism?* The RAMESES II Project https://ramesesproject.org/media/RAMESES_II_What_is_a_mechanism.pdf

Greenhalgh, T., Pawson, R., Wong, G., Westhorp, G., Greenhalgh, J., Manzano, A., & Jagosh, J. (2017g). *What realists mean by context.* https://www.ramesesproject.org/media/RAMESES_II_Context.pdf

Griffiths, S., Weston, L., Morgan-Trimmer, S., Wheat, H., Gude, A., Manger, L., Oh, T. M., Clarkson, P., Quinn, C., Sheaff, R., Clark, M., Sherriff, I., & Byng, R. (2022). Engaging stakeholders in realist programme theory building: Insights from the prospective phase of a primary care dementia support study. *International Journal of Qualitative Methods, 21.* https://doi.org/10.1177/16094069221077521

Groot, G., Waldron, T., Barreno, L., Cochran, D., & Carr, T. (2020). Trust and world view in shared decision making with indigenous patients: A realist synthesis. *Journal of Evaluation in Clinical Practice, 26*(2), 503–514. https://doi.org/10.1111/jep.13307

Groot, G., Waldron, T., Carr, T., McMullen, L., Bandura, L.-A., Neufeld, S.-M., & Duncan, V. (2017). Development of a program theory for shared decision-making: A realist review protocol. *Systematic Reviews, 6*(1), 114. https://doi.org/10.1186/s13643-017-0508-5

Gubrium, A. (2009). Digital storytelling: An emergent method for health promotion research and practice. *Health Promotion Practice, 10*(2), 186–19. https://doi.org/10.1177/1524839909332600

Gubrium, J. F. & Holstein, J. A. (2014). Narrative practice and the transformation of interview subjectivity In Gubrium, J. F., Holstein, J. A., Marvasti, A. B. & Mckinney, K. (eds.) *The Sage handbook of interview research: The complexity of the craft.* SAGE.

Hall, S. M. (2024). Oral Histories and Futures: Researching crises across the life-course and the life-course of crises. *Area, 56*(1), e12904. https://doi.org/10.1111/area.12904

Halvorsrud, K., Rhodes, J., Webster, G. M., Francis, J., Haarmans, M., Dawkins, N., Nazroo, J., & Bhui, K. (2019). Photovoice as a promising public engagement approach: Capturing and communicating ethnic minority people's lived experiences of severe mental illness and its treatment. *BMJ Open Quality, 8,* 665. https://doi.org/10.1136/bmjoq-2019-000665

Hansen, M. B., & Vedung, E. (2010). Theory-based stakeholder evaluation. *American Journal of Evaluation, 31*(3), 295–313. https://doi.org/10.1177/1098214010366174

Hanway, P., Akehurst, L., Vernham, Z., & Hope, L. (2021). The effects of cognitive load during an investigative interviewing task on mock interviewers' recall of information. *Legal & Criminological Psychology, 26*(1), 25–41. https://doi.org/10.1111/lcrp.12182

Harré, R. & Moghaddam, F. M. (2016). *Questioning causality: Scientific explorations of cause and consequence across social context*. Bloomsbury Publishing

Harris, K. (2020). Building capacity in program practitioner realist evaluation through application of CAE principles. *Collaborative Approaches to Evaluation: Principles in Use*, 161–184. https://doi.org/10.4135/9781544344669.N7

Hastings, C. (2021). A critical realist methodology in empirical research: Foundations, process, and payoffs. *Journal of Critical Realism, 20*(5), 458–473. https://doi.org/10.1080/14767430.2021.1958440

Hebbar, P. B. (2023). Implementation of tobacco control policies in India: A realist evaluation. [Doctoral Thesis, Maastricht University]. Maastricht University. https://doi.org/10.26481/dis.20231108ph

Henry, G. T., Julnes, G., & Mark, M. M. (1998). Realist evaluation: An emerging theory in support of practice. *New Directions for Evaluation, 78*, 1–109.

Hergenrather, K. C., Rhodes, S. D., Cowan, C. A., Bardhoshi, G., & Pula, S. (2009). Photovoice as community-based participatory research: A qualitative review. *American Journal of Health Behavior, 33*(6), 686–698. https://doi.org/10.5993/AJHB.33.6.6

Hinds, K., & Dickson, K. (2021). Realist synthesis: A critique and an alternative. *Journal of Critical Realism, 20*(1), 1–17. https://doi.org/10.1080/14767430.2020.1860425

HMG (August2023) International Climate Finance: Overview. HMG (October 2023): https://www.gov.uk/government/publications/uk-international-climate-finance-results-2023/uk-international-climate-finance-results-2023

Hoorens, V. (2014). Positivity bias. In: Michalos AC (Ed.). *Encyclopedia of quality of life and well-being research*. (p. 4938–4941). Springer..

Howe, J. (2022). Delivering evidence-based rural community stroke services: A realist evaluation, University of Nottingham.

Hutcheson, G., & Sofroniou, N. (1999). *The multivariate social scientist: Introductory statistics using generalized linear models*. SAGE.

Ibrahim, M.A. & Spitzer, W.O. (1979). The case control study: The problem and The Prospect. *In the case-control study consensus and controversy* (pp. 139–144). Pergamon.

Indigenous DOHaD Gathering. (2022). Vancouver BC Canada | August 24-26 2022. https://indigenousdohadgathering.org/

Intercollegiate Stroke Working Party. (2016). National Clinical Guideline for Stroke. https://www.hse.ie/eng/about/who/cspd/ncps/stroke/resources/2016-national-clinical-guideline-for-stroke-5th-edition.pdf

International HIV/AIDS Alliance. (2006). Tools together now!: 100 participatory tools to mobilise communities for HIV/AIDS | Participatory Methods. International HIV/AIDS Alliance. https://www.participatorymethods.org/resource/tools-together-now-100-participatory-tools-mobilise-communities-hivaids

Irvine, A. (2011). Duration, dominance and depth in telephone and face-to-face interviews: A comparative exploration. *International Journal of Qualitative Methods, 10*(3), 202–220. https://doi.org/10.1177/160940691101000302

Irvine, F., Roberts, G., & Bradbury-Jones, C. (2008). The researcher as insider versus the researcher as outsider: Enhancing rigour through language and cultural sensitivity. In P. Liamputtong (Ed.), *Doing cross-cultural research: Ethical and methodological perspectives* (pp. 35–48). Springer. https://doi.org/10.1007/978-1-4020-8567-3_3

Itad (2024) https://www.itad.com/

Itzchakov, G., & Grau, J. (2022). High-quality listening in the age of COVID-19: A key to better dyadic communication for more effective organizations. *Organizational Dynamics, 51*(2), 100820. https://doi.org/10.1016/j.orgdyn.2020.100820

Jackson, S. F., & Kolla, G. (2012). A new realistic evaluation analysis method: Linked coding of context, mechanism, and outcome relationships. *American Journal of Evaluation, 33*(3), 339–349. https://doi.org/10.1177/1098214012440030

Jager, A., Papoutsi, C., & Wong, G. (2023a). The usage of data in NHS primary care commissioning: A realist evaluation. *BMC Primary Care, 24*(1), 275. https://doi.org/10.1186/s12875-023-02193-4

Jager, A., Wong, G., Papoutsi, C., & Roberts, N. (2023b). The usage of data in NHS primary care commissioning: A realist review. *BMC Medicine, 21*(1), 236. https://doi.org/10.1186/s12916-023-02949-w

Jagosh, J. (2020). Retroductive theorising in Pawson and Tilley's applied scientific realism. *Journal of Critical Realism, 19*(2), 121–130. https://doi.org/10.1080/14767430.2020.1723301

Jagosh, J., Bush, P. L., Salsberg, J., Macaulay, A. C., Greenhalgh, T., Wong, G., Cargo, M., Green, L. W., Herbert, C. P., & Pluye, P. (2015). A realist evaluation of community-based participatory research: Partnership synergy, trust building and related ripple effects. *BMC Public Health, 15*(1), 725. https://doi.org/10.1186/s12889-015-1949-1

Johnson, T. P., & Van de Vijver, F. J. (2003). Social desirability in cross-cultural research. *Cross-Cultural Survey Methods, 325*, 195–204.

Joseph, J. (2007). Philosophy in international relations: A scientific realist approach. *Millennium: Journal of International Studies, 35*(2), 345–359. https://doi.org/10.1177/03058298070350021401

Kanuha, V. K. (2000). "Being" native versus "going native": Conducting social work research as an insider. *Social Work, 45*(5), 439–447. https://doi.org/10.1093/sw/45.5.439

Karl, K. A., Peluchette, J. V., & Aghakhani, N. (2022). Virtual work meetings during the COVID-19 pandemic: The good, bad, and ugly. *Small Group Research, 53*(3), 343–365. https://doi.org/10.1177/10464964211015286

Kaspar, H., Abegg, A. & Reddy, S. (2023). Of odysseys and miracles: A narrative approach on therapeutic mobilities for ayurveda treatment. *Social Science & Medicine, 334*, 116152. https://doi.org/10.1016/j.socscimed.2023.116152

Keen, S., Lomeli-Rodriguez, M., & Joffe, H. (2022). From challenge to opportunity: Virtual qualitative research during COVID-19 and beyond. *International Journal of Qualitative Methods, 21*, 160940692211050. https://doi.org/10.1177/16094069221105075

Kelling, G.L. & Coles, C.M. (1996) *Fixing broken windows: Restoring order and reducing crime in our communities.* Simon & Schuster.

Koper, C. S. (2006). Just enough police presence: Reducing crime and disorderly behaviour by optimizing patrol time in crime hot spots. *Justice Quarterly, 26*, 649–672. https://doi.org/10.1080/07418829500096231

Kovacs, L., & Corrie, S. (2016). What can realist evaluation tell us about how coaching interventions work? *The Coaching Psychologist, 12*(2), 59–66. https://doi.org/10.53841/bpstcp.2016.12.2.59

Kreuter, F., Presser, S. & Tourangeau, R., (2008). Social desirability bias in CATI, IVR, and web surveys: The effects of mode and question sensitivity. *Public Opinion Quarterly, 72*(5), 847–865. https://doi.org/10.1093/poq/nfn063

Kuha, J., & Jackson, J. (2014). The item count method for sensitive survey questions: Modelling criminal behaviour. *Journal of the Royal Statistical Society: Series C (Applied Statistics), 63*, 321–341. https://doi.org/10.1111/rssc.12018

Kvale, S. (1996). *Interview views: An introduction to qualitative research interviewing.* SAGE.

Kvale, S. & Brinkmann, S. (2009). *Interviews: Learning the craft of qualitative research interviewing*. SAGE.

Lacouture, A., Breton, E., Guichard, A., & Ridde, V. (2015). The concept of mechanism from a realist approach: A scoping review to facilitate its operationalization in public health program evaluation. *Implementation Science, 10*(153), 1–14. https://doi.org/10.1186/s13012-015-0345-7

Langhorne, P., & Baylan, S. (2017). Early supported discharge services for people with acute stroke. *Cochrane Database of Systematic Reviews* (7). https://doi.org/10.1002/14651858.CD000443.pub4

Lawson, S., Mullan, J., Wong, G., Zaman, H., Booth, A., Watson, A., & Maidment, I. (2021). Family carers' experiences of managing older relative's medications: Insights from the MEMORABLE study. *Patient Education and Counseling*. https://doi.org/https://doi.org/10.1016/j.pec.2021.12.017

Lemire, S., Kwako, A., Nielsen, S. B., Christie, C. A., Donaldson, S. I., & Leeuw, F. L. (2020). What is this thing called a mechanism? Findings from a review of realist evaluations. *New Directions for Evaluation, 2020*(167), 73–86. https://doi.org/10.1002/ev.20428

Lemire, S. T., Nielsen, S. B., & Dybdal, L. (2012). Making contribution analysis work: A practical framework for handling influencing factors and alternative explanations. *Evaluation, 18*(3), 294–309. https://doi.org/10.1177/1356389012450654

Lemire, S., Porowski, A., Mumma, K. (2023). How we model matters – Visualizing program theories. *Abt method guide*. Rockville, MD: Abt Associates. https://www.abtglobal.com/insights/events/how-we-model-matters-visualizing-program-theories#:~:text=If%20you%27re%20trying%20to,world%20complexities%20of%20program%20theories.

Lennon-Dearing, R., & Hirschi, M. (2019). A photovoice empowerment intervention for women living with HIV. *Journal of HIV/AIDS & Social Services, 18*(4), 347–366. https://doi.org/10.1080/15381501.2019.1658683

Lennon-Dearing, R., & Price, J. (2018). Women living with HIV tell their stories with photovoice. *Journal of Human Behavior in the Social Environment, 28*(5), 588–601. https://doi.org/10.1080/10911359.2018.1443867

Leon, C.M., Aizpurua, E. & van der Valk, S., (2021). The impact of confidentiality assurances on participants' responses to sensitive questions. *International Journal of Public Opinion Research, 33*(4), 1024–1038. https://doi.org/10.1093/ijpor/edaa039

León, F. R., Lundgren, R., Huapaya, A., Sinai, I., & Jennings, V. (2007). Challenging the courtesy bias interpretation of favorable clients' perceptions of family planning delivery. *Evaluation Review, 31*(1), 24–42. https://doi.org/10.1177/0193841X06289044

Liebenberg, L. (2018). Thinking critically about photovoice: Achieving empowerment and social change. *International Journal of Qualitative Methods, 17*(1), 1–7. https://doi.org/10.1177/1609406918757631

Lindsay, C., Baruffati, D., Mackenzie, M., Ellis, D. A., Major, M., O'Donnell, K., Simpson, S., Williamson, A., Duddy, C., & Wong, G. (2023). A realist review of the causes of, and current interventions to address 'missingness' in health care. *NIHR Open Research, 3*(33). https://doi.org/https://doi.org/10.3310/nihropenres.13431.1

Litorp, H., Mgaya, A., Mbekenga, C. K., Kidanto, H. L., Johnsdotter, S. & Essen, B. (2015). Fear, blame and transparency: Obstetric caregivers' rationales for high caesarean section rates in a low-resource setting. *Social Science & Medicine, 143*, 232–40. https://doi.org/10.1016/j.socscimed.2015.09.003

Little, D. (1991). *Varieties of social explanation: An introduction to the philosophy of social science*. Westview Press.

Liu, X., & Burnett, D. (2022). Insider-outsider: Methodological reflections on collaborative intercultural research. *Humanities and Social Sciences Communications, 9*(1), 314. https://doi.org/10.1057/s41599-022-01336-9

Lo Iacono, V., Symonds, P., & Brown, D. H. K. (2016). Skype as a tool for qualitative research interviews. *Sociological Research Online, 21*(2), 103–117. https://doi.org/10.5153/sro.3952

Lobe, B., Morgan, D., & Hoffman, K. A. (2020). Qualitative data collection in an era of social distancing. *International Journal of Qualitative Methods, 19*, 160940692093787. https://doi.org/10.1177/1609406920937875

Lobe, B., Morgan, D. L., & Hoffman, K. (2022). A systematic comparison of in-person and video-based online interviewing. *International Journal of Qualitative Methods, 21*, 160940692211270. https://doi.org/10.1177/16094069221127068

Loewenson, R., Laurell, A., Hogstedt, C., D'Ambruoso & Shroff, Z. (2014). *Participatory action research in health systems: A methods reader,* Harare, TARSC, AHPSR, WHO, IDRC Canada, EQUINET. https://equinetafrica.org/sites/default/files/uploads/documents/PAR_Methods_Reader2014_for_web.pdf

Loving, T.J. & Agnew, C.R., (2001). Socially desirable responding in close relationships: A dual-component approach and measure. *Journal of Social and Personal Relationships, 18*(4), 551–573. https://doi.org/10.1177/0265407501184007

Macdonald, C. (2012). Understanding participatory action research: A qualitative research methodology option. *Canadian Journal of Action Research, 13*, 34–50. https://doi.org/10.33524/cjar.v13i2.37

Maguire, M. (2007). Crime data and statistics. In M. Maguire, R. Morgan & R Reiner (Eds.). *The Oxford handbook of criminology* (4th Ed.). (pp.241–301), Oxford University Press.

Maidment, I., Lawson, S., Wong, G., Booth, A., Watson, A., McKeown, J., Zaman, H., Mullan, J., & Bailey, S. (2020). Medication management in older people: The MEMORABLE realist synthesis. *Health Service Delivery Research, 8*, 26. https://doi.org/10.3310/hsdr08260

Maidment, I. D., Wong, G., Duddy, C., Upthegrove, R., Oduola, S., Robotham, D., Higgs, S., Ahern, A., & Birdi, G. (2022). REalist synthesis of non-pharmacologicaL interVEntions for antipsychotic-induced weight gain (RESOLVE) in people living with severe mental illness (SMI). *Systematic Reviews, 11*(1), 42. https://doi.org/10.1186/s13643-022-01912-9

Mainland, D. (1958). Notes on the planning and evaluation of research, with examples from cardiovascular investigations. Part II. *American Heart Journal, 55*: 824–837.

Malengreaux, S., Doumont, D., Scheen, B., Van Durme, T. & Aujoulat, I. (2022). Realist evaluation of health promotion interventions: A scoping review. *Health Promotion International, 37*. https://doi.org/10.1093/heapro/daac136

Malterud, K. (2012). Systematic text condensation: A strategy for qualitative analysis. *Scandinavian Journal of Public Health, 40*(8), 795–805. https://doi.org/10.1177/1403494812465030

Mannay, D. (2010). Making the familiar strange: Can visual research methods render the familiar setting more perceptible? *Qualitative Research, 10*(1), 91–111. https://doi.org/10.1177/1468794109348684

Manzano, A. (2016). The craft of interviewing in realist evaluation. *Evaluation, 22*(3), 342–360. https://doi.org/10.1177/1356389016638615

Manzano, A. (2022). Conducting focus groups in realist evaluation. *Evaluation, 28*(4), 406–425. https://doi.org/10.1177/13563890221124637

Manzano, A. (2023). Focus Groups. LIEPP Methods Brief n°37, 2023, 5 p. ffhal-04159342 https://sciencespo.hal.science/hal-04159342

Manzano, A. (2024). User and Stakeholder Involvement in Realist Evaluation. Sciences Po LIEPP Working Paper n°158, January 2024. https://sciencespo.hal.science/hal-04410009

Manzano, A., & Pawson, R. (2014). Evaluating deceased organ donation: A programme theory approach. *Journal of Health Organization & Management, 28*(3), 366–385. https://doi.org/10.1108/JHOM-07-2012-0131

Marchal, B., Kegels, G. & Van Belle, S. (2018). Theory and realist methods. In: Emmel, N., Greenhalgh, J., Manzano, A., Monaghan, M. & Dalkin, S. (eds.) *Doing realist research*. SAGE.

Marchal, B., van Belle, S., van Olmen, J., Hoeree, T., & Kegels, G. (2012). Is realist evaluation keeping its promise? A review of published empirical studies in the field of health systems. *Evaluation, 18*(2), 192–212. https://doi.org/10.1177/1356389012442444

Mark, M. M., Henry, G. T., & Julnes, G. (1998). A realist theory of evaluation practice. *New Directions for Evaluation, 1998*(78), 3–32. https://doi.org/10.1002/ev.1098

Martin, P., & Tannenbaum, C. (2017). A realist evaluation of patients' decisions to deprescribe in the EMPOWER trial. *BMJ Open, 7*(4), e015959–e015959. https://doi.org/10.1136/bmjopen-2017-015959

MAXQDA. (2024). https://www.maxqda.com.

Maxwell, J.A., (2012). *A realist approach for qualitative research*. SAGE.

Mays, N. & Pope, C., (1995). Qualitative research: Rigour and qualitative research. *BMJ 311*(6997), 109–112. https://doi.org/10.1136/bmj.311.6997.109

Mbava, N. P., & Chapman, S. (2020). Adapting realist evaluation for Made in Africa evaluation criteria. *African Evaluation Journal, 8*(1), 11. https://doi.org/10.4102/aej.v8i1.508

McCall, G.J. (1984). Systematic field observation. *Annual Review of Sociology, 10*, 263–282.

McEvoy, P., & Richards, D. (2006). A critical realist rationale for using a combination of quantitative and qualitative methods. *Journal of Research in Nursing, 11*(1), 66–78. https://doi.org/10.1177/1744987106060192

McLaughlin, D. J., Braver, T. S., & Peelle, J. E. (2021). Measuring the subjective cost of listening effort using a discounting task. *Journal of Speech, Language, & Hearing Research, 64*(2), 337–347. https://doi.org/10.1044/2020_JSLHR-20-00086

Mehdipanah, R., Malmusi, D., Muntaner, C., & Borrell, C. (2013). An evaluation of an urban renewal program and its effects on neighborhood resident's overall wellbeing using concept mapping. *Health & Place, 23*, 9–17. https://doi.org/10.1016/j.healthplace.2013.04.009.

Melro, C. M. & Ballantyne, C. T. (2021). Decolonising community-based participatory research: Applying arts-based methods to transformative learning spaces In: Liamputtong, P. (ed.) *Handbook of qualitative cross-cultural research methods. A social science perspective*. Edward Elgar.

Mercier, H., & Sperber, D. (2017). *The enigma of reason*. Harvard University Press.

Merriam, S. B., Johnson-Bailey, J., Lee, M.-Y., Kee, Y., Ntseane, G., & Muhamad, M. (2001). Power and positionality: Negotiating insider/outsider status within and across cultures. *International Journal of Lifelong Education, 20*(5), 405–416. https://doi.org/10.1080/02601370120490

Merton, R. K. (1967). On sociological theories of the middle-range. In: Merton RK (ed.) *On theoretical sociology: Five essays old and new*. The Free Press, 39–72

Merton R. K. (1942/1973). The normative structure of science. In: Merton RK (ed.) *The sociology of science. Theoretical and empirical investigations*. (pp. 267–278). The University of Chicago Press,

Merton, R. K. & Kendall, P. L. (1946). The focused interview. *American Journal of Sociology, 51*(6), 541–557.

Miles, M. & Huberman, M. (1994). *Qualitative data analysis: An expanded sourcebook*. SAGE.

Miller, G. (1997). Introduction: Context and method in qualitative research. In Miller, G. & Dingwall, R. *Context and method in qualitative research*. SAGE.

Milne, B., & Powell, M. (2011). *Investigative interviewing*. Emerald. https://www.academia.edu/download/79733121/powell-investigative-2010.pdf

Mirzoev, T., Etiaba, E., Ebenso, B., Uzochukwu, B., Ensor, T., Onwujekwe, O., Huss, R., Ezumah, N. & Manzano, A. (2020). Tracing theories in realist evaluations of large-scale health programmes in low- and middle-income countries: Experience from Nigeria. *Health Policy & Planning*, *35*(9) 1244–1253 https://doi.org/10.1093/heapol/czaa076

Mozambique-Canada Maternal Health Project (2018) https://maternalhealthmozcan.ca/

Mukumbang, F. C., & van Wyk, B. (2020). Leveraging the photovoice methodology for critical realist theorizing. *International Journal of Qualitative Methods*, 19, https://doi.org/10.1177/1609406920958981

Mukumbang, F. C. (2023). Retroductive theorizing: A contribution of critical realism to mixed methods research. *Journal of Mixed Methods Research*, *17*(1), 93–114. https://doi.org/10.1177/15586898211049847

Mukumbang, F. C., De Souza, D. E., & Eastwood, J. G. (2023). The contributions of scientific realism and critical realism to realist evaluation. *Journal of Critical Realism*, *22*(3), 504–524. https://doi.org/10.1080/14767430.2023.2217052

Mukumbang, F., Marchal, B., Belle, S. & Van Wyk, B. (2020). Using the realist interview approach to maintain theoretical awareness in realist studies. *Qualitative Research 20*(4) 485–515. https://doi.org/10.1177/1468794119881985

Mukumbang, F. C., Marchal, B., Van Belle, S., & Van Wyk, B. (2018). A realist approach to eliciting the initial programme theory of the antiretroviral treatment adherence club intervention in the Western Cape Province, South Africa. *BMC Medical Research Methodology*, *18*(1), 1–16. https://doi.org/10.1186/s12874-018-0503-0

Mukumbang, F. C., & van Wyk, B. (2020). Leveraging the photovoice methodology for critical realist theorizing. *International Journal of Qualitative Methods*, *19*(1), 1–15. https://doi.org/10.1177/1609406920958981

Murphy, E. A. (1976). *The logic of medicine*. Johns Hopkins University Press.

Nakkeeran, N., Sacks, E., Srinivas, P. N., Juneja, A., Gaitonde, R., Garimella, S. & Topp, S. (2021). Beyond behaviour as individual choice: A call to expand understandings around social science in health research. *Wellcome Open Research*, *6*(212), 1–9. https://doi.org/10.12688/wellcomeopenres.17149.1

Ng, C. G., Ting, S. Q., Saifi, R. A., & Kamarulzaman, A. B. (2023). Ethical issues in photovoice studies involving key populations: A scoping review. *Asian Bioethics Review*, 1–21. https://doi.org/10.1007/S41649-023-00264-3

Nichol, A. J., Hastings, C., & Elder-Vass, D. (2023). Putting philosophy to work: Developing the conceptual architecture of research projects. *Journal of Critical Realism*, *22*(3), 364–383. https://doi.org/10.1080/14767430.2023.2217054

Nielsen, S. B., Jaspers, S. Ø., & Lemire, S. (2023). The curious case of realist trials: Oxymoron or methodological unicorn? *Evaluation*, *30*(1), 120–137. https://doi.org/10.1177/13563890231200291

Nielsen, S. B., Lemire, S., & Tangsig. S. (2022). Unpacking context in realist evaluations: Findings from a comprehensive review. *Evaluation*, *28*(1), 91–112. https://doi.org/10.1177/13563890211053032

Norrie, A. (2010). *Dialectic and difference*. Routledge.

Novick, G. (2008). Is there a bias against telephone interviews in qualitative research? *Research in Nursing & Health*, *31*(4), 391–398. https://doi.org/10.1002/nur.20259

Nowell, L. S., Norris, J. M., White, D. E., & Moules, N. J. (2017). Thematic analysis: Striving to meet the trustworthiness criteria. *International Journal of Qualitative Methods*, *16*(1). https://doi.org/10.1177/1609406917733847

O'Rourke, K., Abdulghani, N., Yelland, J., Newton, M., & Shafiei, T. (2022). Cross-cultural realist interviews: An integration of the realist interview and cross-cultural qualitative research methods. *Evaluation Journal of Australasia*, *22*(1), 5–17. https://doi.org/10.1177/1035719x211055229

Office for National Statistics (ONS). (2023). *Crime in England and Wales, quality and methodology information (QMI) report*. ONS. https://www.ons.gov.uk/peoplepopulationandcommunity/crimeandjustice/methodologies/crimeinenglandandwalesqmi

Online Etymology Dictionary. (2023). https://www.etymonline.com/search?q=bias

Oroviogoicoechea, C., & Watson, R. (2009). A quantitative analysis of the impact of a computerised information system on nurses' clinical practice using a realistic evaluation framework. *International Journal of Medical Informatics, 78*(12), 839–849. https://doi.org/10.1016/j.ijmedinf.2009.08.008.

Ospina, S. M., Burns, D., Howard, J. (2021). Navigating the complex and dynamic landscape of participatory research and inquiry. *The Sage handbook of participatory research and inquiry.* SAGE.

Pals, R. A., Olesen, K., & Willaing, I. (2016). What does theory-driven evaluation add to the analysis of self-reported outcomes of diabetes education? A comparative realist evaluation of a participatory patient education approach. *Patient Education and Counseling, 99*(6), 995–1001. https://doi.org/10.1016/j.pec.2016.01.006

Pant, I., Khosla, S., Lama, J. T., Shanker, V., AlKhaldi, M., El-Basuoni, A., Michel, B., Bitar, K., & Nsofor, I. M. (2022). Decolonising global health evaluation: Synthesis from a scoping review. *PLOS Global Public Health, 2*(11), e0000306. https://doi.org/10.1371/journal.pgph.0000306

Paradisi, P., Raglianti, M., & Sebastiani, L. (2021). Online communication and body language. *Frontiers in Behavioral Neuroscience, 15*, 709365. https://doi.org/10.3389/fnbeh.2021.709365

Parlour, R., & McCormack, B. (2012). Blending critical realist and emancipatory practice development methodologies: Making critical realism work in nursing research. *Nursing Inquiry, 19*, 308–321. https://doi.org/10.1111/j.1440-1800.2011.00577.x

Pattyn, V., Álamos-Concha, P., Cambré, B., Rihoux, B., & Schalembier, B. (2022). Policy effectiveness through configurational and mechanistic lenses: Lessons for concept development. *Journal of Comparative Policy Analysis: Research & Practice, 24*(1), 33–50. https://doi.org/10.1080/13876988.2020.1773263

Pawson, R. (1996). Theorizing the interview. *British Journal of Sociology, 47*(2), 295–314. https://doi.org/10.2307/591728

Pawson, R. (2003). Nothing as practical as a good theory. *Evaluation, 9*(4), 471–490. https://doi.org/10.1177/1356389003009004007

Pawson, R. (2013). *The science of evaluation: A realist manifesto.* SAGE. https://doi.org/10.4135/9781473913820

Pawson, R. (2024). *How to think like a realist.* Edward Elgar.

Pawson, R. (2006a). Digging for nuggets: How 'bad' research can yield 'good' evidence. *International Journal of Social Research Methodology, 9*(2), 127–142. https://doi.org/10.1080/13645570600595314

Pawson, R. (2006b). *Evidence-based policy: A realist perspective.* SAGE. http://digital.casalini.it/9781847878199

Pawson, R., Greenhalgh, J., Brennan, C., & Glidewell, E. (2014). Do reviews of healthcare interventions teach us how to improve healthcare systems? *Social Science & Medicine, 114*, 129–137. https://doi.org/10.1016/j.socscimed.2014.05.032

Pawson, R., & Tilley, N. (1994). What works in evaluation research? *The British Journal of Criminology, 34*(3), 291–306. https://doi.org/10.1093/oxfordjournals.bjc.a048424

Pawson, R., & Tilley, Nick. (1997, 2008). *Realistic evaluation.* SAGE. https://doi.org/10.1177/135638909800400213

Pawson, R. & Tilley, N. (2004). *Realist evaluation.* https://cnxus.org/wp-content/uploads/2022/04/RE_chapter.pdf

Pawson, R., Wong, G., & Owen, L. (2011). Myths, facts and conditional truths: What is the evidence on the risks associated with smoking in cars carrying children? *Canadian Medical Association Journal, 183*(10), E680–E684. https://doi.org/10.1503/cmaj.100903

Pawson, R., Wong, G. & Owen, L. (2011) Known knowns, known unknowns, un-known unknowns: The predicament of evidence-based policy. *American Journal of Evaluation, 32*(4), 518–546. https://doi.org/10.1177/1098214011403831

Peelle, J. E. (2018). Listening effort: How the cognitive consequences of acoustic chal-lenge are reflected in brain and behavior. *Ear & Hearing, 39*(2), 204. https://doi.org/10.1097/AUD.0000000000000494

Peters, U. (2022). What is the function of confirmation bias? *Erkenntnis 87*(3): 1351–1376. https://doi.org/10.1007/s10670-020-00252-1

Pino Gavidia, L. A. & Adu, J. (2022). Critical narrative inquiry: An examination of a methodological approach. *International Journal of Qualitative Methods, 21*. https://doi.org/10.1177/16094069221081594

Platt, J. (2012). The history of the interview. In Gubrium, J, Holstein, J, Marvasti, A & McKinney, K (ed.), *The SAGE handbook of interview research: The complexity of the craft (2nd ed)*. (pp. 9–26). SAGE.

Popper, K. (1959). *The logic of scientific discovery*. Hutchinson.

Popper, K. (1963/1989). *Conjectures and refutations*. 5th Edition. Routledge and Kegan Paul.

Popper, K. (1972). *Objective knowledge*. Oxford University Press.

Porpora, D. (2015). *Reconstructing sociology: The critical realist approach*. Cambridge University Press.

Porter, S. (2015). The uncritical realism of realist evaluation. *Evaluation, 21*(1), 65–82. https://doi.org/10.1177/1356389014566134

Pratt, B., Seshadri, T. & Srinivas, P. N. (2020). What should community organisations consider when deciding to partner with researchers? A critical reflection on the Zilla Budakattu Girijana Abhivrudhhi Sangha experience in Karnataka, India. *Health Re-search Policy & Systems, 18*. https://doi.org/10.1186/s12961-020-00617-6

Pratt, B., Seshadri, T. & Srinivas, P. N. (2022a). Overcoming structural barriers to shar-ing power with communities in global health research priority-setting: Lessons from the participation for local action project in Karnataka, India. *Global Public Health, 17*, 3334–3352. https://doi.org/10.1080/17441692.2022.2058048

Pratt, B., Srinivas, P. N. & Seshadri, T. (2022b). How is inclusiveness in health systems research priority-setting affected when community organizations lead the process? *Health Policy & Planning, 37*, 811–821. https://doi.org/10.1093/heapol/czac012

Punton, M. & Vogel, I. (2020). Keeping it real: Using mechanisms to promote use in the realist evaluation of the building capacity to use research evidence program. *New Directions for Evaluation, 2020*(167), 87–100. https://doi.org/10.1002/ev.20427

Punton, M., Vogel, I., Leavy, J., Michaelis, C., & Boydell, E. (2020). Reality bites: Making realist evaluation useful in the real world. Centre for development impact practice paper, 22, 1–13. https://www.ids.ac.uk/publications/reality-bites-making-realist-evaluation-useful-in-the-real-world/

Punton, M., Vogel, I., & Lloyd, R. (2016). *Reflections from a realist evaluation in progress: scaling ladders and stitching theory*. CDI Practice paper, 18, 1–11. https://opendocs.ids.ac.uk/opendocs/bitstream/handle/20.500.12413/11254/CDIPracticePaper_18.pdf;jsessionid=AEC2A5E41EB35647476F7202875DFE3A?sequence=1

Quayle, A. & Sonn, C. (2022). Critical narrative inquiry as psychosocial accompani-ment with Aboriginal communities. In: Liamputtong, P. (ed.) *Handbook of cross-cultural research methods: A social science perspective*. Edward Elgar.

Quraishi, M., Irfan, L., Schneuwly Purdie, M., & Wilkinson, M. L. N. (2022). Doing 'judgemental rationality' in empirical research: The importance of depth-reflexivity when researching in prison. *Journal of Critical Realism, 21*(1), 25–45. https://doi.org/10.1080/14767430.2021.1992735

Radin, B. 2006. *Challenging the performance movement: Accountability, complexity and democratic values*. Georgetown University Press.

Ragin, C. C. (2000). *Fuzzy-set social science*. University of Chicago Press.

RAMESES project website. (2024). https://www.ramesesproject.org/media/RAMESES_II_Working_with_a_librarian.pdf

Rayment-McHugh, S., Adams, D., & McKillop, N. (2021). Introducing a contextual lens to assessment and intervention for young people who engage in harmful sexual behaviour: An Australian case study. *Journal of Children's Services*, *17*(3), 192–204. https://doi.org/10.1108/JCS-06-2021-0024

Redgate, S., Potrac, P., Boocock, E. & Dalkin, S. (2022). Realist evaluation of the football association's post graduate Diploma (PG Dip) in Coach Development, *Sport, Education & Society*, *27*(3), 361–376. https://doi.org/10.1080/13573322.2020.1847066

Reid, S., & Fransman, J. (2021). *Effective consortia working: Literature review and priorities for future research*. https://oro.open.ac.uk/87474/

Renmans, D. (2023). The ResQ approach: Theory building across disciplines using realist evaluation science and QCA. *International Journal of Social Research Methodology*, *26*(4), 469–482. https://doi.org/10.1080/13645579.2022.2052695

Renmans, D., & Pleguezuelo, V. C. (2023). Methods in realist evaluation: A mapping review. *Evaluation & Program Planning*, *97*: 102209. https://doi.org/10.1016/j.evalprogplan.2022.102209

Renmans, D., Sarkar, N., Van Belle, S., Affun-Adegbulu, C., Marchal, B., & Mukumbang, F. C. (2022). Realist evaluation in times of decolonising global health. *The International Journal of Health Planning & Management*, *37*(S1), 37–44. https://doi.org/10.1002/hpm.3530

Ridde, V., Robert, E., Guichard, A., Blaise, P., & Van Olmen, J. (2012). L'approche realist à l'épreuve du reel de l'évaluation des programmes. *The Canadian Journal of Program Evaluation*, *26*(3), 37–59. https://doi.org/10.3138/cjpe.0026.005

Roberts, J. K., Pavlakis, A. E., & Richards, M. P. (2021). It's more complicated than it seems: Virtual qualitative research in the COVID-19 era. *International Journal of Qualitative Methods*, *20*, 160940692110029. https://doi.org/10.1177/16094069211002959

Rohrbasser, A., Wong, G., Mickan, S., & Harris, J. (2022). Understanding how and why quality circles improve standards of practice, enhance professional development and increase psychological well-being of general practitioners: A realist synthesis. *BMJ Open*, *12*(5), e058453. https://doi.org/10.1136/bmjopen-2021-058453

Roller, M. R., & Lavrakas, P. J. (2015). *Applied qualitative research design: A total quality framework approach*. Guilford Publications.

Roulston, K. (2024). Examining the "inside lives" of research interviews. In N. Denzin, Y. Lincoln, M. Giardina, & G. Cannella (Eds.), *The sage handbook of qualitative research* (6th Edition ed.), (pp. 315–331). SAGE.

Royal College of Physicans. (2015). *Post-acute Organisational Audit. Public Report. Phase 2: Organisational audit of post-acute stroke service providers*.

Ruyant, Q. (2021). Semantic realism in the semantic conception of theories. *Synthese*, *198*(8), 7965–7983. https://doi.org/10.1007/s11229-020-02557-8

Rycroft-Malone, J., McCormack, B., Hutchinson, A. M., DeCorby, K., Bucknall, T. K., Kent, B., Schultz, A., Snelgrove-Clarke, E., Stetler, C. B., & Titler, M. (2012). Realist synthesis: Illustrating the method for implementation research. *Implementation Science*, *7*(1), 1–10. https://doi.org/10.1186/1748-5908-7-33

Sackett, D. L. (1979). Bias in analytic research. *Journal Chronic Disease 32*: 51–63.

Salter, K. L., & Kothari, A. (2014). Using realist evaluation to open the black box of knowledge translation: A state-of-the-art review. *Implementation Science*, *9*:115. https://doi.org/10.1186/s13012-014-0115-y

Sanctum Care Group. (2018). Sanctum. Sanctum Group March 13 2018. https://sanctumcaregroup.com/

Santos, M., Sa, A. & Quaresma, J. (2020). Meanings and senses of being a health professional with tuberculosis: An interpretative phenomenological study. *BMJ Open*, *10*, e035873. https://doi.org/10.1136/bmjopen-2019-035873

Saskatchewan Centre for Patient-Oriented Research (SCPOR). (n.d.). *Patient-oriented research level of engagement tool.* https://static1.squarespace.com/static/5c869fd0e666695abe893b3b/t/61b0f04d878a731b75039cdf/1638985805316/PORLET+2021+12+08.pdf

Sayer, A. (1992). *Method in social science: A realist approach.* Routledge.

Sayer, A. (1997). Essentialism, social constructionism, and beyond. *Sociological Review, 45*(3), 453–487. https://doi.org/10.1111/1467-954X.00073

Sayer, A. (2000). *Realism and social science.* SAGE.

Sayer, A. (2011). *Why things matter to people: Social science, values and ethical life.* Cambridge University Press.

Scheibelhofer (2008) Combining narration-based interviews with topical interviews: Methodological reflections on research practices, *International Journal of Social Research Methodology, 11*:5, 403–416. https://doi.org/10.1080/13645570701401370

Scheibelhofer, E. (2023). The interpretive interview. An interview form centring on research participants' constructions *International Journal of Qualitative Methods, 22,* 1–8. https://doi.org/10.1177/16094069231168748

Sedgwick, P. (2014). Non-response bias versus response bias. *BMJ, 348,* 1–2.

Seitz, J., Benke, I., & Madche, A. (2022). *Fatigued by yourself? Towards understanding the impact of self-view designs in virtual meeting software.* https://aisel.aisnet.org/sighci2022/14/

Sharmil, H., Kelly, J., Bowden, M., Galletly, C., Cairney, I., Wilson, C., Hahn, L., Liu, D., Elliot, P., Else, J., Warrior, T., Wanganeen, T., Taylor, R., Wanganeen, F., Madrid, J., Warner, L., Brown, M. & De Crespigny, C. (2021). Participatory action research-Dadirri-Ganma, using yarning: Methodology co-design with aboriginal community members. *International Journal for Equity in Health, 20,* 160. https://doi.org/10.1186/s12939-021-01493-4

Shaw, J., Gray, C. S., Baker, G. R., Denis, J.-L., Breton, M., Gutberg, J., Embuldeniya, G., Carswell, P., Dunham, A., McKillop, A., Kenealy, T., Sheridan, N., & Wodchis, W. (2018). Mechanisms, contexts and points of contention: Operationalizing realist-informed research for complex health interventions. *BMC Medical Research Methodology, 18*(178). https://doi.org/10.1186/s12874-018-0641-4

Sherman, L. W., William, S., Ariel, B., Strang, L.R., Wain, N., Slothower, M., & Norton, A. (2014). An integrated theory of hot spots patrol strategy: Implementing prevention by scaling up and feeding back. *Journal of Contemporary Criminal Justice, 30,* 95–122. https://doi.org/10.1177/1043986214525082

Singer, M. K., Dressler, W., George, S., Baquet, C. R., Bell, R. A., Burhansstipanov, L., Burke, N. J., Dibble, S., Elwood, W., & Garro, L. (2016). Culture: The missing link in health research. *Social Science & Medicine, 170,* 237–246. https://doi.org/10.1016/j.socscimed.2016.07.015

Skelly, A. C., Dettori, J. R., & Brodt, E. D. (2012). Assessing bias: The importance of considering confounding. *Evidence-Based Spine-Care Journal, 3*(01), 9–12. https://doi.org/10.1055/s-0031-1298595

Sloan-Howitt, M. and Kelling, G.L. (1990). Subway graffiti in New York City: "Getting Up" vs. "Meanin It and Cleanin It". *Security Journal, 1,* 131–136.

Smallbone, S. W., Rayment-McHugh, S., & Smith, D. (2013). *Preventing youth sexual violence and abuse in West Cairns and aurukun: Establishing the scope, dimensions and dynamics of the problem.* Griffith University.

Smith, C. (2010). *What is a person?* University of Chicago.

Smith, C., & Elger, T. (2014). Critical realism and interviewing subjects. In P. K. Edwards, J. O'Mahoney, & S.Vincent(Eds.), *Studying organizations using critical realism* (pp. 109–131). Oxford University Press. https://doi.org/10.1093/acprof:oso/9780199665525.003.0006

Sobh, R., & Perry, C. (2006). Research design and data analysis in realism research. *European Journal of Marketing, 40*(11–12), 1194–1209. https://doi.org/10.1108/03090560610702777

Sturges, J. E., & Hanrahan, K. J. (2004). Comparing telephone and face-to-face qualitative interviewing: A research note. *Qualitative Research, 4*(1), 107–118. https://doi.org/10.1177/1468794104041110

Sutton-Brown, C. A. (2014). Photovoice: A methodological guide. *Photography Culture, 7*(2), 169–185. https://doi.org/10.2752/175145214X13999922103165

Tabulawa, R. (2013). *Teaching and learning in context: Why pedagogical reforms fail in Sub-Saharan Africa.* African Books Collective.

Taylor, S. (1982). *Durkheim and the study of suicide.* Red Globe Press.

Teti, M., & van Wyk, B. (2020). Qualitative methods without borders: Adapting photovoice: From a. U.S to South African setting. *International Journal of Qualitative Methods, 19*, https://doi.org/10.1177/1609406920927253

Tilley, N. (2009). *Crime prevention.* Willan Publishing.

Tilley, N., Rayment-McHugh, S., Smallbone, S. W., Wardell, M., Smith, D., Allard, T., … Homel, R. (2014). On being realistic about reducing the prevalence and impacts of youth sexual violence and abuse in two Australian Indigenous communities. *Learning Communities International Journal of Learning in Social Contexts: Special Issue: Evaluation, 14*, 6–26. https://www.cdu.edu.au/sites/default/files/the-northern-institute/10.18793-lcj12014.18714.18702.pdf.

Tilley, N., & Tseloni, A. (2016). Choosing and using statistical sources in criminology: What can the crime survey for England and Wales tell us? *Legal Information Management, 16*(2), 78–90. https://doi.org/10.1017/S1472669616000219

Tolson, D., McIntosh, J., Loftus, L., & Cormie, P. (2007). Developing A managed clinical network in palliative care: A realistic evaluation. *International Journal of Nursing Studies, 44*(2), 183–195. https://doi.org/10.1016/j.ijnurstu.2005.11.027

Trochim, W. M. K. (1989). Outcome pattern matching and program theory', *Evaluation & Program Planning, 12*(4), 355–366. https://doi.org/10.1016/0149-7189(89)90052-9.

Tversky, A., & Kahneman, D. (1988). Rational choice and the framing of decisions. *Decision making: Descriptive, normative, and prescriptive interactions*, 167–192.

Udai, P., & Rao, T. V. (1975). Cross cultural surveys and interviewing (No. WP1975-05-01_00150). *Indian Institute of Management* Ahmedabad, Research and Publication Department.

University of California. (2023). *Exonerations by year: DNA and Non-DNA* https://www.law.umich.edu/special/exoneration/Pages/Exoneration-by-Year.aspx

Uwamahoro, N. S., Forsyth, J., Andre, F., Mandlate, D. A., Gilmore, B., & Muhajarine, N. (2024). Realist evaluation of maternity waiting home intervention models in Inhambane, Mozambique: Protocol for a comparative embedded case study, the Mozambique-Canada maternal health project. *BMJ Open, 14*(3), e075681. https://doi.org/10.1136/bmjopen-2023-075681

Uwamahoro, N. S., McRae, D., Zibrowski, E., Victor-Uadiale, I., Gilmore, B., Bergen, N., & Muhajarine, N. (2022). Understanding maternity waiting home uptake and scale-up within low-income and middle-income countries: A programme theory from A realist review and synthesis. *BMJ Global Health, 7*(9), e009605. https://doi.org/10.1136/bmjgh-2022-009605

Van Belle, S., Abejirinde, I.-O., Ssennyonjo, A., Srinivas, P. N., Hebbar, P., & Marchal, B. (2023). How to develop a realist programme theory using Margaret Archer's structure–agency–culture framework: The case of adolescent accountability for sexual and reproductive health in urban resource-constrained settings. *Evaluation, 29*(3), 259–275. https://doi.org/10.1177/13563890231185167

Van Belle, S., Van De Pas, R. & Marchal, B. (2017). Towards an agenda for implementation science in global health: There is nothing more practical than good (social science) theories. *BMJ Global Health, 2*, e000181. https://doi.org/10.1136/bmjgh-2016-000181

Van Belle, S., Wong, G., Westhorp, G., Pearson, M., Emmel, N., Manzano, A., Marchal, B. (2016). Can "realist" randomised controlled trials be genuinely realist? *Trials, 17*: 313. https://doi.org/10.1186/s13063-016-1407-0

Vareilles, G., Marchal, B., Kane, S., Petrič, T., Pictet, G., & Pommier, J. (2015). Understanding the motivation and performance of community health volunteers involved in the delivery of health programmes in Kampala, Uganda: A realist evaluation. *BMJ Open*, *5*(11), e008614. https://doi.org/10.1136/bmjopen-2015-008614

Vaughn, L. M., & Jacquez, F. (2020). Participatory research methods – Choice points in the research process. *Journal of Participatory Research Methods*. https://doi.org/10.35844/001c.13244

Vésteinsdóttir, V., Joinson, A., Reips, U. D., Danielsdottir, H. B., Thorarinsdottir, E. A., & Thorsdottir, F. (2019). Questions on honest responding. *Behavior Research Methods*, *51*, 811–825. https://doi.org/10.3758/s13428-018-1121-9

Vincent, R., Adhikari, B., Duddy, C., Richardson, E., Wong, G., Lavery, J., Molyneux, S. & Team, T. R. (2022). Working relationships across difference - a realist review of community engagement with malaria research. *Wellcome Open Research*, *7*. https://doi.org/10.12688/wellcomeopenres.17192.1

Vineis, P. (2002). History of bias. *Sozial-und Präventivmedizin 47*: 156–161.

Vogel, I. & Punton, M. (2017). *Building capacity to use research evidence (BCURE) realist evaluation: Stage 2 synthesis report*. ITAD. Hove, United Kingdom. https://www.itad.com/knowledge-product/building-capacity-to-use-research-evaluation-bcure-realist-evaluation-stage-2-synthesis-report/

Vogel, I. & Punton, M. (2018). *Annexes for the final evaluation of the building capacity to use research evidence (BCURE) programme*. ITAD. Hove, United Kingdom. https://www.itad.com/knowledge-product/annexes-for-the-final-evaluation-of-the-building-capacity-to-use-research-evidence-bcure-programme/

Vogl, S. (2013). Telephone versus face-to-face interviews: Mode effect on semistructured interviews with children. *Sociological Methodology*, *43*(1), 133–177. https://doi.org/10.1177/0081175012465967

Von Thiele Schwarz, U., Nielsen, K. M., Stenfors-Hayes, T., & Hasson, H. (2017). Using kaizen to improve employee well-being: Results from two organizational intervention studies. *Human Relations*, *70*(8), 966–993. https://doi.org/10.1177/0018726716677071

Vrij, A., Hope, L., & Fisher, R. P. (2014). Eliciting reliable information in investigative interviews. *Policy Insights from the Behavioral & Brain Sciences*, *1*(1), 129–136. https://doi.org/10.1177/2372732214548592

Vulliamy, G. (1990). Research outcomes: postscript. Doing educational research in developing countries: *Qualitative Strategies*, 169–233.

Waldron, T., Carr, T., McMullen, L., Westhorp, G., Duncan, V., Neufeld, S.-M., Bandura, L.-A., & Groot, G. (2020). Development of a program theory for shared decision-making: A realist synthesis. *BMC Health Services Research*, *20*(1), 59. https://doi.org/10.1186/s12913-019-4649-1

Walshe, C., Ewing, G., & Griffith, J. (2012). Using observation as a data collection method to help understand patient and professional roles and actions in palliative care settings. *Palliative Medicine*, *26*(8), 1048–1054. https://doi.org/10.1177/0269216311432897

Wang, C., & Burris, M. A. (1997). Photovoice: Concept, methodology, and use for participatory needs assessment. *Health Education & Behavior*, *24*(3), 369–387. https://doi.org/10.1177/109019819702400309

Ward, G., & Haigh, M. (2017). Challenges and changes: Developing teachers' and initial teacher education students' understandings of the nature of science. *Research in Science Education*, *47*(6), 1233–1254. https://doi.org/10.1007/s11165-016-9543-9

Warner, S. L. (1965). Randomized response: A survey technique for eliminating evasive answer bias. *Journal of the American Statistical Association*, *60*, 63–69

Warren, E. A., Melendez-Torres, G. J. & Bonell, C. (2022). Are realist randomised controlled trials possible? A reflection on the INCLUSIVE evaluation of a whole-school, bullying-prevention intervention. *Trials*, *23*, 82. https://doi.org/10.1186/s13063-021-05976-1

Webb, E., Campbell, D., Schwartz, R., & Sechrest, L. (2000) *Unobtrusive measures.* SAGE.

Webb, E. J., Campbell, D. T., Schwartz, R. D., & Sechrest, L. (1966). *Unobtrusive measures: Nonreactive research in the social sciences.* Rand Mcnally.

Weiss, C. H. (1995). Nothing as practical as a good theory: Exploring theory-based evaluation for comprehensive community initiatives for children and families, In J. P. Connell, A. C. Kubisch, L. B. Schorr, & C. H. Weiss (Eds.), *New approaches to evaluating community initiatives: Concepts, methods, and contexts* (pp. 65–92). Aspen Institute.

Weiss, C. H. (1997). Theory-based evaluation: Past, present, and future. *New Directions for Evaluation, 76*: 41–55.

Westhorp, G. (2013). Developing complexity-consistent theory in a realist investigation, *Evaluation, 19*(4), 364–382. https://doi.org/10.1177/1356389013505042

Westhorp, G. (2014). *Realistic impact evaluation. An introduction.* A Methods Lab Publication, ODI. in Development, Australian Government Department of Foreign Affairs and Trade. https://odi.org/en/publications/realist-impact-evaluation-an-introduction/

Westhorp, G. (2018). Understanding mechanisms in realist evaluation and research, In N. Emmel, J. Greenhalgh, A. Manzano, M. Monaghan, & S. Dalkin (Eds.), *Doing realist research* (pp. 41–58). SAGE.

Westhorp, G. & Manzano, A. (2017). Realist evaluation interviewing – a 'starter set' of questions. *The RAMESES II Project.* RAMESES_II_Realist_interviewing_starter_questions.pdf (ramesesproject.org)

Westhorp, G., Stevens, K., & Rogers, P. J. (2016). Using realist action research for service redesign. *Evaluation, 22*(3), 361–379. https://doi.org/10.1177/1356389016656514

Williams, E. (2021, February 16-18). *Can a machine think like Ray Pawson?: Potential and perils of machine assisted realist analysis* [Conference session]. The International Conference for Realist Research, Evaluation and Synthesis (REALIST 2021). Online.

Williams V., Boylan A.-M., Nunan D. (2020). Critical appraisal of qualitative research: Necessity, partialities and the issue of bias. *BMJ Evidence-Based Medicine; 25*:9–11. https://doi.org/10.1136/bmjebm-2018-111132

Williams, E., Meggetto, E. & Westhorp, G. (2023). Accountability to Communities and Children in Consortia: Final Report. Charles Darwin University/Save the Children Netherlands. https://resourcecentre.savethechildren.net/pdf/Accountability-to-Children-and-Communities-in-Consortia-Research-Report.pdf/

Wilson, M., & Greenhill, A. (2004). Theory and action for emancipation: Elements of a critical realist approach. In Kaplan B., Truex D.P., Wastell D., Wood-Harper A.T., & DeGross J.I. (Eds.), *Information systems research* (1st Ed, pp. 667–674). Springer.

Wilson, J. Q., & Kelling, G. L. (1982). Broken windows. *The Atlantic Monthly, 249*, 29–38.

Winfred, A., Hagen, E, & George, F. (2021). The lazy or dishonest respondent. *Annual Review of Organizational Psychology & Organizational Behavior, 8*:1,105–137. https://doi.org/10.1146/annurev-orgpsych-012420-055324

Wong, G., Greenhalgh, T., Westhorp, G. & Pawson, R., (2012). Realist methods in medical education research: What are they and what can they contribute?. *Medical Education, 46*(1), 89–96. https://doi.org/10.1111/j.1365-2923.2011.04045.x

Wong, G., Greenhalgh, T., Westhorp, G., & Pawson, R. (2014). Development of methodological guidance, publication standards and training materials for realist and meta-narrative reviews: The RAMESES (realist and meta-narrative evidence syntheses: Evolving standards) project. *Health Services & Delivery Research, 2*(30). https://doi.org/10.3310/hsdr02300

Wong, G., Westhorp. G., Greenhalgh, J., Manzano, A., Jagosh, J., & Greenhalgh, T. (2017). Quality and reporting standards, resources, training materials and information for realist evaluation: The RAMESES II project. *Health Services & Delivery Research, 5*(28). https://doi.org/10.3310/hsdr05280

Wong, G., Westhorp, G., Manzano, A., Greenhalgh, J., Jagosh, J., & Greenhalgh, T. (2016). RAMESES II reporting standards for realist evaluations. *BMC Medicine*, *14*(1), 96. https://doi.org/10.1186/s12916-016-0643-1

Woodgate, R. L., Zurba, M., & Tennent, P. (2017). Worth a thousand words? Advantages, challenges and opportunities in working with photovoice as a qualitative research method with youth and their families. *Forum Qualitative Sozialforschung*, *18*(1). https://doi.org/10.17169/fqs-18.1.2659

Work better together with Mural's visual work platform | Mural. (n.d.). https://www.mural.co/

World Health Organization. (1996). *Maternity waiting homes: A review of experiences.* https://apps.who.int/iris/bitstream/handle/10665/63432/WHO_RHT_MSM_96.21.pdf?sequence=1

Wynn, D., & Williams, C. K. (2012). Principles for conducting critical realist case study research in information systems. *MIS Quarterly: Management Information Systems*, *36*(3), 787–810. https://doi.org/10.2307/41703481

Zibrowski, E., Carr, T., McDonald, S., Thiessen, H., van Dusen, R., Goodridge, D., Haver, C., Marciniuk, D., Stobart, C., Verrall, T., & Groot, G. (2021). A rapid realist review of patient engagement in patient-oriented research and health care system impacts: Part one. *Research Involvement & Engagement*, *7*(1), 72. https://doi.org/10.1186/s40900-021-00299-6

Zurba, M. & Petriello, M. A., Madge, C., Mccarney, P., Bishop, B., Mcbeth, S., Denniston, M., Bodwitch, H., Bailey, M. (2021). Learning from knowledge co-production research and practice in the 21st century. *Sustainability Science, July 7., 17*, 449–467. https://doi.org/10.1007/s11625-021-00996-x

Index

Note: Pages in *italics* represent figures and **bold** indicates tables in the text.